Osteoporosis
Physiological Basis, Assessment, and Treatment

Osteoporosis
Physiological Basis, Assessment, and Treatment

*Proceedings of the Nineteenth Steenbock Symposium
held June 5 through June 8, 1989,
at the University of Wisconsin–Madison, U.S.A.*

Edited by

Hector F. DeLuca, PhD
Steenbock Research Professor
Department of Biochemistry
University of Wisconsin–Madison
Madison, Wisconsin

Richard Mazess, PhD
Professor Emeritus
Department of Medical Physics
University of Wisconsin–Madison
President
Lunar Radiation Corporation
Madison, Wisconsin

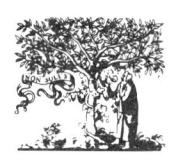

Elsevier
New York • Amsterdam • London

No responsibility is assumed by the Publisher for any injury and/or damage to persons or property as a matter of products liability, negligence, or otherwise, or from any use or operation of any methods, products, instructions, or ideas contained in the material herein. No suggested test or procedure should be carried out unless, in the reader's judgment, its risk is justified. Because of rapid advances in the medical sciences, we recommend that the independent verification of diagnoses and drug dosages should be made. Discussions, views, and recommendations as to medical procedures, choice of drugs, and drug dosages are the responsibility of the authors.

Elsevier Science Publishing Co., Inc.
655 Avenue of the Americas, New York, New York 10010

Sole distributors outside the United States and Canada:
Elsevier Science Publishers B.V.
P.O. Box 211, 1000 AE Amsterdam, The Netherlands

© 1990 Elsevier Science Publishing Co., Inc.

This book has been registered with the Copyright Clearance Center, Inc.
For further information please contact the Copyright Clearance Center, Inc.,
Salem, Massachusetts.

This book is printed on acid-free paper.

Library of Congress Cataloging-in-Publication Data

Steenbock Symposium (19th : 1989 : University of Wisconsin-Madison)
    Osteoporosis: physiological basis, assessment, and treatment.

    1. Osteoporosis—Congresses. I. DeLuca, Hector F., 1930-   . II. Mazess, Richard B. III. Title.
[DNLM: 1. Osteoporosis—congresses. WE 250 S814o 1989]
RC931.O73S74   1989   616.7'16   89-25874
ISBN 0-444-01526-4 (alk. paper)

Current printing (last digit):
10 9 8 7 6 5 4 3 2 1

Manufactured in the United States of America

Contents

Preface ... ix

Participants ... xv

PHYSIOLOGICAL AND CELLULAR BASIS ... 1

The Pathogenesis of Postmenopausal Osteoporosis ... 3
  William A. Peck

Causes of Age-Related Bone Loss and Fractures ... 7
  B. Lawrence Riggs

Therapy Induced Osteoporosis (??? Type III Osteoporosis) ... 17
  Louis V. Avioli

The Metabolic Basis of Osteoporosis ... 23
  B.E.C. Nordin, A.G. Need, H.A. Morris, and M. Horowitz

FRACTURE RISK ... 37

Fracture Patterns ... 39
  L.J. Melton, III

Assessment and Modification of Hip Fracture Risk: Predictions of A Stochastic Model ... 45
  A. Horsman and M.N. Birchall

Fracture Prediction ... 55
  Charles W. Slemenda and C. Conrad Johnston, Jr.

METHODS OF ASSESSMENT 61

Bone Densitometry for Clinical Diagnosis and Monitoring 63
Richard B. Mazess

Quantitative Computed Tomography: Update 1989 87
Harry K. Genant, J.E. Block, P. Steiger, and C.C. Glueer

Bone Histomorphometry 99
F. Melsen, E.F. Eriksen, Le. Mosekilde, Li. Mosekilde, T. Steiniche, and A. Vesterby

Biochemical Assessment of Bone Turnover in Osteoporosis 109
P.D. Delmas

OVERVIEW OF ABSTRACTS PRESENTED ORALLY 119

Overview of Abstracts Presented at the Steenbock Symposium on Osteoporosis: Series 1—8:30 to 10:00—Tuesday, June 6, 1989 121
Lawrence G. Raisz

Overview of Abstracts Presented at the Steenbock Symposium on Osteoporosis: Series 2—8:30 to 10:00—Wednesday, June 7, 1989 123
Charles H. Chesnut III

ESTROGEN 125

Estrogens in Prevention and Treatment of Osteoporosis 127
Robert Lindsay and Jack Tohme

Prevention of Postmenopausal Bone Loss by Long-Term Parenteral Administration of 17β Estradiol: Comparison of Percutaneous and Transdermal Route 137
C. Ribot, F. Tremollieres, and J.M. Pouilles

Prophylaxis of Bone Loss: Long-Term Effects of Continuous and Sequential Estrogen/Progestin Administration and Identification of Women at Risk 147
S. Pors Nielsen, N. Munk-Jensen, E.B. Obel, and O. Barenholdt

A Current Perception of HRT Risks and Benefits 161
T.M. Mack and R.K. Ross

FLUORIDE 179

Benefit-Risk Ratio of Fluoride Therapy in Vertebral Osteoporosis: Comparison of Sodium Fluoride to Monofluorophosphate 181
P.J. Meunier, N. Mamelle, P.D. Delmas, R. Dusan, and J. Dupuis

Fluoride and Calcium Therapy for Osteoporosis Increases Trabecular
Vertebral Bone Density Above the Fracture Threshold   187
   *S.M.G. Farley, V. Perkel, L.A. Tudtud-Hans, M.R. Mariano-Menez, C.R. Libanati,
   E.E. Schulz, and D.J. Baylink*

VITAMIN D   193

**The Basis for 1,25 Dihydroxyvitamin D Therapy in the
Treatment of Osteoporosis**   195
   J.C. Gallagher

**Pathophysiological Study in Women with Postmenopausal osteoporosis
on Long-Term Treatment with Calcitriol**   201
   A. Caniggia, R. Nuti, F. Loré, G. Martini, V. Turchetti, and G. Righi

Benefits/Risks of 1,25-$(OH)_2D_3$ in the Treatment of Osteoporosis   213
   John F. Aloia, Ashok Vaswani, and James K. Yeh

Long-Term Use of 1α(OH)D3 in Involutional Osteoporosis   223
   H. Orimo and M. Shiraki

CALCITONIN   231

Calcitonin: Some Recent Developments   233
   Iain MacIntyre and Mone Zaidi

Secretion, Metabolism, and Action of Endogenous Calcitonin in Human Beings   241
   Hunter Heath III and Robert D. Tiegs

Use of Calcitonin in the Treatment of Postmenopausal Osteoporosis   247
   Charles Nagant de Deuxchaisnes

Intranasal Calcitonin for Prevention and Treatment of Osteoporosis   259
   Kirsten Overgaard, Bente Juel Riis, and Claus Christiansen

Calcitonin and Bone Pain   269
   C. Gennari, D. Agnusdei, and S. Gonnelli

EXERCISE AND CALCIUM   275

Physical Activity and Bone Mass   277
   John A. Eisman, P.J. Kelly, P.N. Sambrook, N.A. Pocock, J.J. Ward, S. Eberl, and M.G. Yeates

Exercise and Bone Mass   285
   Everett L. Smith and Catherine Gilligan

Calcium and Bone Loss in Postmenopausal Women 295
Bess Dawson-Hughes, Elizabeth A. Krall, and Gerard E. Dallal

Calcium Requirements 303
Robert P. Heaney

ADFR 313

ADFR, or Coherence Therapy, for Osteoporosis 315
A.M. Parfitt

BISPHOSPHONATES 321

The Possible Use of Bisphosphonates in Osteoporosis 323
H. Fleisch

The Use of Bisphosphonate in Osteoporosis 331
Olav L.M. Bijvoet, Roelf Valkema, Clemens W.G.M. Löwik, and Socrates E. Papapoulos

ADDENDUM

Do Dermal Losses Explain The Difference Between Absorbed and Excreted Calcium in Normal Subjects on High Calcium Intakes? 339
B.E.C. Nordin

Author Index 341

Subject Index 343

Preface

With the medical advances registered in the last 75 years has come a marked increase in life span. This is resulting in an increasingly aged population, precipitating diseases which are the direct or indirect result of the aging process. No one debates the central concern for diseases such as cancer, heart disease, and circulatory disorders in our aging population. This is understandable because these difficulties are immediately life threatening and account for the greatest number of deaths among our elderly. However, a disease that contributes substantially to morbidity among the elderly is osteoporosis. Furthermore, this disorder not only gives rise to morbidity but also markedly diminishes the quality of life of women after menopause and of both men and women over 65 years of age. Osteoporosis is a diminution of both organic matrix and mineral of the skeleton. When the total amount of bone diminishes to low values, fractures with minimum trauma or spontaneous fractures result, giving rise to symptomatic osteoporosis. In addition, the quality of remaining bone in the elderly may be suspect. Thus, the disease osteoporosis is multifactorial, and has many contributing causes. Some physicians consider osteoporosis a natural consequence of the aging process. However, the fact that some elderly retain strong and relatively dense bone argues against the idea that osteoporosis is an inevitable consequence of aging. We must, therefore, begin to understand what are the factors that play a major role in forming and depositing bone as well as the factors which bring about the resorption and rebuilding of bone. These factors when understood in their fullness will likely provide us with an understanding of management of the bone loss syndrome.

In recent years there have been major advances made in our understanding of calcium physiology and bone structure. We have also made important advances in our methods of measuring bone mass and have accumulated an understanding of the relationship of bone mass with fracture incidence. The discovery of new humoral factors that regulate calcium, phosphorus, and bone have provided new tools with which to understand the disease and with which to treat and/or prevent the disease. Certainly the use of calcitonin, of the new active forms of vitamin D, and replacement estrogen therapy present new possibilities for battling the onset of osteoporosis. It may be possible with further understanding that they can be used in building back skeleton.

The Steenbock Symposium was organized specifically to bring together outstanding clinical investigators to discuss where we are in our understanding of the broad disease of osteoporosis, how do we assess the extent of the disease, what are the risks of diminished bone density and how can this disease be treated or prevented. Work will be presented on the use of estrogens as replacement therapy in the postmenopausal woman, the use of calcitonin to diminish bone pain and also to block bone resorption, and the use of the vitamin D compounds to increase calcium absorption, bone turnover, and to suppress bone loss. Work will also be presented to show the importance of exercise and the need for adequate calcium intakes throughout life. This Symposium will also underline the need for understanding additional factors and new modes of therapy. The Symposium has now been organized into a book which hopefully will reach far beyond the Symposium to educate and/or provide information to the medical world as to how this disease can be managed as of 1989.

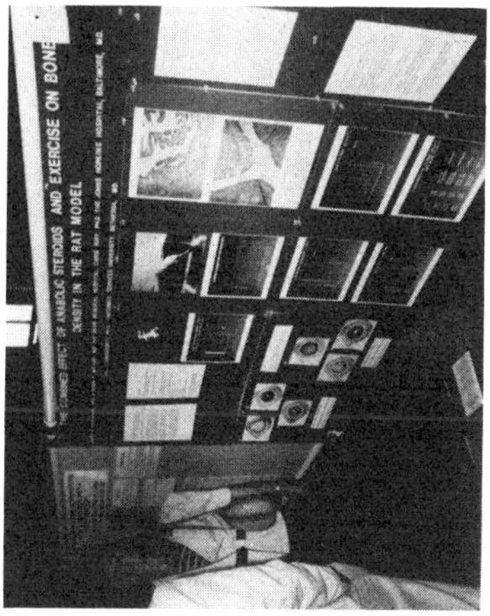
THE COMBINED EFFECT OF ANABOLIC STEROIDS AND EXERCISE ON BONE
DENSITY IN THE RAT MODEL

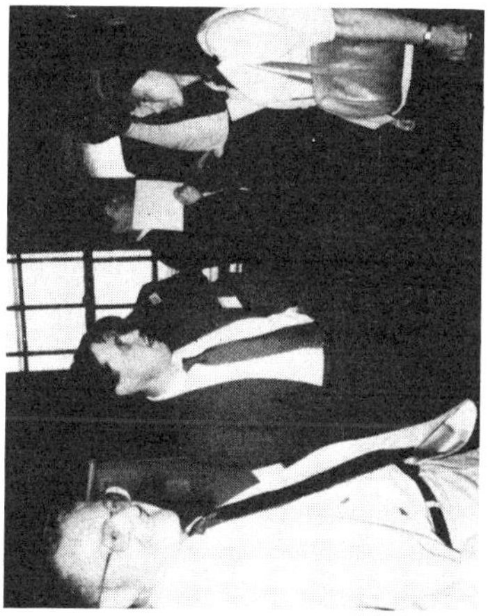

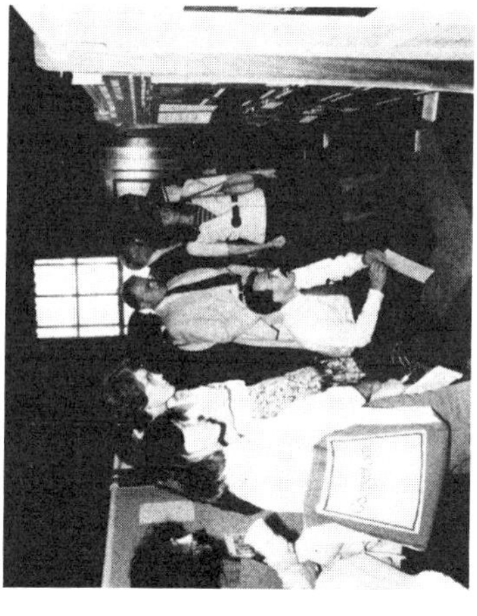

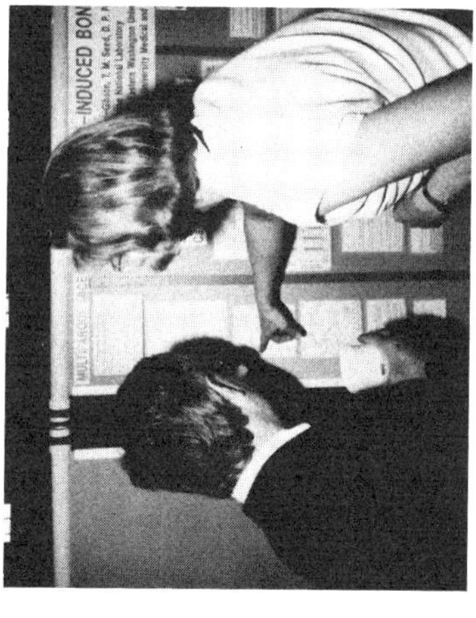

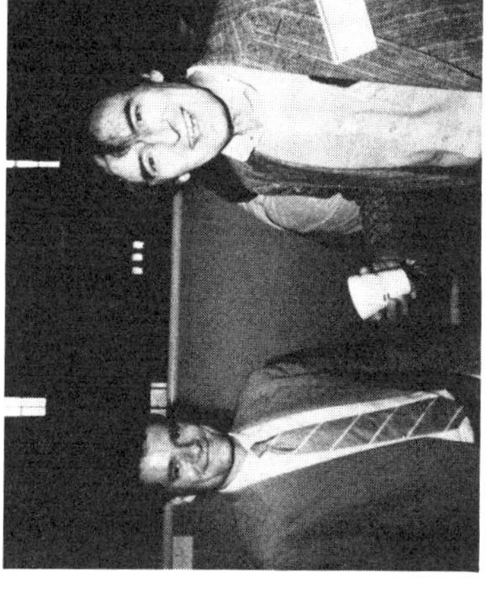

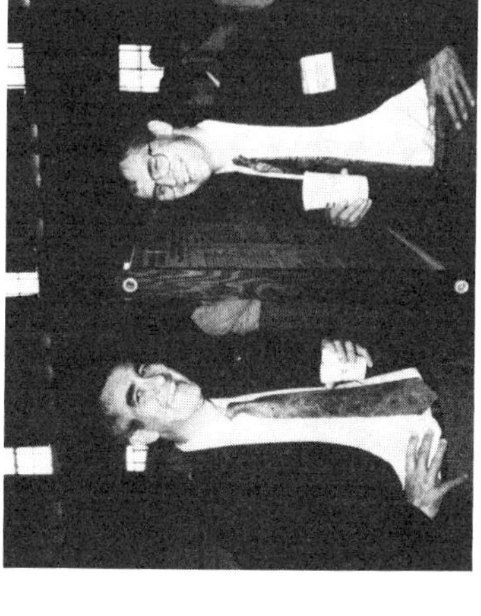

xii

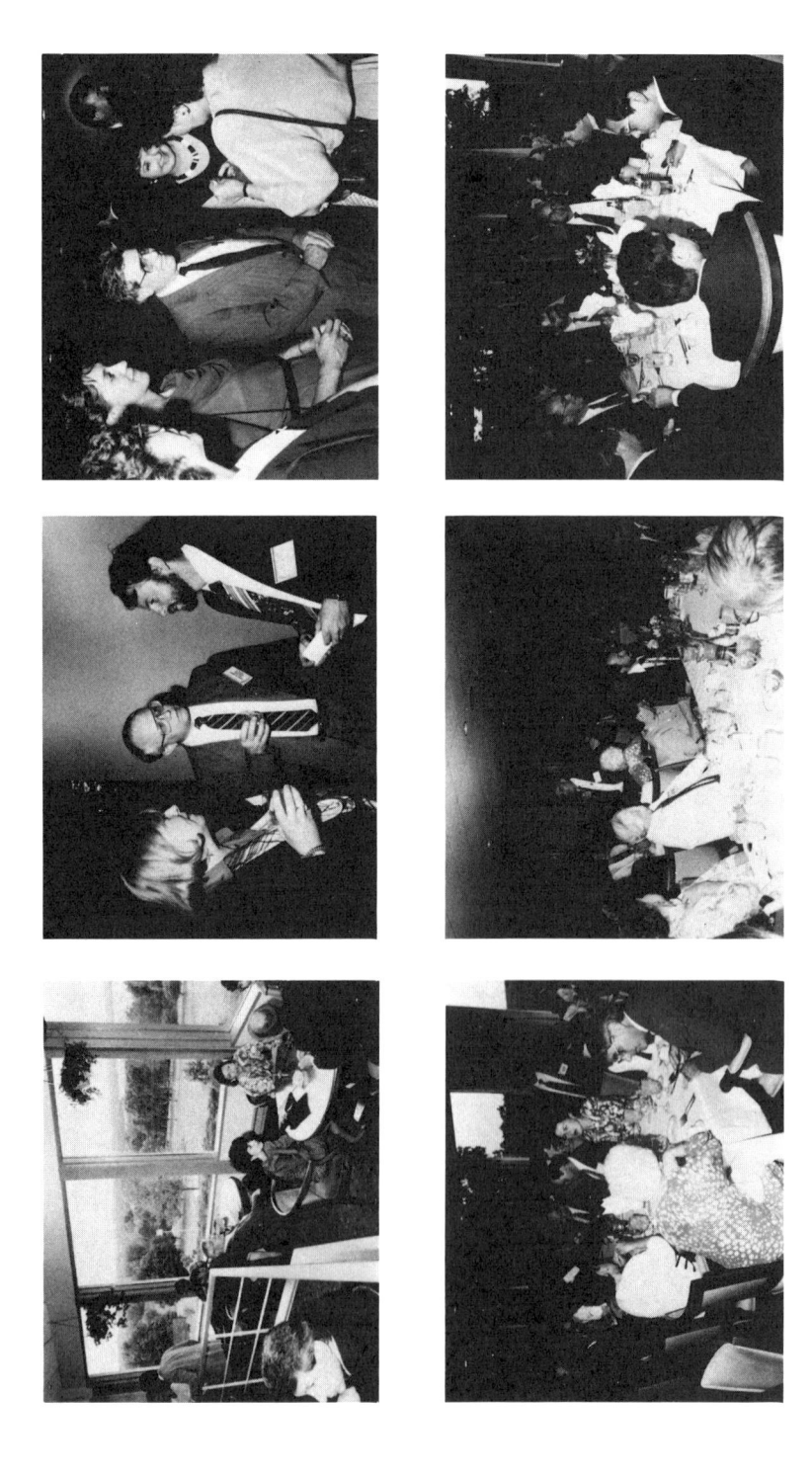

xiii

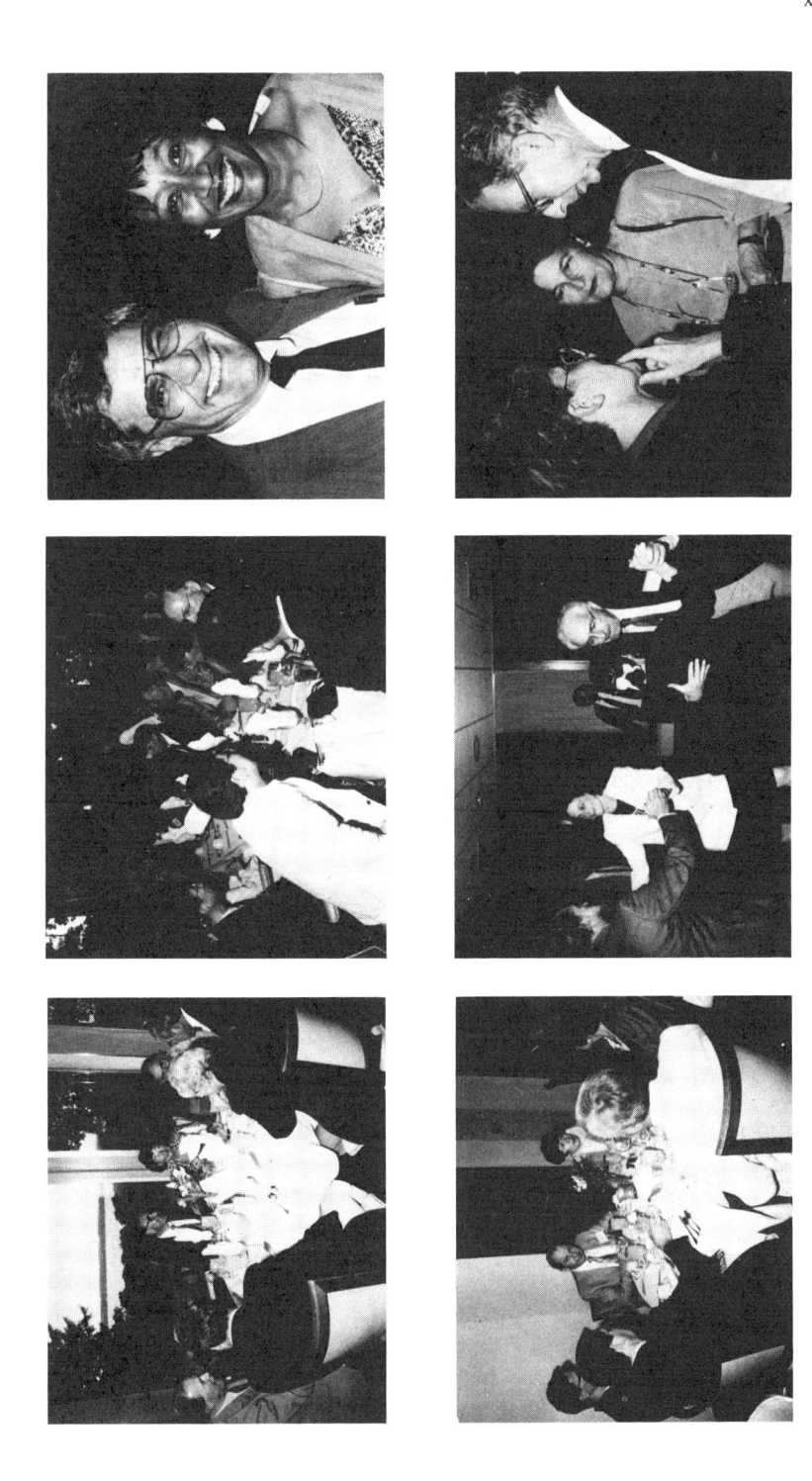

xiv

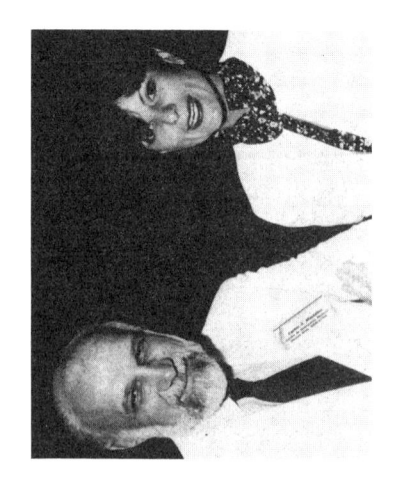

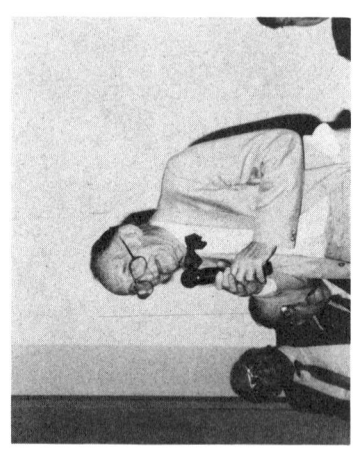

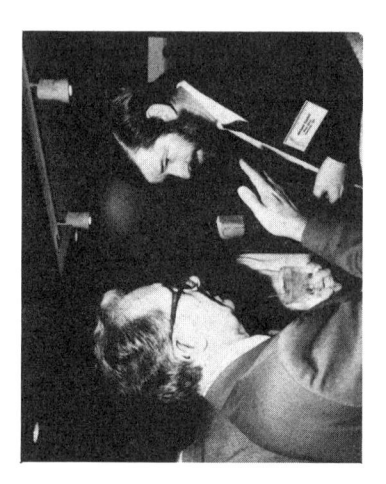

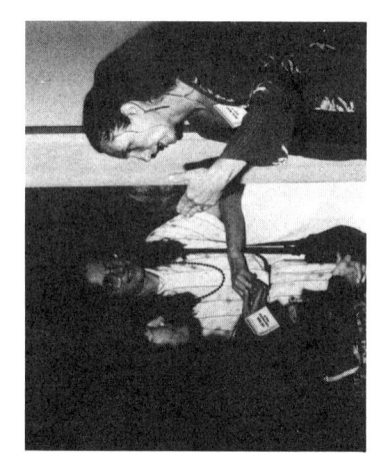

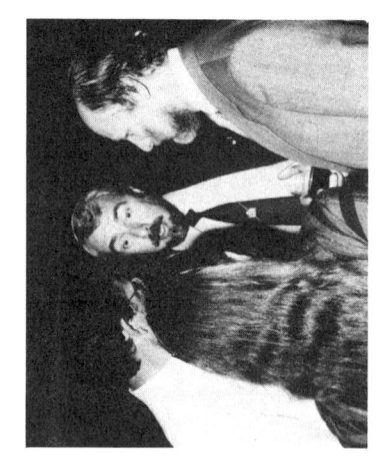

Participants

Adelizzi, Ray
Department of Medicine - Suite 3100
University of Medicine & Dentistry
 of New Jersey (UMDNJ/SOM)
Stratford, NJ 08084 USA

Ainso, Sirje
Sanofi, Inc.
101 Park Avenue
New York, NY USA

Aloia, John
Chairman, Department of Medicine
Winthrop-University Hosital
Mineola, Long Island, NY 11501 USA

Altz-Smith, Mary
103 Bonita Drive
Birmingham, AL 35209 USA

Amano, Atsuo
Pharmaceuticals 2nd Marketing Dept.
Teijin Ltd.
Chiyoda-ku
Tokyo 100, JAPAN

Andon, Mark B.
Research and Development
The Procter & Gamble Company
Cincinnati, OH 45239-8707 USA

Augustine, Matthew
Rorer Central Research
800 Business Center Drive
Horsham, PA 19044 USA

Avioli, Louis V.
Director, Division of Endocrinology
 and Bone Metabolism
The Jewish Hospital of St. Louis
216 South Kingshighway Blvd.
St. Louis, MO 63178 USA

Baim, Sanford
Department of Rheumatology
Rheumatic Disease Center
2015 E. Newport Avenue
Milwaukee, WI 53211 USA

Baker, David L.
Osteoporosis Division
The Monarch Foundation
400 Oak Street
Cincinnati, OH 45219 USA

Balena, Raffaella
Bone and Mineral Division
Henry Ford Hospital
Detroit, MI 48202 USA

Banovac, Kresimir
Orthopedics & Rehabilitation (D-27)
University of Miami
Miami, FL 33101 USA

Barden, Howard
Lunar Radiation
313 W. Beltline Highway
Madison, WI 53713 USA

Bauer, Richard
Department of Medicine
University of Texas Health Science
 Center
San Antonio, TX 78284 USA

Baumgartner, C. John
Endocrinology Minneapolis
6490 Excelsior Blvd.
Minneapolis, MN 55426 USA

Baylink, David J.
Mineral Metabolism (151)
Jerry L. Pettis Veterans Hospital
11201 Benton Street
Loma Linda, CA 92357 USA

Bernstein, Robert M.
Endocrinology, Diabetics &
 Nutrition
531 Harkle Road, Suite A
Santa Fe, NM 87501 USA

Bhattacharyya, Maryka H.
Biological, Environmental, and
 Medical Research Division
Argonne National Laboratory
Argonne, IL USA 60439

Bijvoet, O. L. M.
Department of Clinical Endocrinology
University Hospital
Rijnsburgerweg 10
2333 AA Leiden
THE NETHERLANDS

Bishko, Fred
Department of Medicine Rheumatology
Euclid Clinic Foundation
18599 Lake Shore Blvd.
Cleveland, OH 44119 USA

Bishop, Charles W.
LUNAR Radiation
313 W. Beltline Highway
Madison, WI 53713 USA

Blaylock, William M.
Department of Rheumatology
Lewis-Gale Clinic, Inc.
1802 Braeburn Drive
Salem, VA 24153 USA

Blevins, Thomas C.
Austin Diagnostic Clinic
801 W. 34th Street
Austin, TX 78705 USA

Bloze, Asta E.
Southern California Orthopedic and
 Sports Medical Group
15211 Vanowen Street, Suite 300
Van Nuys, CA 91405-3641 USA

Bock, Lawrence
1079 Hymettus
Leucadia, CA 92024 USA

Bolognese, Michael
19231 Montgomery Village Ave., D11
Gaithersburg, MD 20879 USA

Booher, Delbert L.
Department of Gynecology
Cleveland Clinic Foundation
9500 Euclid Avenue
Cleveland, OH 44195-5158 USA

Brewer, S. J.
Ciba Geigy Pharmaceuticals
General Drugs
Summit, NJ 07901 USA

Briney, Walter G.
Department of Rheumatology
Denver Arthritis Clinic
4545 E. 9th Ave., #510
Denver, CO 80220 USA

Broy, Susan
Department of Medicine
Lutheran General Hospital
1775 Dempster
Park Ridge, IL 60068 USA

Buckley, Lenore
Department of Medicine
University of Vermont
Burlington, VT 05404 USA

Byrd, William J.
Memorial Drive Consultants, Inc.
University Place, Suite 183
124 Mt. Auburn Street
Cambridge, MA 02138 USA

Cameron, E.C.
Department of Medicine
910 W. 10th Avenue
University of British Columbia
Vancouver, BC, CANADA

Caniggia, Angelo
Il Direttore
Instituto di Clinica Medica
University of Siena
53100 Siena
ITALY

Caplan, Robert H.
Department of Internal Medicine
Gunderson Clinic
LaCrosse, WI 54601 USA

Carletti, Enrico
CEF Zaccanti
ITALY

Caulin, Francine
Rorer S.A.
4-rue de la Gare
Levallois, FRANCE 92304

Chandler, Peggy J.
The University of Chicago
 Green 309
5848 S. University Avenue
Chicago, IL 60637 USA

Chesnut, Charles H., III
Director, Osteoporosis Res. Center
University Hospital
University of Washington
Division of Nuclear Medicine
Seattle, WA 98195 USA

Chines, Arkadi
Div. Endocrinology & Metabolism
Jewish Hospital of St. Louis
 at Washington University
St. Louis, MO 63110 USA

Christiansen, Claus
Head, Dept. of Clinical Chemistry
Glostrup Hospital
DK-2600 Glostrup
DENMARK

Clark, Kathleen
Preventive Medicine & Environmental
  Health
University of Iowa
Iowa City, IA 52242 USA

Conley, William R.
320 Juniper Lane
Ann Arbor, MI 48105 USA

Crocker, Laurence G.
1525 Vilas Avenue
Madison, WI 53711 USA

Cyronak, Judith
Marketing
Osteo-Technology, Inc.
55 New York Ave.
Framingham, MA 01701 USA

Dalsky, Gail P.
Osteoporosis Center
Univ. of Connecticut Health Center
Farm Hollow, Suite C-208
Farmington, CT 06032-9984 USA

Danielson, Mikki
Cardiac Rehabilitation &
  Wellness, MOB #108
The Christ Hospital
2123 Auburn Avenue
Cincinnati, OH 45219 USA

Davidai, Giora
610 LaSalle Street, Apt. 7C
Durham, NC 27705 USA

Davidson, James
Internal Medicine/Rheumatology
Monroe Clinic
Monroe, WI 53566 USA

Dawson-Hughes, Bess
Tufts University
Human Nutrition Research Center
  on Aging
711 Washington Street
Boston, MA 02111 USA

Deal, Chad L.
University Hospitals of Cleveland
2073 Abington Road
Cleveland, OH 44106 USA

DeCoteau, W. Earle
Department of Medicine
McMaster University
Box 2000 Station A
Hamilton, Ontario L8N 3Z5
CANADA

Dellanno, Donna
General Drugs - Endocrine
Ciba-Geigy Pharmaceuticals
556 Morris Avenue
Summit, NJ 07901 USA

Delmas, Pierre D.
Unite Inserm 234
Pathologie des Tissus Calcifies
Hopital Edouard Herriot
Pavillon E
Place d'Arsonval
69437 Lyon Cedex 03
FRANCE

DeLuca, Hector F.
Department of Biochemistry
420 Henry Mall
University of Wisconsin-Madison
Madison, WI 53706 USA

Dempster, David W.
Regional Bone Center
Helen Hayes Hospital, Route 9W
W. Haverstraw, NY 10993 USA

Denis, Catherine
Endocrinologie-Gynecologie
Laboratoires Cassenne
Paris 75015 FRANCE

Denton, M. Drue
Osteoporosis Division
Monarch Foundation
400 Oak Street
Cincinnati, OH 45219 USA

Denysyk, Oleh
CIBA-GEIGY
556 Morris Avenue
Summit, NJ 07901 USA

Detter, Jeff R.
Bone Metabolism Unit
601 N. 30th Street, Suite 5730
Creighton University
Omaha, NE 68131 USA

Devogelaer, J. P.
Department of Rheumatology
Saint-Luc University Hospital
Ave Hippocrate 10
Brussels, BELGIUM B-1200

DiMuzio, Michael T.
Division of Diagnostics
Abbott Laboratories
North Chicago, IL 60064 USA

Drinka, Paul
454 Woodside Terrace
Madison, WI 53711 USA

Dubois, Catherine
RUSSEL UCALF/D.M.R.U.
102 et 111, route de Noisy
93230 Romainville, FRANCE

Dutta, S. N.
Div. of Metabolism & Endocrine
  Drug Production, Rm. 14B-03
Food and Drug Administration
5600 Fishers Lane
Rockville, MD 20857 USA

Eash, James R.
Business Development
Rorer International Pharmaceutical
P.O. Box 530
Fort Washington, PA 19034 USA

Eastell, Richard
Dept. Internal Medicine,
  Endocrinology and Metabolism
Mayo Clinic
Rochester, MN 55905 USA

Ebeling, Peter R.
Endocrine Research Unit
Mayo Clinic
Rochester, MN 55905 USA

Eberl, Stefan
Nuclear Medicine Department
St. Vincent's Hospital
Darlinghurst, NSW, AUSTRALIA 2010

Eberle, Robert
Osteoporosis Division
The Monarch Foundation
400 Oak Street
Cincinnati, OH 45219 USA

Eisman, John
Head, Bone and Mineral Research
Garvan Institute of Medical Res.
St. Vincent's Hospital
Darlinghurst NSW 2010
AUSTRALIA

Ethgen, Dominique
Sanofi Recherche
rue du P. J. Blayac
Montpellier, FRANCE 34082

Ettinger, Bruce
Department of Medicine
Kaiser Permenente Medical Center
San Francisco, CA 94115 USA

Fasano, Grace A.
Department of Medicine
Univ. of Chicago Medical Center
Chicago, IL 60637 USA

Fen, Huang
1329 N. Wingra Drive
Madison, WI 53715 USA

Fendrock, Charles
Osteo-Technology, Inc.
Framingham, MA 01701 USA

Finan, Michael J.
Orthopaedic Surgery Associates
1414 W. Lombard St.
Davenport, IA 52804 USA

Fishman, Norman
Suite 410N
222 S. Woodsmill Rd.
Chesterfield, MO 63017 USA

Fleisch, Herbie
Universitat Bern
Pathophysiologisches Institute
CH-3010 Bern
SWITZERLAND

Foldes, A. Joseph
Bone and Mineral Research Laboratory
Henry Ford Hospital
Detroit, MI 48202 USA

Franks, Alan F.
Department of Bone Metabolism
Norwich Eaton Pharmaceuticals
Norwich, NY 13815 USA

Friedl, Karl
P.O. Box 814
Natick, MA 01760 USA

Fudman, Edward
Department of Rheumatology
Austin Diagnostic Clinic
801 W. 34th Street
Austin, TX 78705 USA

Fujita, Takuo
Third Division
Department of Medicine
Kobe University School of Medicine
Kobe, JAPAN 650

Furukawa, Takako
Department of Nuclear Medicine
Kawasaki Medical School
Kurashiki, JAPAN 701-01

Gajardo, Hector
Cuarto Centenario 1262
Santiago, CHILE

Gallagher, J. C.
Section of Endocrinology and
  Metabolism
Creighton University
601 North 30th Street
Suite 5730
Omaha, NE 68131-2197 USA

Gaut, Zane N.
800 Cranford Avenue
Westfield, NJ 07090 USA

Genant, Harry
Department of Radiology
University of California
505 Parnassus, Room M392
San Francisco, CA 94143 USA

Gennari, Carlo
Direttore, Instituto di Semeiotica
  Medica
Universita di Siena
53100 Siena
ITALY

Gerber, Nicholas
Department of Pharmacology
The Ohio State University
Columbus, OH 43210 USA

Gertz, Barry J.
Department of Clinical Research
Merck & Co., Inc.
P.O. Box 2000
WB D-236
Rahway, NJ 07065-0914 USA

Gibbs, Edith
Hologic, Inc.
200 Prospect Street
Waltham, MA 02154 USA

Goodwin, Allan M.
Department of Medicine
Division of Rheumatology
St. Luke's Hospital
Cleveland, OH 44122 USA

Greep, Nancy
5260 El Cedral
Long Beach, CA 90815 USA

Grodberg, Marcus G.
Director of Research
Colgate-Hoyt Laboratories
Canton, MA 02021 USA

Gronow, Michael
Suite 18, 96 Grattan Street
Carlton, Victoria 3053
AUSTRALIA

Han, In Kwon
Mayo Clinic
Endocrine Research Unit
Rochester, MN 55905 USA

Hanamura, Satoshi
2624 Belmont Canyon Road
Belmont, CA 94002 USA

Hansen, James W.
Mead Johnson Research Center (R7)
Evansville, IN 47721-0001 USA

Hanson, Jim
Lunar Radiation
313 W. Beltline Highway
Madison, WI 53713 USA

Harper, Kristine D.
Department of Medicine
University of Rochester School
  of Medicine & Dentistry
1425 Portland Avenue
Rochester, NY 14621 USA

Harrington, J. T.
Department of Rheumatology
Physicians Plus Medical Group
20 S. Park, Suite 301
Madison, WI 53715 USA

Hayes, Wilson C.
Orthopaedic Biomechanics Laboratory
Beth Israel Hospital
330 Brookline Ave.
Boston, MA 02215 USA

Hazum, Eli
Department of Endocrinology
Glaxo Research Laboratories
5 Moore Drive
Research Triangle Park, NC 27709 USA

Heaney, Robert P.
Creighton University
California at 24th Street
Omaha, NE 68178 USA

Heath, Hunter, III
Department of Medicine
Endocrine Research Unit
Mayo Clinic
Rochester, MN 55905 USA

Heileman, John P.
Endocrinology Associates, P.A.
3522 N. 3rd Avenue
Phoenix, AZ 85013 USA

Hinz, James T.
Geriatric Pharmaceutical Corp.
16820 Ridge View Drive
Brookfield, WI 53005 USA

Hodsman, Anthony B.
Department of Medicine
St. Joseph's Health Centre
London, Ontario CANADA N6A 4V2

Holtrop, Mariyke
Department of Medicine
Boston University Medical Center
Boston, MA 02118 USA

Honnens, Jeanne
Pharmaceutical Div. Marketing
Novo-Nordisk A/S
Novo Alle
DK-2880 Bagsvaerd, DENMARK

Horsman, A.
MRC Bone Mineralization Group
Department of Medical Physics
The University of Leeds
Leeds, LS1 3EX
West Yorks, UNITED KINGDOM

Houpt, Joseph B.
Rheumatic Disease Unit
Mount Sinai Hospital
University of Toronto
600 University Avenue, Suite 431
Toronto, Ontario, CANADA M5G 1X5

Ishikawa, Hitoshi
Takeda Chemical Industries, Ltd.
Doshomachi Chuo-Ku
Osaka, JAPAN 541

Jacobsen, Steven J.
Medical College of Wisconsin
P.O. Box 26509
Milwaukee, WI 53226 USA

Jacobson, Don
Department of Medical Physics
Medical College of Wisconsin
8700 West Wisconsin Avenue
Milwaukee, WI 53226 USA

Jamin, Christian
CIBA-GEIGY 2 & 4
rue Lionel Terray
Rueil, FRANCE 92506

Johnson, Gregory M.
LUNAR Radiation
313 W. Beltline Highway
Madison, WI 53713 USA

Johnson, Judy
Department of Medicine, Suite 5730
St. Joseph's Hospital
Creighton University
Omaha, NE 68131 USA

Johnson, William D.
Department of Toxicology
Eli Lilly and Company
Greenfield, IN 46140 USA

Johnston, C. Conrad, Jr.
Department of Medicine
Emerson Hall 421
Indiana University
545 Barnhill Drive
Indianapolis, IN 46223 USA

Johnston, Ian
Suite 10, Cardigan House
96 Gratton Street
Carlton, Victoria 3053
AUSTRALIA

Judge, James
Osteoporosis Center
Farm Hollow
Univ. of Connecticut Health Center
Farmington, CT 06032 USA

Kalchhauser, Georg
Zentralrontgen - Institut
Hanusch - Krankenhaus
Vienna A1140
AUSTRIA

Karlin, Elizabeth
Associated Physicians
4410 Regent Street
Madison, WI 53705 USA

Kasel, Mary
Bone Metabolism Unit, Suite 5730
St. Joseph's Hospital
Creighton University
Omaha, NE 68131 USA

Keller, Carla
UWC - Waukesha County
1500 University Drive
Waukesha, WI 53186 USA

Kelner, Katrina
Science Magazine
1333 H Street, N.W.
Washington, D.C. 20005 USA

Kester, Rita
Center for Metabolic Bone Disorders
Providence Medical Center
4805 NE Glisan
Portland, OR 97213 USA

Khairi, M. Rashid A.
Department of Endocrinology
Endocrine Diagnostics, Inc.
7430 N. Shadeland Ave.
Indianapolis, IN 46250 USA

Kiratli, Jenny B.
Dept. of Preventive Medicine
504 N. Walnut Street
University of Wisconsin-Madison
Madison, Wisconsin 53706 USA

Koch, Karen
Medical Department
Novo-Nordisk A/S, Novo Alle
DK-2880 Bagsvaerd, DENMARK

Kolb, Felix O.
Dept. Medicine/Endocrinology
U.C. Medical Center
9 Starboard Ct.
Mill Valley, CA 94941 USA

Kotowicz, Mark A.
Endocrine Research Unit
Mayo Clinic
Rochester, MN 55905 USA

Kujala, Gregory
Dept. Internal Med./Rheumatology
Rm 2178 HSC-N
West Virginia University
Morgantown, WV 26506 USA

Kumagai, Fumio
Chugai U.S.A., Inc.
520 Madison Avenue
New York, NY 10022 USA

Lampman, James H.
Department of Rheumatology
St. Alexius Medical Center
900 E. Broadway
Bismark, ND 58501 USA

Landau, Moshe
Department of Rheumatology
Hillel Jaffe Memorial Hospital
Hadera, ISRAEL

Larsson, Lasse
Department of Clinical Chemistry
University of Linkoping
S-581 85 Linkoping
SWEDEN

LeBlanc, Lydia K.
Osteoporosis Center
Woman's Hospital
Baton Rouge, LA 70895 USA

LeBoff, Meryl S.
Dept. Endocrinology/Hypertension
Brigham & Women's Hospital
221 Longwood Ave.
Boston, MA 02115 USA

Lee, Martha L.
Department of Rheumatology
Marshfield Clinic
Marshfield, WI 54449 USA

Leone, Mary
Norwich Eaton?

Lieberthal, Alan
Clinical Medicine, S.C.
1218 West Kilbourn Ave., Suite 501
Milwaukee, WI 53233 USA

Lindsay, Robert
Director of Research
Helen Hayes Hospital
Route 9W
West Haverstraw, NY 10993 USA

Lloyd, Tom
Director, Reproductive Endocrinology
  Research Laboratories
Department of Obstetrics and
  Gynecology
Penn State University College of Med.
Hershey, PA 17033 USA

Lofman, Owe
Prevention & Community Medicine
Univ. of Linkoping; Landstinget
Linkoping S-58101
SWEDEN

Lopez-Mendez, Ada
Clinical Immunology & Rheumatology
The Univ. of Alabama at Birmingham
Birmingham, AL 35294 USA

Love, Betsy
Center for Metabolic Bone Disorders
Providence Medical Center
4805 NE Glisan
Portland, OR 97213 USA

Lueg, Mark C.
Osteoporosis Treatment Center
Elmwood Medical Center
1201 S. Clearview Pkwy.
Jefferson, LA 70121 USA

MacIntyre, Iain
Royal Postgraduate Med. School
University of London
Hammersmith Hospital
Du Cane Road
London W12 ONN
ENGLAND

Mack, Thomas
Dept. of Preventive Medicine
USC School of Medicine
2025 Zonal Avenue, PMB B105
Los Angeles, CA 90033 USA

Maenpaa, Pekka H.
Department of Biochemistry
University of Kuopio
P.O. Box 6
SF-70211 Kuopio
FINLAND

Magee, Frank
Animal Research & Basic Sciences
Harrington Arthritis Res. Center
Phoenix, AZ 85015 USA

Mahadevappa, Mahesh
Department of Medical Physics
Medical College of Wisconsin
8700 West Wisconsin Avenue
Milwaukee, WI 53226 USA

Malcolm, Diane
LUNAR PERSON

Mallik, Tilak K.
Department of Endocrinology
Family Health Network
4422 Gen. Meyer Ave., Suite 100
New Orleans, LA 70131 USA

Malluche, Hartmut
MN572 University of Kentucky
  Medical Center
Division of Nephrology Bone &
  Mineral Metabolism
Lexington, KY 40536-0084 USA

Mann, F. A.
Department of Radiology
Mallinckrodt Institute of Radiology
St. Louis, MO 63111 USA

Marinovic, Nash
Dept. of Licensing and Development
Pfizer Inc.
219 E. 42nd Street - 9th Floor
New York, NY 10017 USA

Martens, Kolene
Dept. Bone Metabolism, Suite 5730
St. Joseph's Hospital
Creighton University
Omaha, NE 68131 USA

Marx, Christopher
Scripps Clinic & Research Clinic
10666 North Torrey Pines Road
La Jolla, CA 92037 USA

Masonson, Harvey N.
Clinical Research
Sanofi, Inc.
101 Park Avenue
New York, NY 10178 USA

Matkovich, Velimir
Department of Physical Medicine
  and Medicine
The Ohio State University
Columbus, OH 43210 USA

Mautalen, Carlos A.
Centro de Osteopatias Medicas
Saavedra 189
Beunos Aires, ARGENTINA 1083

Mazess, Richard
LUNAR Radiation
313 W. Beltline Highway
Madison, WI 53713 USA

McCarty, Patricia
Hamilton Carver & Lee
Chicago, IL 60610 USA

McClung, Michael
Center for Metabolic Bone Disorders
Providence Medical Center
4805 NE Glisan Street
Portland, OR 97213 USA

McDonnell, Jessop
1624 - South I Street, #404
Tacoma, WA 98405 USA

McOsker, Jocelyn E.
Department of Bone Metabolism
Norwich Eaton Pharmaceuticals, Inc.
Norwich, NY 13815 USA

Medina, Jeanne
Family Health Plan
12500 W. Bluemound Road
Elm Grove, IL 53122 USA

Mehta, D. M.
Department of Rheumatology
Orthopaedic & Arthritic Hospital
33 Wellesley Street East, Suite 323
Toronto, Ontario, CANADA M4Y 1H1

Mellish, Robert
Regional Bone Center
Helen Hayes Hospital
West Haverstraw, NY 10993 USA

Melsen, Flemming
University Institute of Pathology
Aarhus Amtssygehus
DK-8000 Aarhus C
DENMARK

Melton, L. Joseph, III
Department of Health Sciences
  Research
Section of Clinical Epidemiology
Mayo Clinic
Rochester, MN 55905 USA

Meunier, Pierre J.
Hopital Edouard Herriot
Pavillon F
Unite Inserm 234
Place d'Arsonval - 69437
Lyon Cedex 03, FRANCE

Michael, Roger H.
Orthopaedic Surgery
Union Memorial Hospital
201 E. University Parkway
Baltimore, MD 21218 USA

Milhaud, Gerard
Service de Biophysique
C.H.U. Saint-Antoine
27 Rue de Chaligney
Paris 12e, FRANCE

Millar, Bob
Norland Corporation
Fort Atkinson, WI 53538 USA

Miller, Barbara E.
Department of Bone Metabolism
Norwich Eaton Pharmaceuticals
Norwich, NY 13815 USA

Miller, Henry K.
Women's Clinic and Woman's Hospital
323 East Airport Ave.
Baton Rouge, LA 70806 USA

Miller, Jeffrey L.
1919 Swann Avenue
Tampa, FL 33606 USA

Mizuno, Hatsuhiko
2nd Development Department
Teijin Ltd.
Chiyoda-ku
Tokyo, JAPAN 100

Morgan, Brad
Norland Corporation
Fort Atkinson, WI 53538 USA

Morgan, G. James, Jr.
Rheumatology Desk 200
Dartmouth-Hitchcock Medical Center
Hanover, NH 03755 USA

Moura, Anne-Marie
Department of Endocrinolgy
Roussel-UCLAF
102-111, route de Noisy
93230 Romainville, FRANCE

Mouttet, Ariel
ROUSSEL UCALF/D.M.S.
35, bd des Invalides
75007 Paris, FRANCE

Mueller, Mark
1002 E. South Temple, #405
Salt Lake City, UT 84102 USA

Munoz, Juan M.
R.R. 2, Box 65
Fargo, ND 58102 USA

Musa, Byron U.
1755 Coburg Road, Building 5
Eugene, OR 97401 USA

Myburgh, Kathy H.
MRC/UCT Bioenergetics of
 Exercise
Univ. of Cape Town Med. School
Observatory, Cape Town, S. AFRICA

Myers, Thomas J.
Department of Neurosurgery
Medical College of Wisconsin
Milwaukee, WI 53226 USA

Nagant de Deuxchaisnes, Charles
Service de Rhumatologie
Universite Catholoque de Louvain
Cliniques Universitaires Staint-Luc
1200 Brussels
BELGIUM

Nelson, Donna
Center for Metabolic Bone
 Disorders
Providence Medical Center
4805 Northeast Glisan Street
Portland, OR 97213-2967

Neville, Donna
The Greenbrier Clinic
White Sulphur Springs, WV 24986 USA

Nielsen, Maren
Osteoporosis Detection Center, P.A.
Wichita, KS 67214 USA

Nilsson, Magnus
Karo Bio AB
Huddinge University Hospital, R64
S-14186 Huddinge
SWEDEN

Nishii, Yasuho
Applied Research Laboratories
Research Laboratories
Chugai Pharmaceutical Co., Ltd.
Tokyo, JAPAN 171

Nord, Russ
Norland Corporation
Fort Atkinson, WI 53538 USA

Nordin, B. E. C.
Institute of Medical and Veterinary
 Science
Frome Road
Box 14, Rundle Mall Post Office
Adelaide, SOUTH AUSTRALIA

Nowlin, Nancy S.
Rm. B5112C
Veterans Administration Hospital
Madison, WI 53705 USA

Ohkawa, Hiroyuki
Exploratory Research Labs of Fuji
 Gotemba Research Labs
Chugai Pharmaceutical Co., Ltd.
135, Komakado, 1-Chome
Gotemba 412 JAPAN

Ohzeki, Masahiro
Research Center
Taisho Pharmaceutical Co., Ltd.
24-1, Tahata 3-Chome
Toshimaku, Tokyo 171 JAPAN

Orimo, Hajime
Department of Geriatrics
Faculty of Medicine
University of Tokyo
7-3-1 Hongo, Bunkyo-ku
Tokyo, JAPAN

Orlowski, Ronald C.
2624 Belmont Canyon Road
Belmont, CA 94002 USA

Ostbye, Truls
Dept. of Epidemiology &
  Biostatistics
Kresge Building
University of Western Ontario
London, Ontario N6A 5C1
CANADA

Ostgaard, Roy
Norland Corporation
Rt. 4, Norland Drive
Fort Atkinson, WI 53538 USA

Otomo, Susumu
Research Center
Taisho Pharmaceutical Co., Ltd.
24-1, Tahata 3-Chome
Toshimaku, Tokyo 171, JAPAN

Owen, Perry
Professional Relations Department
Norwich Eaton Pharmaceuticals, Inc.
Norwich, NY 13815 USA

Owens, Jeanna L.
Department of Rheumatology
Oshkosh Clinic
400 Ceape Ave.
Oshkosh, WI 54901 USA

Palummeri, Ernesto
Department of Geriatrics
G. Stuard Hospital-U.S.L. No. 4
Parma, ITALY 43100

Parfitt, A. Michael
Fifth Medical Division
Henry Ford Hospital
2799 W. Grand Blvd.
Detroit, MI 48202 USA

Paris, Jacques
Recherche et Developpement
  pre-Clinique
Laboratoire Theramex
MONACO

Payne, Randy
Norland Corporation
Fort Atkinson, WI 53538 USA

Peck, William A.
Vice Chancellor for Medical Affairs
Washington Univ. School of Medicine
Box 8106
660 S. Euclid Ave.
St. Louis, MO 63110 USA

Pecora, A. M.
Ciba Geigy Pharmaceuticals
General Drugs
Summit, NJ 07901 USA

Perry-Keene, Donald
Department of Endocrinology
Royal Brisbane Hospital
Brisbane, Queensland, AUSTRALIA

Perry-Keene, Isobel
201 Wickham Terrace
Brisbane, Queensland, AUSTRALIA

Peterson, Janis
Marketing Continental Europe
Smith Kline & French Laboratories
B20, 1500 Spring Garden Street
P.O. Box 7929
Philadelphia, PA 19101 USA

Pilbeam, Carol
Department of Endocrinology, AM047
Univ. of Connecticut Health Center
Farmington, CT 06032 USA

Pornel, Bruno
Rue de Roetaert, 68
1180 Brussels, BELGIUM

Pors-Neilsen, Stig
Director, Department of Clinical
  Physiology and Nuclear Medicine
Central Hospital
Hillerod, DENMARK

Posen, Solomon
Department of Medicine
Royal North Shore Hospital,
  St. Leonards
Sydney, NSW
AUSTRALIA

Poteet, Brian
Texas A&M University
College Station, TX USA

Pranger, Martyn H.
New Business Development
Duphar B.V.
Post Box 900
1380 DA Weesp
THE NETHERLANDS

Quinn, Michael J.
Rorer Pharmaceutical
36073 Crompton Circle
Farmington Hills, MI 48331 USA

Raisz, Larry
Endocrinology and Metabolism
University of Connecticut Health
  Center
Farmington, CT 06032 USA

Rayder, Lisa
Worldwide Marketing Research
E. R. Squibb & Sons
P.O. Box 4000
Princeton, NJ 08540 USA

Reed, John
Department of Rheumatology
Fallon Clinic
Worcester, MA 01605 USA

Ribot, C.
Service D'Endocrinologie
Centre Hospitalier Regional
  de Toulouse
C.H.U. Toulouse Purpan
Place du Docteur Baylac
31059 Toulouse Cedex
FRANCE

Riggs, B. Lawrence
Division of Endocrinology and
  Metabolism
Mayo Clinic
Mayo Medical School
Rochester, MN 55905 USA

Robbins, Lana J.
Dept. Medicine, Suite 5730
St. Joseph's Hospital
Creighton University
Omaha, NE 68131 USA

Roberts, Leslie
Providence Medical Center
Portland, OR USA

Rosen, David
Department of Cell Biology
Celtrix Laboratories/Collagen
  Corporation
Palo Alto, CA 94303 USA

Rosini, Sergio
Research-Development
Isituto Farmaceutico Gentili
Pisa 56100, ITALY

Rothschild, Ellen
HPD Medical Department
Building AP30, Abbott Laboratories
One Abbott Park
Abbott Park, IL 60064 USA

Rubinstein, Herbert M.
429 N. Scoville
Oak Park, IL 60302-2260 USA

Russo, Mary Elizabeth
Osteoporosis Center
Woman's Hospital
Baton Rouge, LA 70895 USA

Ryan, Will G.
1753 W. Congress
Chicago, IL 60612 USA

Sacco-Gibson, Nancy
BEM Divison
Argonne National Laboratory
Argonne, IL 60539 USA

Salas, E.
Dept. Rheumatology
Hospital de Alicante
Alicante, SPAIN

Sanchez, Tom
Norland Corporation
Fort Atkinson, WI 53538 USA

Scali, J.
Department of Rheumatology
Durand Central Hospital of
  Buenos Aires
San Pedrito 323 - 6°B
Buenos Aires, ARGENTINA 1406

Schiff, Michael H.
Department of Rheumatology
Denver Arthritis Clinic
4545 E. 9th Ave., #510
Denver, CO 80220 USA

Schilling, Margarita P.
Department of Endocrinology
Osteoporosis Center - Central
  New York
2305 Genesee Street
Utica, NY 13501 USA

Seeman, Ego
Department of Medicine
Austin Hospital Heidelberg 1
Melbourne, Victoria
AUSTRALIA

Sekaran, Chitra
Professional Services
Medical Marketing
Hoffmann-La Roche
340 Kingsland Street
Nutley, NJ 07110-1199 USA

Severson, Arlen R.
Dept. of Biomedical Anatomy
University of Minnesota, Duluth
Duluth, MN 55812 USA

Shaker, Joseph L.
Department of Medicine
St. Luke's Medical Center
St. Luke's Health Science Building
Suite 503
2901 West K. K. River Parkway
Milwaukee, WI 53215 USA

Shoji, Ryuichi
R & D Planning & Coordination
Taisho Pharmaceutical Co., Ltd.
24-1, Tahata 3-Chome
Toshimaku, Tokyo 171, JAPAN

Sleckman, Joseph
Department of Rheumatology
Dakota Clinic
1702 S. University Drive
Fargo, ND 58103 USA

Smith, Everett L.
Director, Biogerontology Lab
Center for Health Sciences
University of Wisconsin
504 Walnut Street
Madison, WI 53705 USA

Smith, Jo-Anne
University of Connecticut -
 Osteoporosis Center
Univ. of Connecticut Health Center
Farm Hollow C-208
Farmington, CT 06032 USA

Smith, Ken T.
Research and Development
Procter and Gamble Co.
Cincinnati, OH 45239-8707 USA

Sohda, Takashi
Tadeda Chemical Industries, Ltd.
17-85, Jusohonmachi 2-chome
Yodogawa-ku
Osaka 532, JAPAN

Sonkin, Lawrence S.
Department of Endocrinology
New York Hospital
Cornell Medical Center
New York, NY 10021 USA

Sowers, MaryFran
Dept. of Epidemiology
Univ. of Michigan
Ann Arbor, MI 48109 USA

Staples, Sarah
222 South Woodsmill Road,
 Suite 410N
Chesterfield, MO 63107 USA

Stein, Karen R.
Cato Research, Ltd.
500 Franklin Square
1829 E. Franklin St.
Chapel Hill, NC 27514 USA

Stein, Ray A.
Hologic, Inc.
200 Prospect Street
Waltham, MA 02154 USA

Stern, Mark
Department of Medicine
Springfield Clinic
1025 South 7th
Springfield, IL 62703 USA

Stern, Paula
Department of Pharmacology
Northwestern University
303 East Chicago Avenue
Chicago, IL 60611 USA

Stillman, Rachel J.
Department of Kinesiology
University of Illinois
Urbana, IL 61801 USA

Szejnfeld, Vera L.
Paulista School of Medicine
Rua Eliseu Visconti 200
Morumbi - São Paulo
BRAZIL

Tamura, Nobuhiko
Sumitomo Pharmaceuticals Co., Ltd.
345 Park Avenue
New York, NY 10154 USA

Tanaka, Akio
Clinical Affairs Dept. 2
Pharmaceutical Products Division
Chugai Pharmaceutical Co., Ltd.
1-9, Kyobashi 2-chome, Chuo-ku
Tokyo 104, JAPAN

Tanaka, Makoto
Clinical Affairs Dept. 2
Pharmaceutical Products Division
Chugai Pharmaceutical Co., Ltd.
1-9, Kyobashi 2-chome, Chuo-ku
Tokyo 104, JAPAN

Tarozzi, Carlo
ITALY

Tesar, Rogene
Bone Densitometry & Nutrition
  Services
Austin Diagnostic Clinic
Austin, TX 78705   USA

Tilyard, Murray
Department of General Practice
Medical School, University of
  Otaso
Dunedin, NEW ZEALAND

Trahiotis, Margaret
Osteoporosis Center
Farm Hollow-C-208
Univ. Connecticut Health Center
Farmington, CT 06032   USA

Tremollieres, Florence
Department of Endocrinology
Metabolic Bone Disease Unit
Centre Hospitalo-Universitaire
Toulouse 31059, FRANCE

Tsuda, Masao
Biology Laboratories
Takeda Chemical Industries, Ltd.
17-85, Jusohonmachi 2-chome
Yodogawa-ku
Osaka, JAPAN 532

Uskokovic, Milan R.
Chemistry Research
Hoffmann-La Roche, Inc.
Nutley, NJ 07110   USA

VanHooke, Janeen L.
Department of Biochemistry
University of Wisconsin-Madison
Madison, WI 53706   USA

Vialle-Valentin, Catherine
Bone Metabolism/Product Development
Norwich Eaton Pharmaceuticals, Inc.
P.O. Box 191
Norwich, NY 13815-0191   USA

Vickery, Brian H.
Department of Endocrine Physiology
SYNTEX Research
3401 Hillview Avenue
Palo Alto, CA 94304   USA

Villanueva, Antonio R.
Animal Research & Basic Sciences
Harrington Arthritis Res. Center
Phoenix, AZ 85015   USA

Votano, Joseph R.
Expert Image Systems
35 Medford Street
Somerville, MA 02143   USA
University Inn

Wallis, Lila A.
Department of Medicine
Cornell University Medical College
New York, NY 10021   USA

Wardlaw, Gordon
Department of Medical Dietetics
The Ohio State University
Columbus, OH 43210   USA

Weinstein, Allan
Iatro Med, Inc.
2850 South 36th Street
Phoenix, AZ 85040   USA

Weissman, Peter
8700 N. Kendall Drive
Miami, FL 33176   USA

Wiita, Brinda U.
Clinical Research Department
Reid-Rowell, Inc.
901 Sawyer Road
Marietta, GA 30062   USA

Williams, Clair C.
Department of Medicine
The Wellesley Hospital
Suite 302, Elsie K. Jones Bldg.
160 Wellesley Street, East
Toronto, Ontario M4Y 1J3
CANADA
C
Williams, Fred
Pacific Biomedical Corporation
9705 SW Sunshine Court, Suite 400
Beaverton, OR 97005   USA

Wisneski, Leonard A.
Department of Endocrinology
6410 Rockledge Drive, Suite 308
Bethesda, MD 20817   USA

Yamada, Kozo
Business Coordination Department
Chugai Pharmaceutical Co., Ltd.
1-9, Koyobashi 2-chome, Chuo-ku
Tokyo 104, JAPAN

Yu-Yahiro, Janet A.
Department of Orthopaedics
The Union Memorial Hospital
201 E. University Parkway
Baltimore, MD 21218 USA

Zanchetta, Jose R.
Montevideo 928, P.B. "A"
Buenos Aires 1019
ARGENTINA

Zaccanti, Carlo (Lunar)
CEF Zaccanti
Bologna, ITALY

Zeiders, Robert S.
Department of Medicine
Carle Clinic Association
602 W. University Avenue
Urbana, IL 61801 USA

Zummer, Michel
Department of Rheumatology
Hopital Maisonneuve-Rosemont
5415 De L'Assomption
Montreal, Quebec CANADA H1T 2M4

PHYSIOLOGICAL AND CELLULAR BASIS

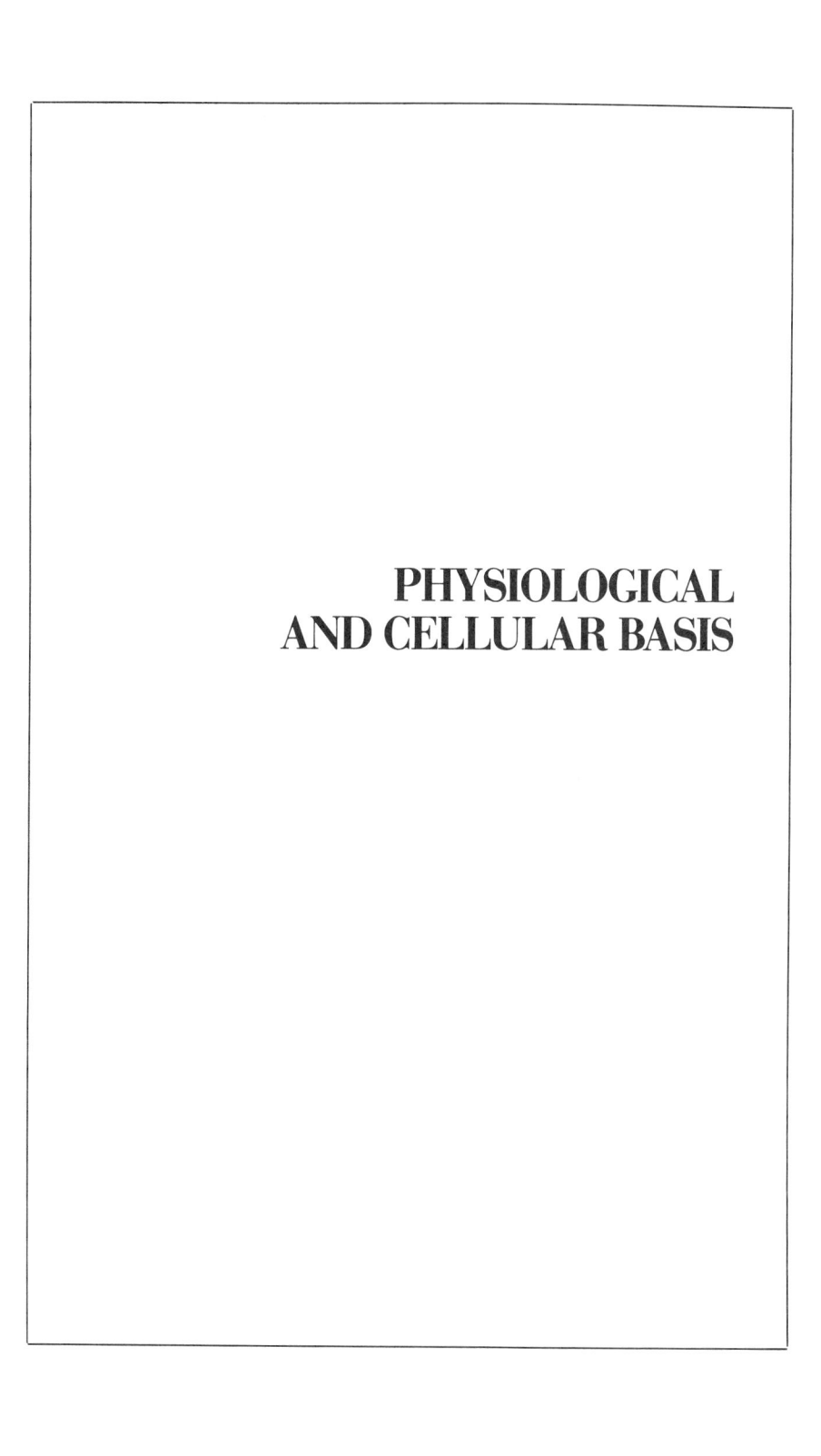

The Pathogenesis of Postmenopausal Osteoporosis
William A. Peck
Washington University School of Medicine, St. Louis, Missouri

Since the pioneering observations of Fuller Albright [1], the concept of estrogen deficiency as the agency of postmenopausal osteoporosis has become solidly entrenched. Estrogen deficiency is now known to be the dominant if not sole contributor to the well-recognized acceleration of bone loss that occurs in many women during the first five to ten postmenopausal years, and may contribute to the more gradual bone loss thereafter. Bone loss also accompanies premenopausal estrogen deficiency states, caused for example by anorexia nervosa [2], excessive athleticism [3] or prolactinoma [4]. Estrogen therapy prevents postmenopausal bone loss, and does so at relatively low doses [See reference 5 for review]. Furthermore, some, but not all observers have found higher bone mass among premenopausal users of oral contraceptives than among nonusers. [6,7].

Estrogen deficiency rapidly induces the initiation of bone remodeling at previously quiescent bone surfaces, and may enhance the resorptive and formative phases of active remodeling loci. (See reference 8 for review). The fact that bone is lost from virtually all measurable skeletal sites indicates the presence of a general remodeling imbalance. Initiation of new remodeling units and a widened gap between resorption and formation at each site signify skeletal "double jeopardy," culminating in a substantially increased rate of bone loss.

From these data, it appears that estrogen functions as a suppressor of remodeling initiation, a modulator of resorption, and perhaps a promoter of bone formation [8]. It might be argued that enhanced rates of bone formation during estrogen deficiency merely reflect coupled responses to primary increases in resorption. Indeed, biochemical indices of resorption and formation point to a close coupling of the two processes in time, if not in degree.

The mechanisms whereby estrogen deficiency jeopardizes and sufficiency protects the skeleton under physiological circumstances have been subject to vigorous inquiry. Available data suggest two principal possibilities; first, that estrogen acts indirectly, via humoral systems that influence remodeling; and second, that estrogen acts directly on bone cells, affecting one or more of the steps in the complex sequence of remodeling events. Among the indirect (humoral) mechanisms of estrogen action which have received most experimental support are two; promotion of calcitonin secretion [9] and enhancement of 1,25 dihydroxy vitamin D_3 production [10].

The best studied of these theoretical mechanisms is the role of calcitonin in transducing the skeletal effects of estrogen. Available data are conflicting, because of important interstudy methodological differences [11-16]. Antibody characteristics, immunoassay procedures, extraction methods (e.g. yielding assays for calcitonin monomer or whole plasma activity) and testing methods are among the variables which have fueled these conflicts. Consequently, it cannot yet be regarded as factual that the production of biologically active calcitonin is a determinant of postmenopausal bone homeostasis. Estrogen also increase circulating "free" 1,25 hydroxy vitamin D_3 thereby possibly enhancing intestinal calcium absorption and perhaps bone formation [10].

It should be stressed that these possible humoral effects are not likely candidates to explain the dramatic loss of bone following estrogen deficiency, since one would expect a concomitant, compensatory modulation of parathyroid hormone secretion, and no net change in bone homeostasis. Circulating levels of bioactive parathyroid hormone drift upward with advancing age, in association with an apparent decline in renal 1 alpha hydroxylase reserve and reduced intestinal calcium absorption, but these changes do not occur soon after the menopause and do not correlate with rapid bone loss [17-20]. It may well be that very different mechanisms underly the bone loss of estrogen deficiency in its early or more severe form and that which is associated with the aging process.

It was a consistent failure to demonstrate the presence of operational estrogen receptors in bone tissue that supported an indirect mode of estrogen action on bone. Recently, however, two groups of investigators, one using cells cultured from human bone tissue [21] and the other cultures of osteosarcoma cells, have demonstrated the presence of estrogen binding activity [22]. Considerable circumstantial evidence indicates that this binding may be to functioning estrogen receptors. In the human bone cell system 17 beta estradiol has been shown to induce progesterone receptors and, moreover, mRNA for estrogen receptors has been identified [21]. In various osteosarcoma cell lines, 17 beta estradiol at low concentrations, but not the biological inactive 17 alpha estradiol, promotes mRNA for collagen and transforming growth factor beta (TGF beta), increases alkaline phosphatase activity and enhances the accumulation of insulin-like growth factors 1 and 2 [22-24]. 17 beta estradiol also enhances osteoblast proliferation and collagen synthesis in isolated non-transformed rodent bone cells [25], and causes various other biochemical changes in bone tissue *in vitro* [26]. Furthermore, the effect of estrogen on cell replication appears to be mediated by insulin-like growth factors, at least in part [27,28].

These data suggest that estrogen is a direct agonist of osteoblast activity. Since estrogen has been regarded mainly as an inhibitor of remodeling and resorption, the significance of its putative action on osteoblasts remains obscure. An action of estrogen on osteoblastic cells is not at odds with an inhibitory effect on resorption, since lining cells of osteoblast origin appear to function as transducers of activating messages; parathyroid hormone, 1,25 dihydroxy vitamin D_3, Interleukin 1 and other resorption promoters appear to interact primarily with lining cells, eliciting the production of intermediary stimulators of osteoclast formation and activity (See reference 29 for review). The nature of the intermediary stimulators is as yet unknown. Activation may involve a decrease in the synthesis TGF beta, a known suppressor of osteoclast formation and activity, by osteoblastic cells. It may also involve enhanced production of prostoglandins of the E series (PGE). Estrogen, therefore, could act either by stimulating TGF beta or inhibiting PGE production by bone lining cells of osteoblast origin. Alternatively, osteoblastic cells may elaborate a more specific regulator of osteoclasts [30].

Recently described studies indicate that Interleukin 1 may participate in the skeletal actions of estrogen. Interleukin 1 is a potent stimulator of bone resorption, and is elaborated by bone marrow and possibly bone cells [29]. It is believed to be one of the factors in malignancy-associated bone loss and perhaps bone loss accompanying local inflammation [29].

Pacifici et.al. found a close positive correlation between Interleukin 1 production by blood monocytes in vitro and the rate of bone turnover in osteoporotic subjects [31]. Furthermore, cross sectional studies disclosed a sharp transmenopausal increase in blood monocyte Interleukin 1 production [32]. Although the capacity of monocytes to release Interleukin 1 decreased progressively after menopause, the decline was slower in osteoporotic than in non-osteoporotic subjects. Prospective studies have shown that sex hormone therapy (cyclic estrogen/progestogen treatment) rapidly restores elevated monocyte Interleukin 1 release to premenopausal levels in osteoporotic and non-osteoporotic subjects [32].

The significance of changes in blood monocyte Interleukin 1 production is unknown. Blood monocyte activity may reflect similar events in the skeletal compartment; accordingly, estrogen deficiency would enhance the potential for bone cells or bone marrow elements to release this powerful stimulator of bone resorption. Alternatively, monocyte Interleukin 1 production may be secondary to more fundamental metabolic changes induced by estrogen deficiency.

In summary, estrogen deficiency is the dominant if not the exclusive cause of bone loss in the postmenopause, and is a likely contributor to aging associated bone loss as well. Evidence exists for both indirect and direct actions of estrogen on the skeleton; the discovery of estrogen receptors in bone cells and of a variety of biochemical responses of bone cells to estrogen suggests the importance of direct effects. It must be stressed that osteoporosis is a multifactorial disease; premenopausal and aging associated determinants combined with the impact of estrogen dificiency determine the ultimate likelihood of a sufficiently low bone mass to place the postmenopausal woman at risk for fracture.

REFERENCES

1. Albright, F., Burnett, O.H., Lepe, O., Parsons, W. J.Clin.Endocrin. 1:711-716, 1941.
2. Rigotti, N.A., Nussbaum, S.R., Herzog, D.B., Neer, R.M. N. Engl. J. Med. 11:1601, 1984.
3. Marcus, R., Cann, C., Madrig. P. Ann. Intern. Med. 102:158-163, 1985.
4. Klibanski, A., Neer, R.M., Beitins, I.Z., Ridgeway, E.C., Servas, N.T. and McArthur, J.W. N.Engl.J.Med. 313:1511-1514, 1980.
5. Barzel, U. Am.J.Med. 85:847-850, 1988
6. Lindsay, R., Tohme, J., Karders, B. Contraception, 34:333-340, 1986.
7. Lloyd, T., Buchanan, J.R., Ursino, G.R., Myers, C., Woodward, G. and Halbert, D.R. Am.J.Obstet.Gynecol. 160:402-404, 1989.
8. Lindsay, R. Sex Steroids in the Pathogenesis and Prevention of Osteoporosis, pp.353-358 in Osteoporosis: Etiology, Diagnosis and Management, 1988, ed. B.L. Riggs and L.J. Melton III, Raven Press, NY., 1988.
9. Deftos, L.J., Weisman, M.H., Williams, G.W., Karpl, D.B. Frunar, A.M., Davidson, B.J., Parthemore, J.G., Judd, H.L. N.Engl.J.Med. 302:1551-1353, 1980.
10. Cheema, C., Grant, B.F., Marcus, R. J.Clin.Invest. 83:537-542, 1989.
11. Tiegs, R.D., Body, J.J., Barta, J.M., Heath, III, H. J.Bone Min.Res. 1:339-349, 1986.
12. Hillyard, C.J., Stevenson, J.C. and Macintyre, I. Lancet ii; 961-961, 1978.
13. Stevenson, J.C., Abeyasekara, G., Hillyard, C.J., Phang, K.J., Macintyre, I., Campbell, S., Lane, G., Townsend, P.T., Young, O. and Whitehead, M.I. Eur.J.Clin.Invest. 13:481-487, 1983.
14. Reginster, J.Y., Deroisy, R., Albert, A., Denis, D., Lecart, M.P. Collette, J. and Franchimont, P. J.Clin.Endo.Metab. 68:223-226, 1989

15. Body, J.J., Struelens, M., Borkowski, A., Mandart, G. J.Clin.Endo.Metab. 68:223-226, 2989.
16. Hurley, D.L., Tiegs, R.D., Barta, J., Laakso, K., Heath III, H. J.Bone Min.Res. 4:89-95, 1989.
17. Gallagher, J.C., Riggs, B.L., Jerpbak, C.M. and Arnavel, C.D. J.Lab.Clin.Med. 95:373-385, 1980.
18. Gallagher, J.C., Riggs, B.L., Eisman, J., Hamstra, A., Arnavel, S.B., Deluca, H.F. J.Clin.Invest 64:729-736, 1979.
19. Tsai, K.S., Heath, III, H., Kumar, R., and Riggs, B.L. J.Clin.Invest. 73:1668-1672, 1984.
20. Nordin, B.E.C., Wilkinson, R., Marshall, D.H., Gallagher, J.C., Williams, A. and Peacock, M. Calcif.Tiss.Res. 21 (Suppl.) 442-451, 1976.
21. Erikson, E.F., Colvard, D.S., Berg, N.J., Graham, M.L., Mann, K.G. Spelsberg, T.C., Riggs, B.L. Science 241:84-86, 1988.
22. Komm, B.S., Terpening, C.M. Benz, D.J., Graeme, KA. Gallegos, A. Korc, M., Greene, G.L., O'Malley, B.W., Haussler, M.R. Science 241:81-83, 1988.
23. Gray, T.K., Flynn, T.C., Gray, K.M., Nabell, L.M. Proc.Natl.Acad.Sci. 84:pp.6267-6271, 1987.
24. Gray, T.K., Mohan, T.A., Linkhart and Baylink, D.J. Biochem.Biophy. Res.Comm. 158:407-412.Vol.2, 1989.
25. Ernst, M. Schmid, Ch., Froesch, E.R. Proc.Natl.Acad.Sci. 86:2307-2310, 1988.
26. Somjen, D., Weisman, Y., Harell, A., Berger, E., Kaye, A.M. Proc.Natl.Acad.Sci. 86:3361-3365, 1989.
27. Ernst, M. and Froesch, E.R. Biochem.Biophy.Res.Comm. 151:142-147, 1988.
28. Ernst, M., Schmid, C., Frankenfeldt, C. and Froesch, E.R. Calcif.Tissue Int. 42(Suppl.), abstract 117, 1988.
29. Peck, W.A. and Woods, W.L. The Cells of Bone, pp.1-44 in Osteoporosis: Etiology, Diagnosis and Management, ed. B.L. Riggs and L.J. Melton III, Raven Press, NY., 1988.
30. Dickson, E.R., and Scheven, A.A. Biochem.Biophy.Res.Comm. 159:1383-1390, 1989.
31. Pacifici, R., Rifas, L., McCracken, R., Vered, I., McMurtry, C., Avioli, L.V., Peck, W.A. Proc.Natl.Acad.Sci. 86:2398-2402, 1989.
32. Pacifici, R., Rifas, L., McCracken, R., Vered, I., McMurtry, C., Avioli, L.V., Peck, W.A. Proc.Natl.Acad.Sci. 86:2398-2402, 2989.

Causes of Age-Related Bone Loss and Fractures

B. Lawrence Riggs

Division of Endocrinology and Metabolism, Mayo Clinic and Mayo Foundation, Rochester, Minnesota

ABSTRACT

Age-related osteoporosis is a multifactorial disorder resulting in increased bone fragility and fractures due to bone loss. The major causes of age-related bone loss are decreased calcium absorption resulting in secondary hyperparathyroidism and increased bone turnover, decreased osteoblastic activity, and, if possible, late effects of sex steroid deficiency. Because age-related bone loss has occurred over many decades before fractures begin to occur, intervention programs aimed at preventing age-related osteoporosis must be begun early.

INTRODUCTION

Involutional osteoporosis is the common, primary form of the form of the disease that occurs with increasing frequency after middle age. It is one of the most important medical disorder affecting the elderly and, because of the high incidence of fractures and their huge costs, its prevention is one of the major unresolved public health problem facing America today.

CAUSES OF FRACTURES

The morbid event in osteoporosis is fracture. Operationally, there are three independent causes of these fractures--decreased bone density, qualitative changes in bone structure, and trauma from falls. Of these, by far the most important is decreased bone density [1]. Bone strength is determined by absolute bone density, regardless of age. In the absence of severe trauma, fractures do not occur until bone density has fallen below the fracture threshold which is about 1.0 g/cm^2 for both the vertebrae and the proximal femur [2] (Fig. 1). Interestingly, this fracture threshold corresponds to the lower limit of values found in young adulthood suggesting that any degree of bone loss from peak values is pathological. With further decreases in bone density, the incidence of hip fractures and the prevalence of vertebral fractures increase further [3] (Fig. 1). Low bone density, therefore, is a necessary, but not a sufficient, cause of fracture, and the risk of fracture is a probabilistic function of a given level of bone density.

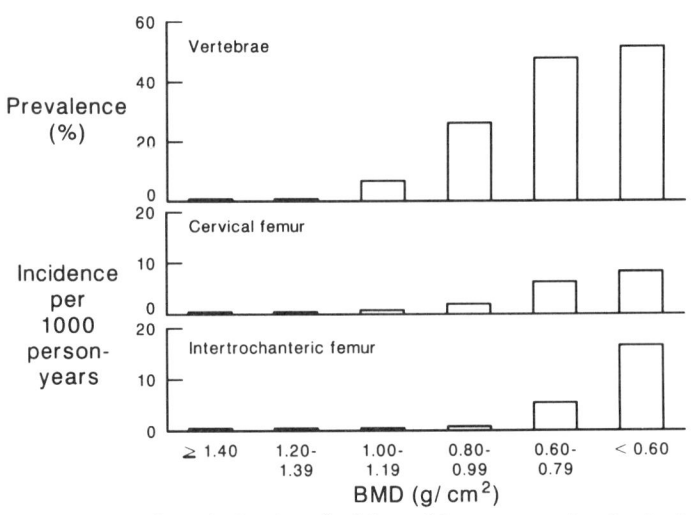

Figure 1. Occurrence of vertebral and proximal femoral fractures at various levels of vertebral and proximal femur bone mineral density (from Riggs and Melton [3], with permission of the New England Journal of Medicine).

The second cause is qualitative changes in bone structure [4] that result in a degree of bone fragility greater than would be predicted from the degree of bone loss. Possible causes of qualitative changes in bone structure with aging that could impair bone strength are listed in Table I.

Table I. Qualitative Defects in Bone That May Increase Bone Fragility.

    Accumulation of microfractures

    Fatigue damage

    Loss of trabecular connectivity

    Failure to complete secondary mineralization

    Histologic osteomalacia

The third cause is trauma due to falls. With their low bone mass, fractures occur in the elderly at levels of trauma that would rarely cause injury in young persons. Indeed, the most common cause of fractures in the elderly is a fall from a standing position. Moreover, the elderly have an increased propensity to fall because of failing eyesight, arthritis, neurological diseases, muscle weakness, drop attacks, hypotensive drug use and other causes. At least one-third of elderly persons have one or more falls each year [5].

Also, the trauma of falls is increased in elderly persons because their impaired coordination and slowed reflexes decrease their ability to break the impact of falls [5]. The type of fall also may be important. Cummings [6] has suggested that posterior falls with a landing on the buttocks are particularly likely to cause hip fractures.

TYPES OF FRACTURE SYNDROMES

On the basis of evidence that is summarized elsewhere [3,7], Riggs and Melton have suggested that involutional osteoporosis can be divided into two separate syndromes (Table II). Superimposed on bone loss from these two syndromes are the effects of sporadically occurring factors that affect some, but not other individuals such as tobacco and alcohol abuses, use of drugs or occurrence of diseases that affect bone mass, and activity status [3].

Table II. The Two Types of Involutional Osteoporosis.

	Type I	Type II
Age (yr)	51-75	>70
Sex ratio (F:M)	6:1	2:1
Type of bone loss	Mainly trabecular	Trabecular and cortical
Rate of bone loss	Accelerated	Not accelerated
Fracture sites	Vertebrae (crush) and distal radius	Vertebrae (multiple wedge) and hip
Main causes	Factors related to menopause	Factors related to aging

Although the concept of two syndromes of involutional osteoporosis is not accepted by everyone, it may be serve a useful role in the examination of pathogenesis in decision making regarding therapy.

Type I (postmenopausal) osteoporosis characteristically affects women within 15 to 20 years after menopause and results from an exaggeration of the postmenopausal phase of accelerated bone loss. This syndrome is characterized by disproportionate loss of trabecular bone (Fig. 2), which results in fractures of the vertebrae and distal forearm (Colles' fracture), skeletal sites that contain large amounts of trabecular bone. The vertebral fractures usually are the "crush" type associated with deformation and pain. Accelerated bone loss occurring in type I osteoporosis is three times greater than normal in trabecular bone, but only slightly greater than normal in cortical bone. There is increased bone turnover, and bone resorption increases more than bone formation.

The major cause of type I osteoporosis is estrogen deficiency. However, only a relatively small subset of postmenopausal women develop type I osteoporosis, although all postmenopausal women are relatively estrogen deficient. Thus, some additional factor must interact with estrogen deficiency to determine individual susceptibility. The possibilities include impaired coupling of formation to resorption, increased local production of interleukin-1, or another factor that increases bone resorption, prolongation of the phase of accelerated bone loss, or some combination of these factors.

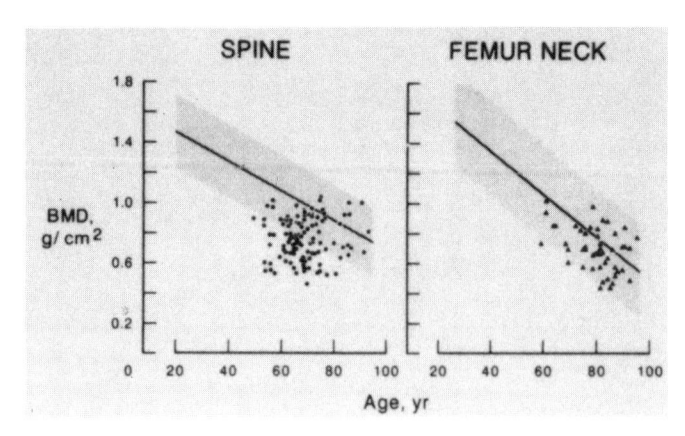

Figure 2. Bone mineral density values for lumbar spine and femoral neck. The line represents the regression on age and the cross hatched area the 90% confidence range for normal women without osteoporosis. The solid circles represent values for osteoporotic women with vertebral fractures and the solid triangles values for osteoporotic women with hip fracture. From Riggs and Melton [3] with permission of the New England Journal of Medicine.

Type II (age-related) osteoporosis occurs in both elderly men and women and is manifested mainly by hip and vertebral fractures, although fractures of the proximal humerus, proximal tibia, and pelvis also are common. Bone loss occurs gradually over many decades. In the vertebrae, this results in gradual thinning of the trabeculae causing the multiple wedge type of vertebral fractures leading to dorsal kyphosis ("dowager's hump"). Type II osteoporosis is believed to be due to factors related to the aging process.

This review will not discuss type I osteoporosis further and will be confined to causes of type II osteoporosis.

AGE-RELATED BONE LOSS

Age is by far the most important determinant of bone mass. Indeed, if the age of a healthy woman is known, it is possible to predict the bone density with a standard deviation of only about 10% [2] (Fig. 3).

Age-related bone loss probably begins in the fourth decade in both sexes and continues throughout life, or at least into extreme old age. This process occurs at a rate of about 1% per year and is slightly greater in trabecular than in cortical bone. In women, a transient phase of accelerated bone loss due to estrogen-deficiency occurs at the menopause and lasts about 4 to 8 years. This results in a loss of about 15% to 20% of trabecular bone and about 10% to 15% of cortical bone [3]. These losses are superimposed on the slow, age-related bone loss occurring in both sexes and, along with a smaller peak bone mass, account for the smaller bone mass in women and for their greater susceptibility to osteoporotic fractures. Riggs and Melton [3,7] have suggested that this slow, age-related phase of bone loss is the underlying cause of type II osteoporosis.

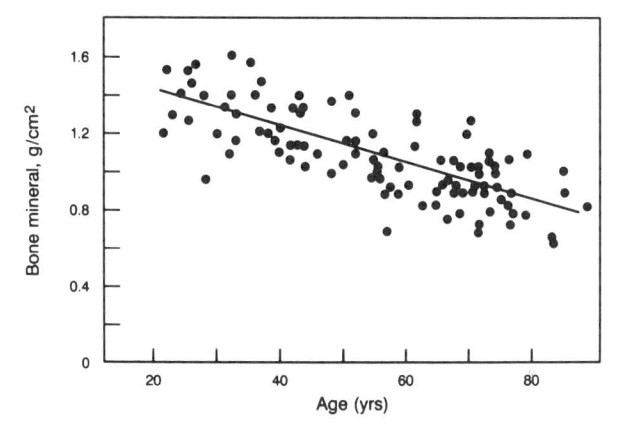

Figure 3. Effect of age on bone mineral density of the lumbar spine in 117 normal women assessed by dual photon absorptiometry (from Riggs et al. [8], with permission of the Journal of Clinical Investigation).

EFFECT OF AGE ON BONE TURNOVER

Bone remodeling occurs at discrete foci throughout the skeleton called basic multicellular units or BMUs [9]. At the beginning of each remodeling cycle, osteoclasts appear on previously inactive bone and, over a period of several weeks, construct a tunnel in cortical bone or a lacuna on the surface of trabecular bone. The osteoclasts are then replaced by osteoblasts, which over a period of three to four months, fill in the resorption cavity to create a new structural unit of bone.

Changes in bone mass are determined by the interaction of two independent processes affecting bone remodeling--the rate of bone turnover and the remodeling balance between bone resorption and bone formation [9]. The rate of bone turnover, the amount of old bone replaced by new bone per unit of time, is determined by the total number of BMUs in the skeleton at any given time. As assessed by bone histomorphometry, this is about 4% per year in normal young adults. However, in these normal young adults, there is a tight coupling of the resorption and formation phases so that changes in turnover over relatively wide ranges do not result in changes in bone mass. Bone loss implies an imbalance, "uncoupling", in the remodeling process so that there is either an increase in the resorptive phase or a decrease in the formative phase.

The elderly were formerly believed to have a decrease in bone turnover [10-12]. More recent evidence, however, suggests that they may have an increase. Some investigators have found age-related increases in serum levels of biochemical markers for bone turnover such as bone Gla-protein (BGP, osteocalcin) [13-15] and bone alkaline phosphatase [14], whereas others have not [16-18]. Whole body retention of diphosphonate, another index of bone turnover, increases with aging [19]. Although previous histomorphometric studies had indicated that older women had decreased remodeling, more recent ones employing tetracycline double labeling have suggested that, in fact, it is increased [20-22].

Despite the apparent increase in the number of new BMUs with age, there is evidence that the formative phase of the remodeling cycle is impaired. Lips and Meunier [2] found an age-related decrease in wall thickness of trabecular packets which is incontrovertible evidence of decreased bone formation at the BMU level. Thus, the elderly have a remodeling imbalance;

at each BMU, the osteoblasts fail to replace completely the bone resorbed by the osteoclasts. In the presence of a remodeling imbalance, the higher the rate of turnover, i.e., the greater number of BMUs in the skeleton, the greater the rate of bone loss.

FACTORS CONTRIBUTING TO AGE-RELATED BONE LOSS

Although it is customary to attribute bone loss to "aging", this very probably reflects the aggregate effects of several age-related processes that regulate bone cell function rather than bone cell senescence. The factors that are most likely to contribute to age-related bone loss are discussed below.

Decreased Calcium Absorption

As assessed by radioactive isotopes of calcium, absorption decreases with aging in both sexes, especially after age 65 [23-25]. The decreases have been most prominent when smaller amounts of calcium carrier have been employed, suggesting that the defect may be limited to active calcium transport, a process regulated mainly by the physiologically active vitamin D metabolite, 1,25-dihydroxyvitamin D ($1,25(OH)_2D$). The impaired calcium absorption appears to be the result of two defects--increased resistance of the intestine to $1,25(OH)_2D$ action and, later in life, impaired conversion of the major circulating form of vitamin D, 25-hydroxyvitamin D ($25[OH]D$) to $1,25(OH)_2D$.

Although several smaller studies, including [25] one by our group have reported lower serum levels of $1,25(OH)_2D$ with aging, the largest study [26] and a recent study by us [27], have shown that serum $1,25(OH)_2D$ increases up to age 65 and then decreases or levels off. Because $1,25(OH)_2D$, the major factor regulating calcium absorption, is increasing while active calcium absorption is decreasing, this is strong evidence for resistance of the intestine to the action of $1,25(OH)_2D$. In this regard, it is of interest that intestinal $1,25(OH)_2D$ receptors have been found to be decreased in aged rats [29]. Experimental studies testing this hypothesis should now be undertaken.

The decrease in serum $1,25(OH)_2D$ levels after age 65 appears to be due to reduced activity of the renal $25(OH)D$ 1α-hydroxylase enzyme, which is rate limiting for $1,25(OH)_2D$ production in response to physiological needs. Decreased enzyme activity has been demonstrated directly in aged rats [30] and indirectly in elderly women [31] by measuring the response of serum $1,25(OH)_2D$ levels to infusion of synthetic PTH (1-34), a potent stimulator of enzyme activity.

Other Age-Related Hormonal Changes

Numerous investigators have shown that immunoreactive parathyroid hormone increases with age. These past data are difficult to interpret, however, because the reduction in glomerular filtration rate with aging may decrease clearance of COOH-terminal fragments of parathyroid hormone, thereby increasing circulating levels of immunoreactive species of parathyroid hormone that are not bioactive. Recently, more specific measurements have clearly demonstrated that parathyroid function, in fact, does increases with aging. Urinary cyclic AMP [13,31] and nephrogenic cyclic AMP excretion [32], both measures of biologic action of parathyroid hormone, increase with age. Although bioactive PTH, assessed by the cytochemical bioassay, did not increase with age [33], higher values in the elderly were found with the renal membrane assay for adenylate cyclase after immunoextraction of serum [34], a more precise method for detecting small increases. Moreover, serum intact PTH, as assessed by either a NH_2-terminal-specific radioimmunoassay [35] or by the two-site immunoradiometric assay [27] increased by about 50% over life. Increased secretion of parathyroid hormone with aging is the probable cause of the increase in bone turnover previously described and, because of the coexistence of an age-related imbalance in bone remodeling, would lead to increased bone loss.

A contributory causal role of calcitonin, a potent antiresorptive hormone, has also been suggested. Patients who have undergone total thyroidectomy and who are presumably calcitonin deficient have lower bone density values than controls [36]. Several groups have shown that women have lower plasma levels of immunoreactive calcitonin than men at all ages [37,38]. Although Deftos et al. [38] reported that these levels decrease with age in both sexes, Body and Heath [39], using a method highly sensitive for monomeric calcitonin, could not confirm this finding; they did, however, confirm lower values in women.

Serum 25(OH)D, an indicator of vitamin D stores, declines moderately in the elderly [40,41] due to impaired vitamin D absorption, decreased exposure to sunlight, decreased photo dermal conversion of precursors to vitamin D, and, in some, poor nutrition. In some elderly subjects, particularly in those who are housebound with poor nutrition, histological osteomalacia may occur [42-46] (Table III). In those series that are the largest, that have the least referral bias, and that use the most rigorous histomorphometric criteria, the incidence still is appreciable in the 10 to 20% range. In addition to its effect on decreasing bone strength, vitamin D deficiency may worsen the age-related bone loss.

Table III. Proportion of Patients with Hip Fracture Whose Bone Biopsy Meet Criteria for Histologic Osteomalacia.

Series	Country	Affected, %
Aaron et al., 1974	U.K.	34
Sokoloff et al., 1978	U.S.A.	26
Lund et al., 1982	Denmark	25
Peacock and Horton, 1987	U.K.	15
Johnston et al., 1987	U.S.A.	10

Decreased Osteoblast Function

The decrease in bone formation at the cellular level that has been documented by histomorphometry, may be due to impaired regulation of osteoblast activity caused by abnormalities in either systemic or local growth factors. Serum levels of both growth hormone and insulin-like growth factor-I (IGF-I, somatomedin C), which mediates the effect of growth hormone on bone and cartilage, decline with age [47]. It is more likely, however, that the decreased osteoblast function results from impaired production of growth factors by bone cells. At least 12 local regulators of growth, produced by bone, cartilage, or marrow cells, have been identified [48]. The most important of these appear to be IGF-I, IGF-II (now known to be identical to skeletal growth factor [49]), and transforming growth factor-β. Undoubtedly, future research will be directed at defining these possible abnormalities directly.

Sex Steroid Deficiency

As discussed earlier, women have a transient acceleration of bone loss following menopause and, thereafter, resume a slow rate of bone loss that is presumed to be due to only age-related processes. However, the possibility that this slow bone loss has a component of estrogen deficiency cannot be excluded. There is indirect evidence that estrogen antagonizes the effect of PTH on bone [50] and this would be expected to potentiate the effect of the age-related secondary hyperparathyroidism. Indeed, Quigley et al. [51] have reported that estrogen treatment slows bone loss in women who are up to 20 years postmenopausal. This important question needs further study. Although men do not undergo the equivalent of menopause, gonadal function does decline in a substantial subset of aging men [52], and it is possible that this contributes to their bone loss.

SUMMARY AND CONCLUSIONS

Osteoporosis and fractures in the elderly are common in the elderly and probably result from processes that involve the entire population of aging men and women. These processes involve slow bone loss acting over many decades. Osteoporosis is more common in elderly women than in elderly men as a result of the rapid bone loss occurring in the decade following menopause many years earlier. The slow phase of bone loss, although age-related, probably results from the summation of several age-related processes, the most important of which are summarized in Fig. 4. Because osteoporosis is more difficult to treat than to prevent, it will be important in the future to define these causal processes better and to intervene to correct them before fractures due to osteoporosis develop.

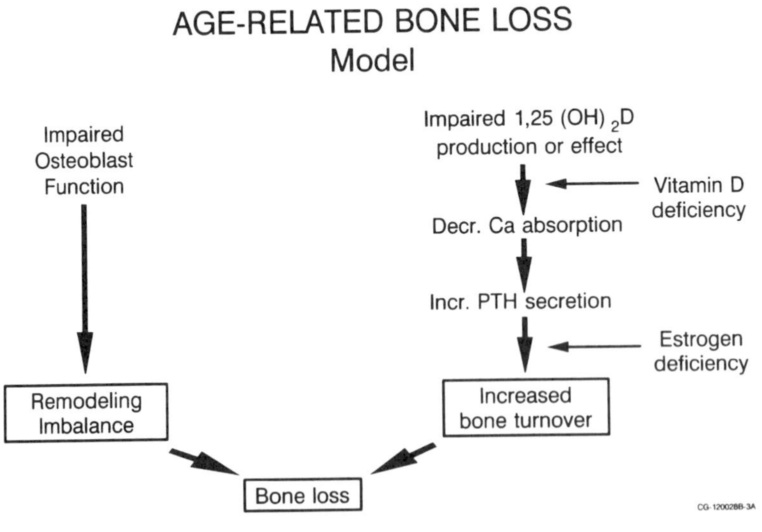

AGE-RELATED BONE LOSS
Model

Figure 4. Model for causes of age-related bone loss.

REFERENCES

1. L.J. Melton III and B.L. Riggs, in: The Osteoporotic Syndrome, L.V. Avioli, ed. (Grune & Stratton, New York 1983) pp. 47-72.
2. B.L. Riggs, H.W. Wahner, W.L. Dunn, R.B. Mazess, K.P. Offord and L.J. Melton III, J. Clin. Invest. 67, 328-335 (1981).
3. B.L. Riggs and L.J. Melton III, N. Engl. J. Med. 314, 1676-1686 (1986).
4. R.P. Heaney, Osteoporosis 1, 281-287 (1987).
5. L.J. Melton and B.L. Riggs, Clin. Geriatr. Med. 1, 1-15 (1985).
6. S.R. Cummings, J.L. Kelsey, M.C. Nevitt and K.J. O'Dowd, Epidemiol. Rev. 7, 178-208 (1985).
7. B.L. Riggs and L.J. Melton III, Am. J. Med. 75, 899-901 (1983).
8. E. Seeman, R. Kumar, G.G. Hunder, M. Scott, H. Heath III and B.L. Riggs, J. Clin. Invest. 66, 664-669 (1980).
9. A.M. Parfitt, Calcif. Tissue Int. 28, 1-5 (1979).
10. W.A. Merz and R.K. Schenk, Acta Anat. 76, 1-15 (1970).
11. H.M. Frost, Clin. Endocrinol. Metab. 2, 257-275 (1973).
12. F. Melsen and L. Mosekilde, Calcif. Tissue Res. 26, 99-102 (1978).
13. P.D. Delmas, D. Stenner, H.W. Wahner, K.G. Mann and B.L. Riggs, J. Clin. Invest. 71, 1316-1321 (1983).
14. R.J. Duda, Jr., J.F. O'Brien, J.A. Katzmann, J.M. Peterson, K.G. Mann and B.L. Riggs, J. Clin. Endocrinol. Metab. 66, 951-957 (1988).
15. S. Epstein, J. Poser, R. McClintock, C.C. Johnston, Jr., G. Bryce and S. Hui, Lancet 1, 307-310 (1984).
16. P.A. Price, J.G. Parthemore, L.J. Deftos and S.K. Nishimoto, J. Clin. Invest. 66, 878-883 (1980).
17. R.A. Melick, W. Farrugia and K.J. Quelch, Aust. NZ J. Med. 15, 410-416 (1985).
18. B.D. Catherwood, R. Marcus, P. Madvig and A.K. Cheung, Bone 6, 9-13 (1985).
19. I. Fogelman and R. Bessent, J. Nucl. Med. 23, 296-300 (1982).
20. S. Vedi, J.E. Compston, A. Webb and J.R. Tighe, Metab. Bone Dis. Rel. Res. 5, 69-74 (1983).
21. R. Eastell, P.D Delmas, S.F. Hodgson, E.F. Eriksen, K.G. Mann and B.L. Riggs, J. Clin. Endocrinol. Metab. 67, 741-748 (1988).
22. E. Dahl, K.P. Nordal, J. Halse and A. Attramadal, Bone and Min. 3, 369-377 (1988).
23. J.R. Bullamore, J.C. Gallagher, R. Wilkinson, B.E.C. Nordin and D.H. Marshall, Lancet 2, 535-537 (1970).
24. C.C. Alevizaki, D.G. Ikkos and P. Singhelakis, J. Nucl. Med. 14, 760-762 (1973).
25. J.C. Gallagher, B.L. Riggs, J. Eisman, A. Hamstra, S.B. Arnaud and H.F. DeLuca, J. Clin. Invest. 64, 729-736 (1979).
26. S. Epstein, G. Bryce, J.W. Hinman, O.N. Miller, B.L. Riggs, S.L. Hui and C.C. Johnston, Jr., Bone 7, 421-425 (1986).
27. R. Eastell, N.E. Vieira, A.L. Yergey, H.W. Wahner, M.N. Silverstein, R. Kumar and B.L. Riggs. Submitted to the American Federation for Clinical Research Meeting, September 9-14 (1989).
28. R.L. Horst and T.A. Reinhardt, J. Bone Min. Res. 2, 200 (1987).
29. H.J. Armbrecht, T.V. Zenser and B.B. Davis, J. Clin. Invest. 66, 1118-1123 (1980).
30. K.-S. Tsai, H. Heath III, R. Kumar and B.L. Riggs, J. Clin. Invest. 73, 1668-1672 (1984).
31. K.L. Insogna, A.M. Lewis, B.A. Lipinski, C. Bryant and D.T. Baran, J. Clin. Endocrinol. Metab. 53, 1072-1075 (1981).
32. R. Marcus, P. Madvig and G. Young, J. Clin. Endocrinol. Metab. 58, 223-230 (1984).
33. P.W. Saphier, T.C.B. Stamp, C.R. Kelsey and N. Loveridge, Bone and Min. 3, 75-83 (1987).
34. M.S. Forero, R.F. Klein, R.A. Nissenson, K. Nelson, H. Heath III, C.D. Arnaud and B.L. Riggs, J. Bone Min. Res. 2, 363-366 (1987).

35. G. Young, R. Marcus, J.R. Minkoff, L.Y. Kim and G.V. Segre, J. Bone Min. Res. 2, 367-374 (1987).
36. M.T. McDermott, G.S. Kidd, P. Blue, V. Ghaed and F.D. Hofeldt, J. Clin. Endocrinol. Metab. 56, 936-939 (1983).
37. H. Heath III and G.W. Sizemore, J. Clin. Invest. 60, 1135-1140 (1977).
38. L.J. Deftos, M.H. Weisman, G.W. Williams, et al., N. Engl. J. Med. 302, 1351-1353 (1980).
39. J.-J. Body and H. Heath III, J. Clin. Endocrinol. Metab. 57, 897-903 (1983).
40. J.L. Omdahl, P.J. Garry, L.A. Hunsaker, W.C. Hunt and J.S. Goodwin, Am. J. Clin. Nutr. 36, 1225-1233 (1982).
41. K.-S. Tsai, H.W. Wahner, K.P. Offord, L.J. Melton III, R. Kumar and B.L. Riggs, Calcif. Tissue Int. 40, 241-243 (1987).
42. J.E. Aaron, J.C. Gallagher, J. Anderson, L. Stasiak, E.B. Longton, B.E.C. Nordin and M. Nicholson, Lancet 1, 229-233 (1974).
43. L. Sokoloff, Am. J. Surg. Pathol. 2, 21-30 (1978).
44. B. Lund, O.H. Sorensen, B. Lund, F. Melsen and L. Mosekilde, Acta Orthop. Scand. 53, 251-254 (1982).
45. L.D. Hordon and M. Peacock, Bone and Min. 2, 413-426 (1987).
46. C.C. Johnston, M. Peacock and P.J. Meunier, in: Osteoporosis (Norhaven A/S, Viborg, Denmark 1987) pp. 317-320.
47. A. Bennett, H.W. Wahner, B.L. Riggs and R.L. Hintz, J. Clin. Endocrinol. Metab. 59, 701-704 (1984).
48. M. Centrella and E. Canalis, Endocr. Rev. 6, 544-551 (1985).
49. S. Mohan, J. Jennings, T. Linkhardt, J. Wergedal and D. Baylink, J. Bone Min. Res. 3, 598 (1988).
50. R.P. Heaney, Am. J. Med. 39, 877-880 (1965).
51. M.E. Quigley, P.L. Martin, A.M. Burnier and P. Brooks, Am. J. Obstet Gynecol. 156, 1516-1523 (1987).
52. C. Foresta, G. Ruzza, R. Mioni et al., Horm. Res. 19, 18-22 (1984).

Therapy Induced Osteoporosis (??? Type III Osteoporosis)

Louis V. Avioli

Division of Bone and Mineral Diseases, Washington University School of Medicine, The Jewish Hospital of St. Louis, St. Louis, Missouri

ABSTRACT

A variety of structurally unrelated pharmacological agents, when administered chronically, can result in alterations in calcium homeostasis and osteopenia. This "Type III" form of acquired osteoporosis is often attended by changes in circulating levels of parathyroid hormone, vitamin D metabolites, and osteocalcin, as well as defects in calcium absorption and the renal conservation of calcium. Appropriate alterations in polypharmacy profiles (especially for the elderly) with substitution of drugs, decreasing drug dosages, together with the incorporation of remedial therapeutic agents and serial bone mass monitoring with non-invasive procedures appear mandatory since it is considerably easier to maintain bone mass than it is to replace it!

Osteoporotic syndromes caused by either normal cessation of ovarian function and/or progressive senescence have been variably characterized as either "postmenopausal," "senile," "Type I," "Type II," "inactive," "active," "high-turnover," "low-turnover," and "involutional" [1,2]. This confusing and apparent redundant array of terminologies is usually offered as a means of categorizing the osteoporotic syndrome(s), and is frequently used to imply the need for specific theapeutic modes [2]. While acknowledging the potential utility of categorizing osteoporotic syndrome(s), we should not ignore the additional complications which result either from the abuse of over-the-counter drugs, such as vitamins A or D and phosphate binding antiacids, or drugs prescribed by physicians for a variety of acquired maladies (Table I).

TABLE I. Pharmacological Agents Which Adversely Effect Calcium and/or Skeletal Metabolism

Glucocorticoid drugs
Thyroid hormone preparations
Anticonvulsants
Anticoagulants
Phosphate-binding antiacids
Cytotoxic agents
Phenothiazine derivatives
Lithium
GnRH-LHRH agonists or antagonists
Tetracycline
Loop Diuretics
? Aluminum containing antiacids

Drug therapy can and often does result in a variety of disturbances in mineral metabolism either indirectly by altering calcium absorption and/or excretion, and the release, metabolism and/or skeletal response to the calcitropic hormones, or by direct inhibition of bone cell function as well as collagen production and mineralization. The resultant "Type III" osteoporotic syndrome(s) can be attended by normal or elevated values for blood parathyroid hormone, normal or low values for 25OHD, normal, low or elevated circulating 1,25(OH$_2$)D, decreased or increased calcium absorption and either hyper- or hypocalciuria. Thus, when considering either "Type I" or "Type II" osteoporotic syndromes and their respective classic biochemical profiles for blood calcium, phosphate, vitamin D metabolites and parathyroid hormone [1,2] in patients on medications known to produce osteopenia (Table I), the potential alterations in both histological presentation and diagnostic tests by the drug-induced Type III syndrome should be acknowledged.

Although there is uniform belief that chronic exposure to supraphysiological levels of glucocorticoids leads almost inevitably to significant bone loss and an increased prevalence of rib and vertebral fractures [3-5], there is still considerable contention regarding the effect of "low-dose glucocorticoid therapy" (LDGC) on bone [6-8]. In patients receiving prednisolone in doses ranging from 4 to 10 mg/day, Reid et al., demonstrated a close negative correlation between total body calcium and steroid doses [6]. Nagant de Deuxchaisnes et al., reported that the bone mass of the appendicular skeleton of premenopausal women was unaffected by the administration of LDGC (i.e., prednisone, 7.5 mg/day), whereas, postmenopasual women on the same dose of glucocorticoids lost twice as much bone as did age-matched postmenopausal women who were not taking glucocorticoids [8]. Sambrook et al., reported that prednisolone doses of 8.0 ± 3.2 mg/day were not associated with significantly increased axial or appendicular bone loss in 84 women (mean age 56.0 ± 13.7 yrs) with rheumatoid arthritis; although prednisolone doses of 10.3 ± 4.7 in 27 males of similar ages resulted in significantly increased rates of bone loss. They concluded that LDGC (5-7.5 mg prednisolone/day) is relatively safe but that dosages greater than 10 mg/day should be avoided [7]. Although alternate day glucocorticoid therapy can mitigate undesirable effects of daily glucocorticoid therapy on growth suppression, hypothalamic-pituitary-adrenal axis suppression and infections, alternate steroid regimens do not reduce the osteopenic effects recorded with daily steroid regimens [3]. Therapeutic attempts to counteract the effects of steroids on bone with "triple" drug (sodium fluoride, calcium, and vitamin D) have proved unrewarding [9]. However, 25OHD in doses of 40-100 µg/d, plus 500 mg of elemental calcium daily, significantly improves parameters of mineral and bone metabolism although hypercalciuria inevitably occurs on this regimen [10]. Others have shown [11] that calcium supplementation alone in doses of 1 gram of elemental calcium/day is effective in decreasing bone loss in patients on steroid regimens ranging from 6-160 mg prednisone (median dose, 15 mg/day) for 0.2-35 years (median duration 3 yrs); favorable responses have also been recorded in studies utilizing vitamin D and thiazides [12], and calcitonin [13]. The APD diphosphonate in doses of 150 mg/day combined with 1 gram of elemental calcium daily [14] is also effective. Since plasma testosterone levels are often suppressed in males receiving pharmacological doses of glucocorticoids [15], testosterone replacement therapy is also recommended. The recent discovery of deflazacort, a diene derivative of prednisolone with similar anti-inflammatory potencies to prednisone [16] and less pronounced effects on calcium metabolism [17], led to its use in patients requiring steroid therapy. The results to date are quite provocative with reports of significantly less vertebral and pelvic bone loss when compared to comparable doses of prednisone [18,19], and no deleterious effect on the statural growth of children [20]!

Disturbances in calcium and bone metabolism, well-documented in patients with thyroid disease and elevated blood levels of thyroid hormones

[21], have also been recorded in patients on thyroid replacement therapy [22-25]. Despite a mild hyperthyroxinemia, serum triiodothyronine levels are characteristically normal and patients asymptomatic [22-25]. Recent evidence suggests that thyroid replacement therapy (especially L-thyroxine) using previously accepted doses may have long-term adverse effects on bone [26,27]. Studies in patients treated with contemporary L-thyroxine preparations reveal that 80% of patients ingesting 125 µg or more per day were "overdosed" as detected by thyrotrophin response to thyrotrophin-releasing hormone [26]. It is suggested that because of increased bioavailability of L-thyroxine thyroid hormone preparations, replacement doses should approximate 100 µg/day or 1.7 µg/kg body weight [26]; patients requiring thyroxine for suppression (i.e., goiter, cold nodules, thyroid cancer) will require more than 125 µg/day. It should also be recognized that, especially in postmenopausal females, L-thyroxine dosage requirements decrease with age [27]. In order to minimize undesired skeletal effects of overly-zealous thyroxine replacement therapy, doses of thyroid hormone administered to hypothyroid patients should be adjusted so that serum TSH, measured by the new highly sensitive assays, is within the normal range [28].

Since initial reports of "anticonvulsant osteomalacia" appeared in European literature in 1968, alterations in calcium and skeletal metabolism in both children and adults on anticonvulsant medications have been recorded worldwide [3]. The clinical severity of the bone disease varies considerably, ranging from subclinical decreases in bone mass detectable only by the most sensitive non-invasive methods, to marked hypocalcemia and severe osteopenia with multiple recurrent bone fractures [29]. A trend toward increased skeletal demineralization has been associated with the length of anticonvulsant therapy [29], although it has been reported a "steady state" is achieved in adults [29] with a greater effect of prolonged therapy on the growing child. Therapeutic regimens with vitamin D metabolites have mitigated the effects of the anticonvulsant medications [3]; obviously, the treatment of choice is gradual withdrawal of anticonvulsant drugs especially in patients free of seizures for 2-3 years [30,31].

Glucocorticoids, thyroid supplements, and anticonvulsants presumably are well-established as bone "toxins" when used indiscriminately or in inappropriately large doses. We must also recognize that heparin anticoagulants [32] do result in osteoporosis whereas sodium warfarin drugs do not adversely affect the skeleton [33], despite reports of impaired carboxylation of osteocalcin in warfarin-treated patients [34] and decreased serum osteocalcin levels in patients treated with the vitamin K antagonist, phenprocoumon [35]. Lithium treatment results in elevations in circulating parathyroid hormone [36], hypercalciuria and increased calcium absorption [37], and a decrease in bone mineral content [38], alterations which can occur as early as 3 months following treatment with oral lithium doses of 28 mEq/day [38]. Although chronic administration of thiazide diuretics may, in fact, decrease the risk of skeletal fracture [39], "loop" diuretics, such as furosemide, should prove harmful to calcium homeostasis because of the hypercalciuria-induced by this drug [40,41].

Cytotoxic chemotherapy with drugs like vincristine and cyclophosphamide alter dental development leading to enamel and dentinal hypoplasia [42,43]. Similar findings should ultimately occur in patients treated with methotrexate for either malignant disorders or rheumatoid arthritis [44]. Chemotherapy will result in a loss of skeletal mass either because of a direct toxic effect of the agent on calcifying tissue [42,43], or because of the induction of gonadal damage and decreased levels of gonadal hormones [45,46]. "Medical gonadectomy," induced by GnRH antagonist or agonist treatment for prostatic cancer, the premenstrual syndrome [47], polycystic ovarian syndrome [48], and endometriosis [49], could [50], and does [49], result in bone loss, although the loss of bone appears to be reversible [49]. Finally, studies in laboratory animals suggest that either cyclosporin A [51,52], theophylline-like drugs [53,54], and phenothiazine derivatives [55], will also interfere with calcium homeostasis in humans if used chronically.

Recognition of the potential adverse effects of a variety of seemingly unrelated medications on mineral and skeletal metabolism, and the appropriate use of either modified treatment regimens and/or drugs which protect the skeleton in situations where potentially harmful medications cannot be changed or their doses altered, coupled with serial measurements of bone mass at predetermined intervals should help to minimize a Type II osteoporotic complication in patients with either Type I or Type II osteoporosis. It is far more practical and easier to direct our efforts toward preventing bone loss these days when attempts to increase bone mass so often prove futile.

REFERENCES

1. B.L. Riggs and L.J. Melton III, New Engl. J. Med. 314, 1676-1686 (1986).
2. R. Civitelli, S. Gonnelli, F. Zacchei, S. Bigazzi, A. Vattimo, L.V. Avioli, and C. Gennari, J. Clin. Invest. 82, 1268-1274 (1988).
3. T.J. Hahn and L.V. Avioli in: Endocrinology, Vol. 2, L.J. DeGroot, ed. (W.B. Saunders Co., Philadelphia 1989) pp. 1085-1110.
4. A.D. Adinoff and J.R. Hollister, New Engl. J. Med. 309, 265-268 (1983).
5. A.G. Need, Aust. N. Z. J. Med. 17, 267-272 (1987).
6. D.M. Reid, N.S.J. Kennedy, M.A. Smith, P. Tothill, G. Nuki, Brit. Med. J. 285, 330-332 (1982).
7. P.N. Sambrook, J.A. Eisman, G. David Champion, M.G. Yeates, N.A. Pocock, and S. Eberl, Arthritis Rheum. 30, 72-728 (1987).
8. C. Nagant de Deuxchaisnes, J.P. Devogelaer, W. Esselinckx, B. Bouchez, G. Depresseux, C. Rombouts-Lindemans and J.P. Huax in: Glucocorticoid effects and their biological consequences, L.V. Avioli, C. Gennari and B. Imbimbo, eds., (Plenum Press, New York 1984) pp. 209-239.
9. H. Rickers, Aa. Deding, C. Christiansen, and P. Rodbro, Calcif. Tissue Int. 36, 169-273 (1984).
10. T.J. Hahn, L.H. Halstead, S.L. Teitelbaum, and B.H. Hahn, J. Clin. Invest. 64, 655-665 (1979).
11. I.R. Reid, and H.K. Ibbertson, Amer. J. Clin. Nutr. 44, 287-290 (1986).
12. J.R. Condon, C.E. Dent, J.R. Nassim, A. Hilb, E.M. Stainthorpe, Postgrad. Med. J. 54, 249-252 (1978).
13. J.D. Ringe and D. Welzel, Euro. Clin. Pharmacol. 33, 35-39 (1987).
14. I.R. Reid, C.J. Alexander, A.R. King, H.K. Ibbertson, Lancet I, 143-146 (1988).
15. I.R. REid, H.K. Ibbertson, J.T. France, J. Pybus, Brit. Med J. 291, 574 (1985).
16. B. Lund, C. Egsmose, S. Jorgensen, and M.R. Krogsgaard, Calcif. Tissue Int. 41, 316-320 (1987).
17. T.J. Hahn, L.R. Halstead, B. Strates, B. Imbimbo, and D.T. Baran, Calcif. Tissue Int. 31, 109-115 (1980).
18. C. Gennari and B. Imbimbo, Calcif Tissue Int. 37, 592-593 (1985).
19. V. LoCascio, E. Bonucci, B. Imbimbo, P. Ballanti, D. Tartarotti, G. Galvanini, L. Fuccella, and S. Adami, Calcif. Tissue Int. 36, 435-438 (1984).
20. S. Balsan, D. Steru, A. Bourdeau, R. Grimberg, and G. Lenoir, Calcif. Tissue Int. 40, 303-309 (1987).
21. G. Benker, N. Breuer, R. Windeck, and D. Reinwein, J. Endocrinol. Invest. 11, 61-69 (1988).

22. K. Banovac, M. Paple, M.S. Bilsker, M. Zakarija, J. M. McKenzie, Arch. Intern. Med. 149, 809-812, (1989).
23. J-M. Coindre, J-P. David, L. Riviere, J-F. Goussot, P. Roger, A. de Mascarel, P.J. Meunier, Arch. Intern. Med. 146, 48-53 (1986).
24. T.L. Paul, J. Kerrigan, A.M. Kelly, L.E. Braverman, D.T. Baran, JAMA 259, 3137-3141 (1988).
25. M.D. Fallon, H.M. Perry III, M. Bergfeld, D. Droke, S.L. Teitelbaum, L.V. Avioli, Arch. Intern. Med. 143, 442-444 (1983).
26. J.V. Hennessey, J.E. Evaul, Y-C. Tseng, K.D. Burman, and L. Wartofsky, Ann. Int. Med. 105, 11-15 (1986).
27. L. Wartofsky, Thyroid Today XI, 1-11 (1988).
28. D.S. Ross, Mayo Clin. Proc. 63, 1223-1229 (1988).
29. H.S. Barden, R.B. Mazess, R.W. Chesney, P.G. Rose, and R. Chun, Metab. Bone Dis. Rel. Res. 4, 43-47 (1982).
30. N. Callaghan, A. Garrett, and T. Goggin, New Engl. J. Med. 318, 942-946 (1988).
31. T.A. Pedley, New Engl. J. Med. 318, 982-984 (1988).
32. H.T. Griffiths, D.T.Y. Liu, Postgrad. Med. J. 60, 424-425 (1984).
33. L.D. Piro, M.P. Whyte, W.A. Murphy, and S.J. Birge, J. Clin. Endocrinol. Metab. 54, 470-473 (1982).
34. R.K. Menon, D.S. Gill, M. Thomas, P.B.A. Kernoff, and P. Dandona, J. Clin. Endocrinol. Metab. 64, 59-61 (1987).
35. P. Pietschmann, W. Woloszczuk, S. Panzer, P. Kyrle, and J. Smolen, J. Clin. Endocrinol. Metab. 66, 1071-1074 (1988).
36. L.E. Mallette, K. Khouri, H. Zengotita, B.W. Hollis, and S. Malini, J. Clin. Endocrinol. Metab. 68, 654, 660 (1989).
37. J.H. Lazarus, C.J. Davies, J. S. Woodhead, D.A. Walker, G.M. Owen, Mineral Electrolyte Metab. 13, 63-66 (1987).
38. C. Christiansen, P.C. Baastrup and I. Transbol, Neuropsychobiology 6, 280-283 (1980.
39. W.A. Ray, W. Downey, M.R. Griffin, L.J. Melton III, Lancet I, 687-690 (1989).
40. H. Toft, J. Roin, Brit. Med. J. 1, 437-438 (1971).
41. C.G. Duarte, Metabolism 17, 867-876 (1968).
42. R.I. Macleod, R.R. Welbury, J.V. Soames, J. Royal Society Med. 80, 207-209 (1987).
43. A.K. Adatia, J. Royal Society Med. 80, 784-785 (1987).
44. P. Tugwell, K. Bennett, and M. Gent, Ann. Int. Med. 107, 356-366 (1987).
45. S.A. Rivkees, J.D. Crawford, JAMA 259, 2123-2125 (1988).
46. I.C. Henderson, New Engl. J. Med. 318, 443-444 (1988).
47. K.N. Muse, N.S. Cetel, L.A. Futterman, and S.S.C. Yen, New Engl. J. Med. 311, 1345-1349 (1984).
48. T.J. McKenna, New Engl. J. Med. 318, 558-562 (1988).
49. M.R. Henzl, S.L. Corson, K. Moghissi, V.C. Buttram, C. Beroqvist, and J. Jacobson, New Engl. J. Med 318, 485-489 (1988).
50. J.A. Gudmundsson, S. Ljunghall, C. Bergquist, L. Wide, and S.J. Millius, J. Clin. Endocrinol. Metab. 65, 159-163 (1987).
51. C. Movsowitz, S. Epstein, M. Fallon, F. Ismail, and S. Thomas, Endocrinology 123, 2571-2577 (1988).
52. M. Schlosberg, C. Movsowitz, S. Epstein, F. Ismail, M.D. Fallon, and S. Thomas, Endocrinology 124, 2179-2184 (1989).
53. R.L. Prince, K.J. Monk, G.N. Kent, I. Dick, P.J. Thompson, Mineral Electrolyte Metab. 14, 262-265 (1988).
54. S.J. Whiting and H.L. Whitney, J. Nutrition 117, 1224-1228 (1987).
55. T. Komoda, A. Nagata, M. Kiyoki, M. ,iura, I. Koyama, Y. Sakagishi, and M. Kumegawa, Calcif. Tissue Int. 42, 58-62 (1988).

The Metabolic Basis of Osteoporosis

B.E.C. Nordin,*‡ A.G.Need,* H.A. Morris,* and M. Horowitz**

Division of Clinical Chemistry, Institute of Medical and Veterinary Science
‡*Department of Pathology, University of Adelaide,*
**Department of Medicine, Royal Adelaide Hospital, Adelaide, South Australia*

ABSTRACT

   To define the metabolic basis of osteoporosis, we have compared the biochemical profiles of normal pre- and postmenopausal women on the one hand, and normal and osteoporotic postmenopausal women on the other. The rise in plasma calcium at the menopause is largely or wholly due to a rise in the complexed fraction which in turn is secondary to the rise in plasma bicarbonate. The associated rise in obligatory (fasting) urinary calcium is greater than would be predicted from the rise in filtered load and therefore represents a fall in tubular reabsorption of calcium in the kidneys. The reduced tubular reabsorption of calcium may result from the increase in the complexed fraction or the loss of a direct oestrogen effect on tubular handling of calcium. Hormone replacement therapy restores the premenopausal status. The osteoporotic (crush fracture) cases are characterised by a further increase in obligatory calcium loss, which is largely or wholly tubular, associated with malabsorption of calcium (in small part accounted for by reduced serum 1,25D), which combined with the high urinary calcium, accounts for the high urinary hydroxyproline. The latter can be suppressed by calcium supplementation in those with normal calcium absorption and by calcium with calcitriol in those with impaired calcium absorption. Osteoporotic women also have significantly lower serum albumin and dehydroepiandrosterone and thinner skin than age-matched controls; these could be markers of decreased bone formation and explain their favourable response to anabolic steroid therapy.

INTRODUCTION

   Osteoporosis is a disorder in which the amount of bony tissue in the bone ("bone density") is below the young normal range determined at the same skeletal site in subjects of the same sex [1]. Its clinical significance arises from the increase in fracture risk which it entails, but bone density is a continuous variable and the inverse relationship between bone density and fracture risk extends into the normal range [2]. Thus any definition must be arbitrary; the choice of the young normal lower limit as the "cut-off point" is consistent with the practice in other branches of biology and medicine and has the merit that osteoporosis defined in this way involves approximately a twofold increase in fracture risk [2].

   Osteoporosis can be and has been classified in many ways. It can be classified by pathogenesis (oestrogen deficiency, alcohol excess, corticosteroid administration, hyperparathyroidism, etc) or by the type of fracture with which it is associated (Type I with vertebral and wrist fractures and Type II with hip fracture [3]) but these classifications are not mutually exclusive and therefore of limited value. It is perhaps simplest to classify it initially by severity, as is done with hypertension (simple and accelerated), and then to consider pathogenesis. We therefore apply the label "simple osteoporosis" to subjects whose bone density, though below the normal range, is within the reference range for age and sex and site of measurement, and "accelerated osteoporosis" to those whose bone density is low by comparison with others of the same age and sex measured at the same skeletal site [4]. We are aware of the crucial importance of peak bone density. The term "accelerated osteoporosis" does not necessarily imply that this state has been reached by accelerated bone loss; it could have been arrived at because the subject started from a lower peak bone density [5].

To describe the metabolic basis of osteoporosis, one therefore needs to look at the metabolic status of those with simple osteoporosis compared with normal subjects, and of those with accelerated osteoporosis compared with those with simple osteoporosis. To reduce the number of variables involved, we shall concentrate on postmenopausal osteoporosis and confine ourselves to two types of comparison - that between normal pre- and postmenopausal women and that between normal postmenopausal women and those with crush fractures of the spine who, at least as a group, have less bone than age-matched controls at most if not all skeletal sites [6-9].

NORMAL PRE- AND POSTMENOPAUSAL WOMEN

Most workers probably agree that the total plasma calcium rises at the menopause [10-16], and that this is accompanied by very significant elevations of fasting urinary calcium, hydroxyproline and plasma alkaline phosphatase [13,14] (and probably BGP [17]). These events are associated with an increase in bone resorption and a secondary but presumably incomplete compensatory increase in bone formation, as judged by bone histology [6-8] and kinetic studies [18]. The controversy arises over the interpretation of these events. The prevailing view is probably that the increase in bone turnover results from the loss of an antiresorptive action of oestrogen on bone [19,20] (which is supported by the discovery of oestrogen receptors in bone [21]) and that all the other manifestations are secondary to this primary event. If there is a fall in calcium absorption [22], which is somewhat controversial [23], it is attributed to secondary depression of PTH and consequent depression of 1,25D production [24]. There is also a school of thought which brings calcitonin into the story, claiming that oestrogen deficiency depresses calcitonin levels and leads to bone resorption by this route [25]. Advocates of these models invoke the fall in plasma and urinary calcium, alkaline phosphatase and urinary hydroxyproline and convincing inhibition of bone loss which follow oestrogen administration, but these observations are all equally compatible with the concept that the primary events occur outside the bone and that the bone events are secondary.

The "direct effect" model assumes that the rise in plasma calcium at the menopause takes place in the ionized fraction. Alhough there is one report of elevated ionized calcium (not corrected to pH 7.4) in postmenopausal women [15] most of the latest work points the other way to at least three recent studies have failed to show any difference in ionized calcium concentration (corrected to pH 7.4) between pre- and postmenopausal or between young and old women [11,12,16] and our observations point the same way (Table I). We have also calculated the calcium fractions in the plasma by a method described elsewhere [26]. In 47 perimenopausal women, the total plasma calcium was 0.07 mmol/L higher than in 52 premenopausal women (p<0.001; Fig. 1) made up of 0.02 mmol/L in the ionized calcium (ns), 0.02 mmol/L in the protein-bound fraction (p<0.05) and 0.03 mmol/L (p<0.001) in the complexed fraction. The rise in complexed calcium is due to a rise

TABLE I: Measured total and ionized calcium (mmol/L ± SE) in normal pre- and postmenopausal women

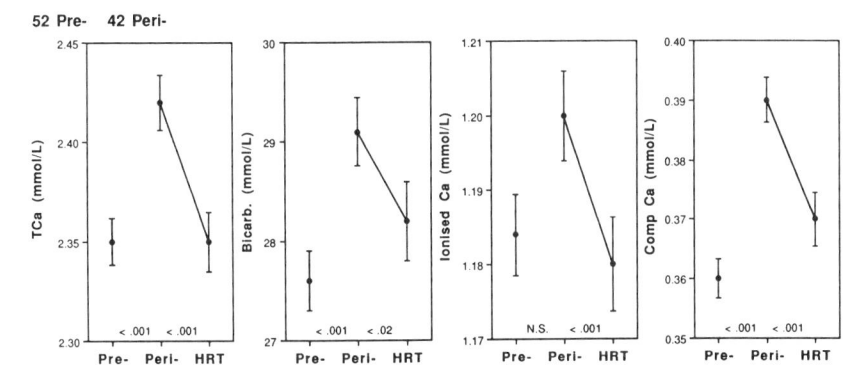

Source	Total Ca Pre-	Total Ca Post-	p	Ionized Ca Pre-	Ionized Ca Post-	p
Adelaide SMAC II; Radiometer	(62) 2.31±.012	(62) 2.44±.0083	<.001	(62) 1.22±.0038	(62) 1.23±.0049	ns
Sokoll [12] Nova 7	(83) 2.29±.0080	(319) 2.32±.0045	<.01	(83) 1.27±.0033	(319) 1.27±.0020	ns
Marshall [15] AutoAnal; Nova	(62) 2.36±.012	(90) 2.43±.0074	.001	(62) 1.17±.0051	(90) 1.20±.0043	<.001
Endres [16] SMAC-24; Radiometer	(31) 2.38±.01	(30) 2.45±.01	<.05	(31) 1.23±.01	(30) 1.24±.01	
Price [11] SMAC Radiometer	(27) 2.30±.07 (27) 2.30±.09	(44) 2.34±.09 (44) 2.33±.09	<.05	(27) 1.23±.03 (27) 1.23±.03	(44) 1.24±.03 (44) 1.22±.03	ns

FIG. 1: Plasma calcium, bicarbonate and calcium fractions in untreated pre- and peri-menopausal women, and after hormone replacement therapy in the latter. Note the rise of each variable and its fall in response to hormone therapy.

in plasma bicarbonate (which has been described before [27,28]) and it makes a major contribution to the elevation in total calcium that occurs at the menopause (Fig. 1). The rise of nearly 10% in the complexed calcium is of course much larger than could be accounted for by a primary change of less than 2% in the ionized fraction.

If there is in fact no change in plasma ionized calcium at the menopause, it would explain why the serum PTH [29] and 1,25D [30] do not change. Nor does oestrogen therapy seem to alter serum PTH despite the fall in total plasma calcium which it produces [31]; its positive effect on serum 1,25D is probably accounted for by an elevation of vitamin D-binding protein

[31,32]. However, a fall in measured ionized calcium (not corrected to pH 7.4) has been reported on hormone replacement therapy [31] and we see the same in the calculated ionized fraction but it is associated with a disproportionate fall in the complexed fraction (due to a fall in the plasma bicarbonate) which accounts for most of the fall in total calcium (Fig. 1). However, the calculation assumes a blood pH of 7.4 and would not be valid if the pH changed - nor would ionized calcium measurements corrected to pH 7.4. Thus changes in plasma bicarbonate play an important role in the plasma calcium changes at the menopause and on hormone therapy. These bicarbonate effects could be metabolic or respiratory in origin. We are inclined to favour the latter because it is known that oestrogen potentiates the positive effect of progesterone on the respiratory centre [33]. Only a very small rise in pCO at the menopause would be required to explain the rise in plasma bicarbonate of about 1 mmol/L and a mild respiratory acidosis might account for the bone resorption both at the menopause and in later life. On the other hand, a mild metabolic alkalosis with a small rise in blood pH would explain the elevation of total calcium very elegantly because of its positive effect on calcium binding by the various ligands involved. There is in fact one report that venous pH was marginally higher in post- than premenopausal women but we do not know what importance to attach to venous pH measurements [12].

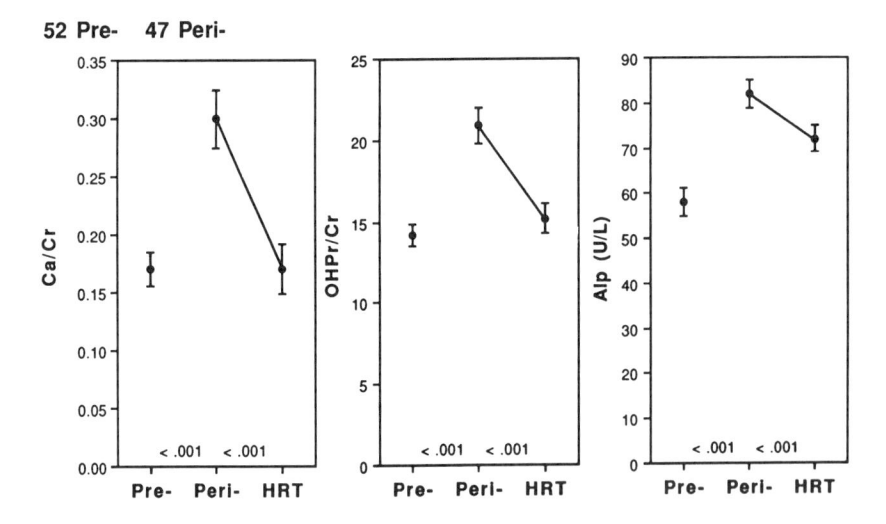

FIG. 2: Fasting urinary calcium and hydroxyproline and plasma alkaline phosphatase in the same subjects as Fig. 1. Note the rises in all variables at the menopause and their fall on hormone therapy.

Associated with these changes in the plasma, there are rises in Ca/Cr, OHPr/Cr and plasma alkaline phosphatase, all reversible by hormone replacement therapy (HRT) (Fig.2).

We have hitherto assumed that the rise in urinary calcium at the menopause could be accounted for by the rise in filtered load [13]. With the development of methodology for the calculation of the ultrafiltrable calcium fraction (which paradoxically is almost certainly more precise than direct measurement after ultrafiltration), we are now able to examine more closely the relationship between filtered and excreted calcium using the calculated ultrafiltrable calcium as the filtered load. The basis for this approach was provided by the calcium infusions performed in Leeds many years ago [34] which established the normal relationship between ultrafiltrable calcium and calcium excretion shown. The regression line was calculated on the basis of a Tm model by Marshall [35] and can be expressed in the following equation:

$$TmCa = \frac{UFCa - Ca_e}{1 - [0.08(\log(\frac{UFCa}{Ca_e}))]}$$

where UFCa is the filtered load of calcium in units per unit volume of GF and Ca_e is the calcium excretion in the same units (i.e. Ca/Cr x plasma creatinine).

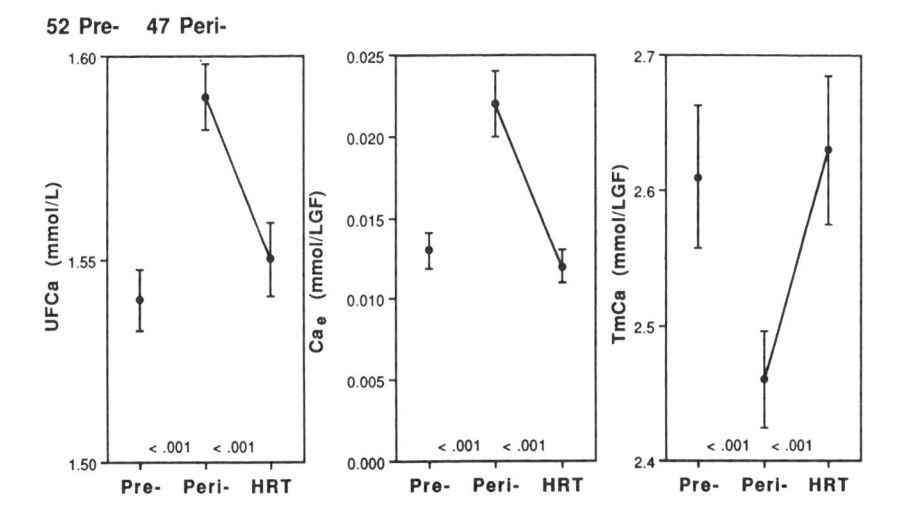

FIG. 3: Ultrafiltrable calcium, calcium excretion relative to GFR and TmCa in the same units (same subjects as Figs. 1 and 2). Note fall in TmCa at the menopause and its rise on therapy.

We have used this formula to calculate TmCa in the same pre- and perimenopausal women (Fig. 3). The filtered load (UFCa) rises very significantly at the menopause and falls on HRT. Calcium excretion in mmol/L of GF also rises at the menopause and falls on HRT, but the urinary changes are greater than would be expected for the changes in filtered load in each direction. Thus tubular reabsorption of calcium falls at the menopause. This would be compatible with a reduction in PTH activity but serum PTH does not appear to change at the menopause nor can we find any change in TmP [36]. The effect of hormone replacement therapy on the filtered and excreted calcium in symptomatic perimenopausal women is also shown in Fig. 3. Because the fall in urine calcium is greater than would be expected from the fall in filtered load, the TmCa rises to the premenopausal level.

These observations suggest that the rise in urine calcium at the menopause may be a primary event, i.e. that urinary calcium is being "pulled out" of the body rather than "pushed out". This is in turn supported by another observation, namely the strong positive correlation between fasting urinary calcium and urinary sodium in postmenopausal women [13,37].

To understand the significance of this, it has to be appreciated that the oft-quoted relationship between urinary sodium and calcium (in which 1 mmol of calcium is associated with about 100 mmol of sodium [13,37]) is fully expressed only in states of calcium deficiency, i.e. on low calcium diets or in the fasting state. This is illustrated in Table II. In 444 24-hour urine collections from normal postmenopausal women, the urine calcium was significantly related to the sodium in those whose calcium intakes were below 1000 mg daily, but not in those with intakes over 1000 mg. It must be appreciated that the correlation between urinary calcium and urinary sodium has little to do with the calcium/sodium ratio in the diet. If the calcium intake is high, some of the surplus absorbed calcium will appear in the urine regardless of sodium intake or output, i.e. calcium is "pushed" out of the body. If the calcium intake is low (as on a low calcium diet or in the fasting state), calcium is "pulled" out of the body at a rate determined largely by tubular reabsorption, which in turn is largely determined by the sodium load. All healthy persons are in sodium balance; what goes in goes out. This means that sodium output is virtually independent of calcium intake in the steady state. The same is not true of calcium. All healthy persons are not necessarily in calcium balance; there is a reservoir of calcium in the skeleton to be drawn on as required. The correlation between urine sodium and calcium must therefore be due to the effect of sodium on calcium rather than vice versa. Thus sodium takes calcium out of the body, leading to bone resorption if the necessary calcium replacement is not supplied from the diet. The result is a strong positive correlation between the fasting urine calcium and hydroxyproline in postmenopausal women and barely significant in premenopausal women (Table III). This is hardly what would be expected if the postmenopausal calcium loss were being "pushed" out by an increase in bone resorption, but just what would be expected if the calcium were being "pulled" out. There is even a strongly positive correlation between urine sodium and hydroxyproline (Table III) which cannot possibly be the result of bone resorption; there is not enough sodium in bone to explain this relationship.

TABLE II: Correlations with 24-hour urinary calcium in 444 normal postmenopausal women

	n					R	t	p
Ca intakes over 1,000 mg	174	24 Ca =	0.066	x	24 P		2.6	<0.02
			-0.041	x	24 Cr		0.4	ns
			+0.0026	x	24 Urea		1.0	ns
			+0.0041	x	24 Na		1.2	ns
			+1.30 mmol			0.34		<0.001
Ca intakes below 1,000 mg	270	24 Ca =	0.072	x	24P		3.4	<0.001
			-0.022	x	24 Cr		0.3	ns
			+0.0023	x	24 Urea		1.2	ns
			+0.0090	x	24 Na		3.9	<0.001
			+0.45 mmol			0.48		<0.001

TABLE III: Internal correlations between fasting urine calcium, sodium and hydroxyproline in 52 normal pre- and 302 normal postmenopausal women within 10 years of menopause

	Pre-	r	p	Post-	r	p	p (diff)
Ca/Cr on Na/Cr							
Slope	0.0067	0.44	<0.001	0.0089	0.42	<0.001	<0.001
Intercept	0.1	-	<0.001	0.14	-	<0.001	<0.001
OHPr/Cr on Ca/Cr							
Slope	8.4	0.19	ns	16.5	0.40	<0.001	<0.001
Intercept	12.7	-	<0.001	16.0	-	<0.001	<0.001
OHPr/Cr on Na/Cr							
Slope	0.030	0.01	ns	0.24	0.27	<0.001	<0.001
Intercept	13.8	-	<0.001	17.3	-	<0.001	<0.001

So important is the latter relationship that simple restriction of salt intake lowers hydroxyproline output in postmenopausal women (Table IV). Even in premenopausal women, salt loading increases hydroxyproline output [37]. It appears that hydroxyproline excretion (and presumably bone resorption) can be turned on and off simply by manipulating salt intake.

TABLE IV: Effect of varying salt intakes on urine hydroxyproline/creatinine (μmol/mmol) in normal pre- and postmenopausal women

	Premenopausal (9) Goulding [37]	Postmenopausal (31) Adelaide
Diet Ca	200 mg	Free
Specimen	24-hr urines	Fasting urines
OHPr/Cr on high or free Na	27 ± 6	19.1 ± 0.8
OHPr/Cr on 70 mmol Na	19 ± 3	17.0 ± 1.0
p	<0.01	<0.01

It should be noted in this context that the rise in urine calcium at the menopause is much more apparent in the fasting urine than in the 24-hour excretion. This is illustrated in Fig. 4 which shows evening and morning Ca/Cr values in pre- and postmenopausal women. There is no difference between the two groups in the evening but an obvious difference in the morning. The feature of the postmenopausal group is their failure to reduce their urine calcium overnight. This is compatible with the fact that the difference in 24-hour calcium output between pre- and postmenopausal women on a free diet is only about 10% (and barely significant) whereas the rise in fasting urine calcium is about 50% and highly significant (Table V).

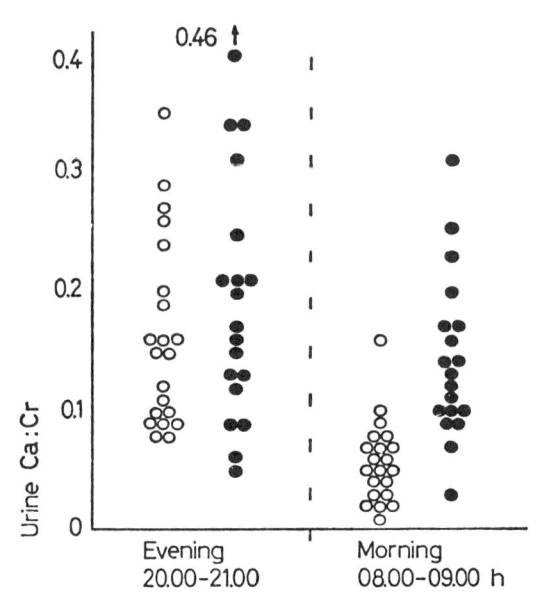

FIG. 4: Evening and morning (fasting) urinary calcium/creatinine ratios (mg/mg) in normal pre-[o] and post-[●] menopausal women. Note that urine calcium falls overnight in pre- but not postmenopausal women.

TABLE V: 24-hour and fasting urine calcium in normal pre- and postmenopausal women (below age 60)

	Premenopausal	Postmenopausal	p	Change
24-hr calcium (mmol SE)	(76) 3.58 ± 0.33	(337) 4.2 ± 0.12	<0.05	+12%
24-hr creatinine (mmol/L ± SE)	(76) 10.14 ± 0.49	(337) 10.13 ± 0.11	ns	
24-hr Ca/Cr	(76) 0.36 ± 0.035	(337) 0.41 ± 0.011	<0.05	+11%
Fasting Ca/Cr	(52) 0.17 ± 0.015	(118) 0.26 ± 0.014	<0.001	+53%

The train of events which best explains all these observations is that extra loss of calcium starting at the menopause in the urine (particularly at night perhaps) is the significant primary event which activates bone resorption (and subsequently bone formation) and thereby raises the urine hydroxyproline (and subsequently the alkaline phosphatase). This postulated sequence is supported by the positive effect of thiazide diuretics on bone mass [38] since a primary effect of thiazides is to lower urine calcium by an action on the kidney.

ACCELERATED OSTEOPOROSIS

The above considerations regarding simple postmenopausal osteoporosis can be applied with equal force to accelerated osteoporosis in postmenopausal women, i.e. to women with crush fractures of the vertebrae. These women, as a group, have very significantly lower bone density at all measured sites than women of the same age without crushed vertebrae [5,40]. This does not mean that they all fall below the lower reference limit for their age and sex - the reference ranges are wide at all sites - but it does mean that their bone densities are almost invariably below the mean for their age. It is clear that crush fracture patients taken as a group can be regarded as examples of accelerated osteoporosis and comparisons between them and women without crush fractures therefore provide information about the metabolic profile of accelerated osteoporosis.

The measured and derived variables in normal and osteoporotic postmenopausal women aged 61-75 years are shown in Figs. 5-9. Their mean ages are not significantly different but the osteoporotics are three years further from the menopause. The total plasma calciums do not differ between the two groups but the lower albumin in the osteoporotics (p<0.001) conceals their significantly higher calculated ultrafiltrable calcium which is made up of equal rises (about 0.01 mmol/L) in the ionized and complexed fractions (Fig.5). There is also a significantly higher fasting urine calcium in the osteoporotics (p<0.001) (even after correction for sodium) and significantly higher urinary hydroxyproline (p<0.05) and plasma alkaline phosphatase (p<0.1) (Fig. 6). The higher obligatory urinary calcium in the osteoporotics could simply result from their increased filtered load, but the difference in urinary calcium between the groups is out of proportion to the difference in filtered load indicating that there is a difference in tubular reabsorption of calcium between them (Fig. 7).

102 N   116 OP   Age 61-75

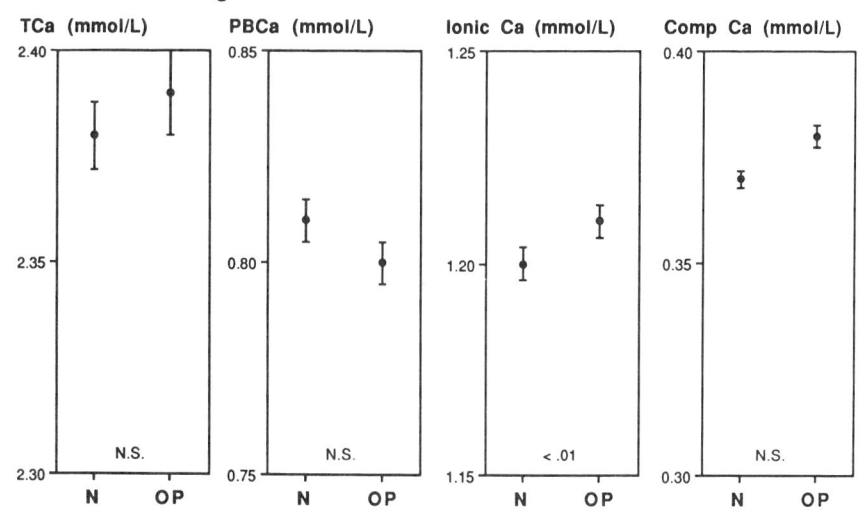

FIG. 5: Total plasma calcium and its fractions (calculated) in normal and osteoporotic postmenopausal women. Note significant difference in ionized calcium.

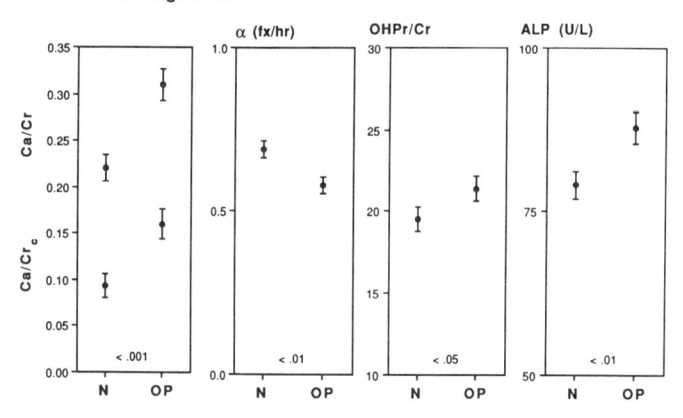

FIG. 6: Fasting urinary Ca/Cr (lower pair after correction for sodium), radiocalcium absorption, urinary hydroxyproline and plasma alkaline phosphatase in normal and osteoporotic women. Note significant differences in all variables.

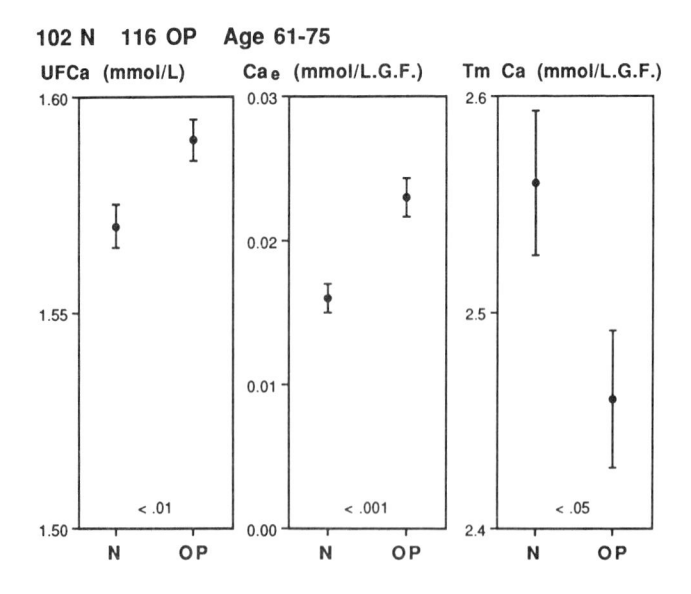

FIG. 7: Ultrafiltrable calcium, calcium excretion relative to GFR and TmCa in the same units in normal and osteoporotic postmenopausal women. Note that the increased calcium excretion in the osteoporotics is out of proportion to the rise in filtered load as indicated by their reduced TmCa.

There is again a highly significant correlation between urinary sodium and calcium with similar regression coefficients in the two groups (again about 1 mmol of calcium excreted for each 100 mmol of sodium) but the intercept of the regression slope on the Y-axis is significantly higher in the osteoporotics than in the normals because their filtered load is higher or because their tubular reabsorption is lower - or both (Table VI). There is also a highly significant correlation between fasting urinary calcium and hydroxyproline in both groups but there is more hydroxyproline excreted for each unit of calcium in the osteoporotics than in the normals (Table VI). It seems that there is some other factor raising bone resorption in accelerated osteoporosis in addition to the calcium loss in the urine.

TABLE VI: Relationships between Ca/Cr, Na/Cr, OHPr/Cr and calcium absorption in 102 normal and 116 osteoporotic postmenopausal women aged 61-75

	Normal	r	p	Osteoporotic	r	p
Ca/Cr on Na/Cr	y = .0099x + .095	.39	<.001	y = .0088x + .179	.39	<.001
OHPr/Cr on Ca/Cr	y = 14.8x + 16.3	.28	<.001	y = 16.2x + 16.8	.33	<.001
OHPr/Cr on Ca Abs	y = -4.9x + 22.9	.16	ns	y = -7.9 + 26.3	.24	<.02

This other factor is almost certainly the reduced absorption of calcium, which is the principal additional feature of the osteoporotic patients (Fig. 7). This malabsorption of calcium has been observed by other workers [24] but whereas they generally attribute it to low serum 1,25D levels resulting from increased bone resorption, we find that it is mainly due to gastrointestinal resistance to the action of calcitriol [39]. The present set again shows that the significant reduction in calcium absorption in osteoporotics (Fig. 6) is not accounted for by a corresponding reduction in serum 1,25D (Fig. 8).

If malabsorption of calcium were the cause of the accelerated bone resorption in these patients, one would expect to find an inverse correlation between calcium absorption and urinary hydroxyproline as is in fact the case in both groups though only significant in the osteoporotics (Table VI). On multiple linear regression in the whole set, hydroxyproline is a positive function of urine calcium (p<0.001) and a negative function of radiocalcium absorption (p<0.002) with a multiple R of 0.39 (p<0.001). A simple way of illustrating the positive relationship between hydroxyproline and urine calcium and the negative relationship between hydroxyproline and radiocalcium absorption is to subtract the Ca/Cr from the radiocalcium fractional absorption (both of which happen to be in comparable units) to yield a quotient which is a function of the difference between the calcium absorbed and the obligatory calcium excreted. This empirical quotient is very significantly inversely related to the urinary hydroxyproline (p<0.001).

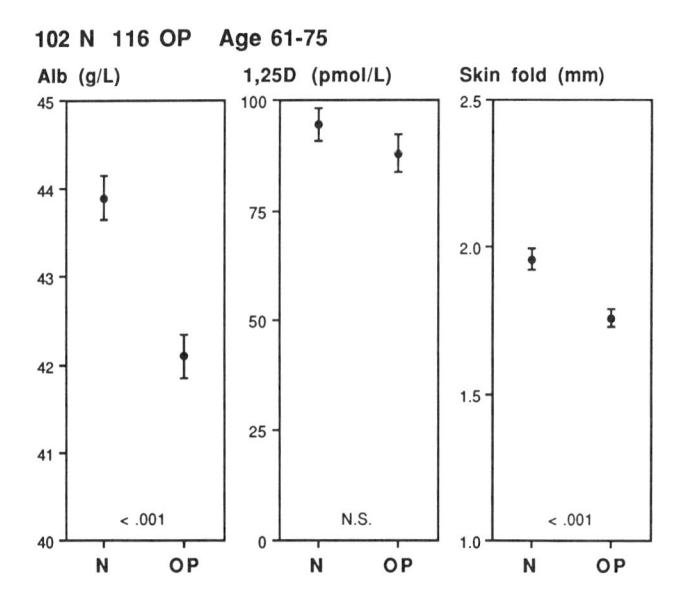

FIG. 8: Plasma albumin, serum calcitriol and skinfold thickness in normal and osteoporotic postmenopausal women. Note significant difference in albumin and skinfold but not in calcitriol.

In choosing between the alternative models for accelerated osteoporosis (primary event in bone or primary event outside bone), the response to therapy is highly relevant. The morning urinary hydroxyproline is suppressed by evening calcium administration in osteoporotic women with normal calcium absorption [40] and by calcium combined with calcitriol in those with malabsorption of calcium [41]. These intervention studies make it very much more likely that the urinary calcium loss and the malabsorption of calcium are primary events responsible for the high bone resorption rather than secondary events resulting from it. This model is also supported by evidence of a protective action of thiazide diuretics against hip fracture [42] since their action is to enhance the tubular reabsorption of calcium.

Finally, it is possible that an additional abnormality in these osteoporotic women is some impairment of bone formation. It is difficult to be definitive about this in biochemical terms because the markers of bone formation (alkaline phosphatase and BGP) are both elevated in these patients. Nonetheless, they display certain abnormalities which point to a depression of protein synthesis, notably significantly reduced plasma albumin and skinfold thickness (Fig. 8) and serum DHA [43] which point in this direction. These variables also fall with age in normal women [13] but they appear earlier in women with accelerated osteoporosis. Depression of bone formation is also implied by a number of histological studies on osteoporotic women [7,8,44]. It is this aspect of the osteoporotic process which probably accounts for the positive response to anabolic steroid therapy which is another feature of these cases [45].

These apparently disparate abnormalities in accelerated osteoporosis are perhaps internally related. Thus we have evidence that the "resistance" to 1,25D, which is largely responsible for the calcium malabsorption, is in its turn related to the plasma albumin level. Perhaps the key to accelerated osteoporosis is that it occurs in women in whom these various risk factors happen to be combined, or perhaps there is some underlying unifying principle which still escapes us.

CONCLUSIONS

The metabolic abnormalities associated with bone loss in postmenopausal women are compatible with a calcium deficiency model, according to which the loss of bone is essentially due to loss of calcium in the urine, possibly secondary to reduced tubular reabsorption of calcium. The more severe bone loss in women with accelerated osteoporosis can be explained by the same model, since they display a further increase in obligatory urinary calcium associated with malabsorption of calcium in the digestive tract - from whatever cause. An additional risk factor in these latter patients may be a relative impairment of bone formation, which renders them more vulnerable to any loss of bone they may experience during phases of negative calcium balance - possibly every night - because they cannot put bone back as fast as it is removed.

REFERENCES

1. Nordin BEC. Calcif Tissue Int 40, 57-58 (1987)
2. Nordin BEC, Chatterton BE, Walker CJ, Wishart J. Med J Aust 146, 300-304 (1987)
3. Riggs BL, Melton J. Am J Med 75, 899-901 (1983)
4. Nordin BEC, Crilly RG, Smith DA in Metabolic Bone and Stone Disease, BEC Nordin, ed. (Churchill Livingstone, Edinburgh 1984) pp 1-70
5. Nordin BEC, Wishart JM, Horowitz M, Need AG, Bridges A, Bellon M. Bone and Mineral 5, 21-23 (1988)
6. Nordin BEC, Aaron J, Speed R, Crilly RG. Lancet ii, 277-280 (1981)
7. Meunier PJ in Osteoporosis, BL Riggs, LJ Melton, eds. (Raven Press, New York 1988) pp 317-332
8. Parfitt AM in Osteoporosis, BL Riggs, LJ Melton, eds. (Raven Press, New York 1988) pp 45-93
9. Genant HK, Ettinger B, Harris ST, Block JE, Steiger P in Osteoporosis, BL Riggs, LJ Melton, eds. (Raven Press, New York 1988) pp 221-249
10. Young MM, Nordin BEC. Lancet ii, 118-120 (1967)
11. Price RI, Gutteridge DH, Barnes MP et al, in Osteoporosis, C Christiansen, JS Johansen, BJ Riis, eds. (Osteopress, Copenhagen 1987) pp 177-179
12. Sokoll LJ, Dawson-Hughes B. Calcif Tissue Int 44, 181-185 (1989)
13. Nordin BEC, Polley KJ. Calcif Tissue Int 41, S1-S60 (1987)
14. Stepan JJ, Pospichal J, Presl J, Pacovsky V. Bone 8, 279-284 (1987)
15. Marshall RW, Francis RM, Hodgkinson A. Clin Chim Acta 122, 283-287 (1982)
16. Endres DB, Morgan CH, Garry PJ, Omdahl JL. J Clin Endocrinol Metab 65, 724-731 (1987)
17. Delmas PD, Stenner D, Wahner HW, Mann KG, Riggs BL. J Clin Invest 71, 1316-1321 (1983)
18. Heaney RP, Recker RR. J Lab Clin Med 92, 964-979 (1978)
19. Jasani C, Nordin BEC, Smith DA, Swanson I. Royal Soc Med 58, 441-444 (1965)
20. Heaney RP. Am J Med 39, 877-880 (1965)

21. Eriksen EF, Colvard DS, Berg NJ, et al. Science 241, 84-86 (1988)
22. Heaney RP, Recker RR, Saville PD. J Lab Clin Med 92, 953-963 (1978)
23. Nordin BEC. Calcium. J Food Nutrition 42, 67-82 (1986)
24. Gallagher JC, Riggs BL, Eisman J, Hamstra A, Arnaud SB, DeLuca HF. J Clin Invest 64, 729-736 (1979)
25. Stevenson JC, Abeyasekera G, Hillyard CJ, Phang KG, MacIntyre I. Lancet i, 693-695 (1981)
26. Nordin BEC, Need AG, Hartley TF, Philcox JC, Wilcox M, Thomas DW. Clin Chem 35, 14-17 (1989)
27. Hodgkinson A, Selby PL, Burrows AW. Maturitas 5, 25-30 (1983)
28. McPherson K, Healy MJR, Flynn FV, Piper KAJ, Garcia-Webb P. Clin Chim Acta 84, 373-397 (1987)
29. Sokoll LJ, Morrow FD, Quirbach DM, Dawson-Hughes B. Clin Chem 34, 407-410 (1988)
30. Falch JA, Oftebro H, Haug E. J Clin Endocrinol Metab 64, 836-841 (1987)
31. Selby PL, Peacock M, Barkworth SA, Brown WB, Taylor GA. Clin Sci 69, 265-271 (1985)
32. Crilly RG, Marshall DH, Horsman A, Nordin BEC, Bouillon R in Osteoporosis: Recent Advances in Pathogenesis and Treatment, HF DeLuca et al, eds. (University Park Press, Baltimore 1981) pp 359-367
33. Brodeur P, Mockus M, McCullough R, Grindlay Moore L. J Appl Physiol 60, 590-595 (1986)
34. Peacock M, Nordin BEC. J Clin Path 21, 353-358 (1968)
35. Marshall DH in Calcium, Phosphate and Magnesium Metabolism, BEC Nordin, ed. (Churchill Livingstone, Edinburgh 1976) pp 257-297
36. Bijvoet OLM. Clin Sci 37, 23-26 (1969)
37. Goulding A, Everitt HE, Cooney JM, Spears GFS in Recent Advances in Clinical Nutrition 2, ML Wahlqvist, AS Truswell, eds. (Libbey, London 1986) pp 99-108
38. Wasnich RD, Benfante RJ, Yano K, Heilbrun L, Vogel JM. N Engl J Med 309, 344-347 (1983)
39. Morris HA, Nordin BEC, Fraser V, Hartley TF, Need AG, Horowitz M in Vitamin D: Chemical, Biochemical and Clinical Update, AW Norman et al, eds. (Gruyter, Berlin 1985) pp 996-997
40. Horowitz M, Need AG, Philcox JC, Nordin BEC. Am J Clin Nutr 39, 857-859 (1984)
41. Need AG, Horowitz M, Philcox JC, Nordin BEC. Mineral Electrolyte Metab 11, 35-40 (1985)
42. Holbrook TL, Barrett-Connor E, Wingard DL. Lancet ii, 1046-1049 (1988)
43. Nordin BEC, Robertson A, Seamark RF et al. J Clin Endocrinol Metab 60, 651-657 (1985)
44. Carasco G, deVernejoul MC, Sterkers Y, Morieux C, Kuntz D, Miravet. Calcif Tissue Int 44, 173-175 (1989)
45. Need AG, Chatterton BE, Walker CJ, Steurer TA, Horowitz M, Nordin BEC. Maturitas 8, 275-280 (1986)

FRACTURE RISK

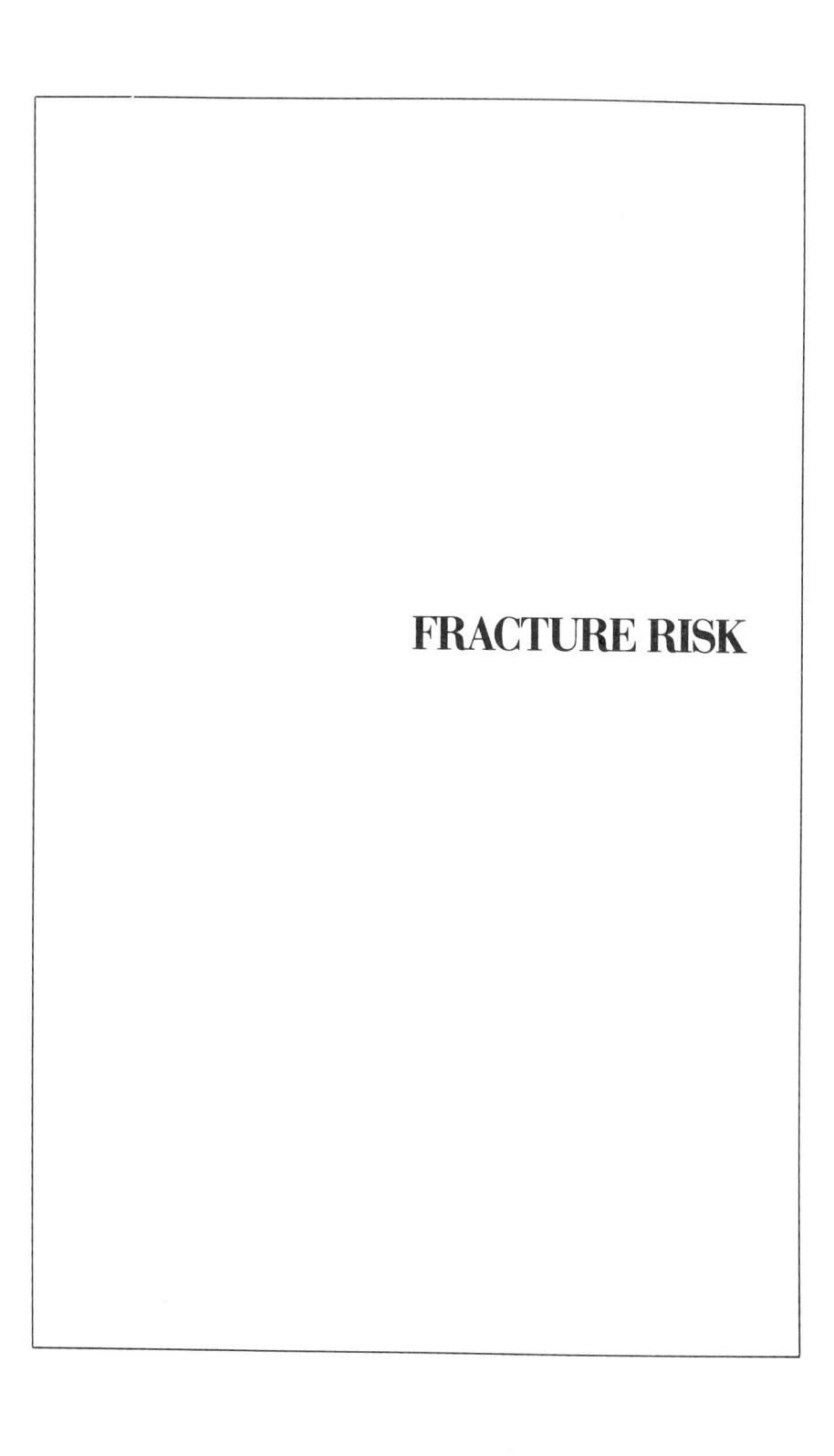

Fracture Patterns

L.J. Melton, III

Mayo Clinic and Foundation, Rochester, Minnesota

ABSTRACT

Fracture patterns provide clues to underlying pathophysiology. The age-related rise in fracture incidence is generally related to declining bone mass and more severe falls, but the pattern is not the same for each type of fracture. This heterogeneity is a stimulus to produce more insightful models of osteoporosis natural history.

INTRODUCTION

Fracture incidence in the community is bimodal by age. Fractures are common among young people, where they are more frequent in boys than girls and usually result from significant trauma; incidence rates rise again later in life but with a different pattern (Figure 1). These "age-related" fractures are more frequent in women than men and typically result from nonviolent trauma, usually a fall [1]. Metaphyseal sites are most often affected. By tradition, the proximal femur (hip), vertebrae and distal forearm are considered age-related fracture sites [2], but fractures of the pelvis [3], proximal humerus [4], shaft and distal femur [5,6] and ankle [7] should be included as well when they occur without violent trauma.

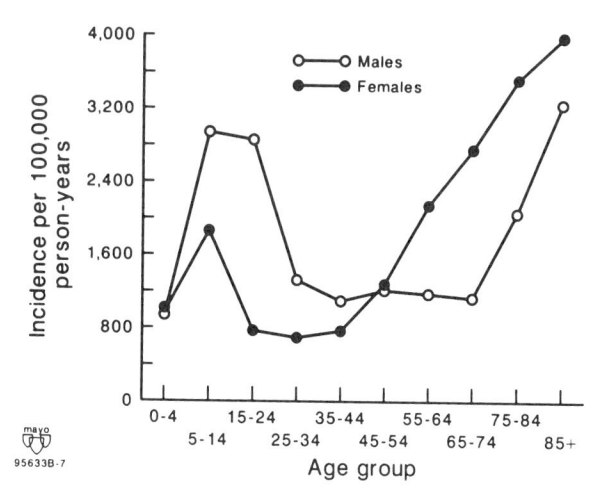

FIG. 1. Average annual age- and sex-specific incidence of all limb fractures among Rochester, Minnesota residents. From Garraway et al. [1], with permission.

RELATION OF FRACTURES TO BONE MASS AND FALLS

These age-related (≈ osteoporotic) fractures are generally attributed to bone loss that compromises the biomechanical integrity of the skeleton, although an increase in serious falls also plays a role. The frequency of falls rises with age and is greater among women than men [8]. A third or more of elderly individuals may experience a fall each year, and up to half of those over 80 years of age. The frequency of falls per se cannot entirely account for the fracture pattern in the community because the incidence of fractures rises with age at a much faster rate than the incidence of falls; and some fractures, especially of the vertebrae, are not associated with falls [2]. Moreover, there is evidence that young people have fewer fractures than might be expected from their bone mass levels, while older individuals have more than expected [9]. These observations might be accounted for by a declining capacity to dissipate the kinetic energy of a fall, leading to an age-related increase in the degree of trauma actually experienced [10]. In epidemiologic parlance, falls are a necessary cause of most age-related fractures, but they are not a sufficient cause as demonstrated by the fact that most falls do not result in a fracture. Even among the elderly, only 5-6% of falls lead to fractures and only 1% end in a hip fracture [8,11].

As the likelihood of falling rises with age, bone strength declines. Over life, women lose about one-third of their original cortical (compact) bone, which forms the shafts of the limb bones and comprises up to 80% of the skeleton; they may lose half of their trabecular (cancellous) bone that accounts for the remaining 20%; men lose about two-thirds of these amounts [12]. Although bone architecture and bone quality influence bone strength, the main determinant is bone mass; and any decline in bone mass results in a disproportionately greater loss of bone strength [13]. Consequently, age-related bone loss leads to an increased risk of fractures (Figure 2).

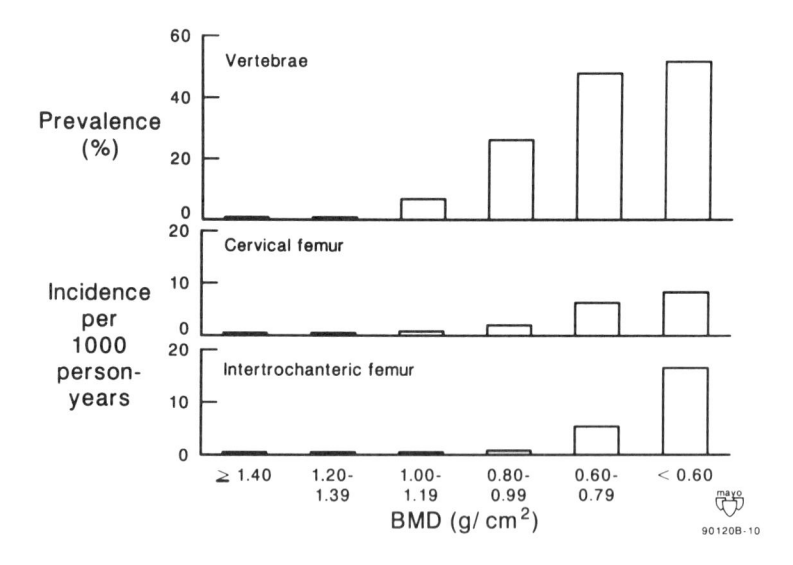

FIG. 2. Estimated prevalence of vertebral fractures by lumbar spine bone mineral density (BMD) and estimated incidence of cervical and intertrochanteric hip fractures by cervical and intertrochanteric BMD, respectively, among Rochester, Minnesota women ≥ 35 years of age. From Riggs and Melton [14], with permission.

Population-based studies have shown a gradient of continuously increasing hip fracture incidence associated with declining bone mineral density in the proximal femur [15], rising Colles' fracture incidence with decreasing bone mass in the radius [16,17], and higher vertebral fracture incidence [18] and prevalence [19] with lessened bone density in the spine. Several prospective studies show, in addition, that bone mass predicts the risk of fractures generally [20-22]. Even among individuals with low bone mass, however, the risk of fracture is relatively low. For example, in women with the lowest 5% of femoral bone mass, the incidence of hip fractures is estimated at only about 2% per year [15]. Thus, osteoporosis is also a necessary but not sufficient cause of most age-related fractures [10].

HETEROGENEITY OF FRACTURE SYNDROMES

Within the general epidemiologic pattern of rising fracture incidence with age, however, there are distinctions which may have etiologic significance. Hip fracture rates increase exponentially throughout life (Figure 3), as do those for fractures of the proximal humerus, pelvis and distal femur, albeit less dramatically [23]. All are considered manifestations of Type II (age-related) osteoporosis, which occurs commonly in elderly women and men and is characterized by loss of both cortical and trabecular bone at a rate similar to that in the general population [14].

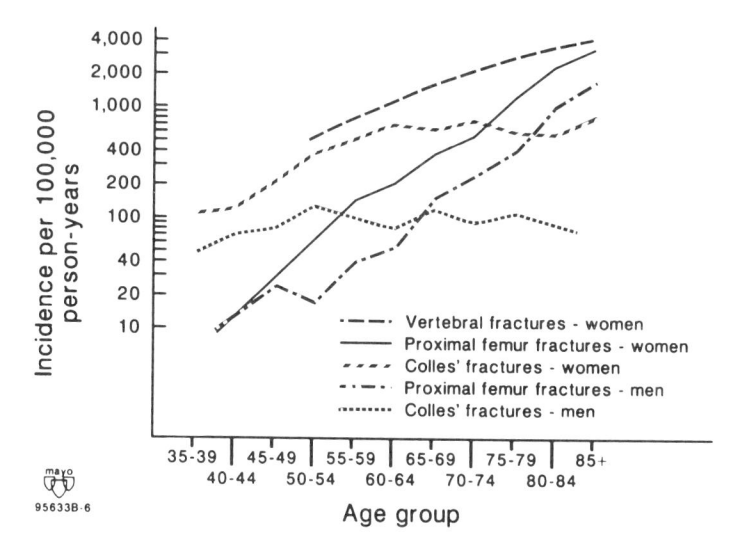

FIG. 3. Age- and sex-specific incidence of Colles' fractures contrasted with that of vertebral and hip fractures among Rochester, Minnesota residents. From Melton [2] with permission.

Incidence rates for distal forearm fractures (Figure 3) and ankle fractures are higher in the perimenopausal period, but then level off. While no explanation for this is known, possibilities include 1) a perimenopausal increase in osteoclast-mediated trabecular bone loss, 2) a transient increase in cortical porosity or 3) a shift in the nature of falls related to a slowing of gait speed [24]. Distal forearm fractures and postmenopausal vertebral crush fractures are hypothesized to be manifestations of Type I (postmenopausal) osteoporosis, which occurs in a relatively small proportion of women and even less commonly in men and is characterized by accelerated and disproportionate loss of trabecular bone [14].

This striking difference in the epidemiologic features of Colles' fractures and hip fractures has parallels elsewhere [25]. The exponential increase in hip fracture incidence with aging in both sexes recalls exponentially increasing incidence rates for a number of other complex chronic conditions (Figure 4). These common degenerative diseases have been termed "Gompertzian" (after the British actuary, Benjamin Gompertz, who first described the exponential nature of mortality) and they have certain characteristics in common (Table I). Thus, hip fractures, the characteristic clinical manifestation of Type II osteoporosis, increase exponentially in incidence, reflecting the Gompertzian model of a degenerative disease with early onset and insidious progression until a symptomatic threshold is reached after a long latent period. Such diseases are typically multifactorial and affect the majority of the population.

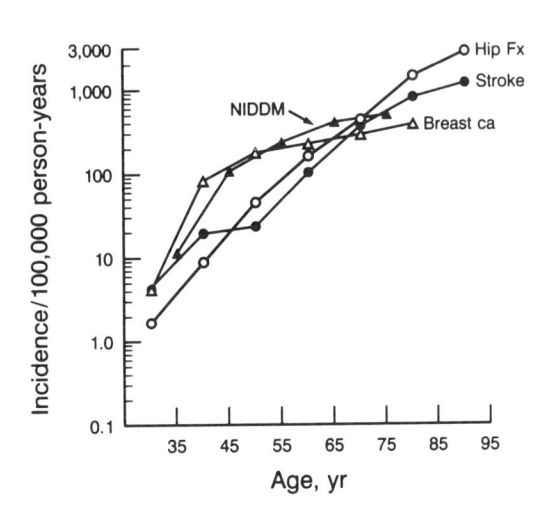

FIG. 4. Age-specific incidence of hip fracture, stroke, breast cancer and non-insulin-dependent diabetes mellitus (NIDDM) among Rochester, Minnesota women.

TABLE I. Characteristics of the two kinds of chronic disease, modified from Fries [25].

Gompertzian (Exponential increase with aging)	Non-Gompertzian (Non-exponential relation with age)
Universal propensity	Specific individuals affected
Early onset with insidious progression	More acute onset with variable progression
Symptom threshold late in life	Symptoms early but remissions may occur
Multiple risk factors	Specific pathophysiology
No single cause so unamenable to therapy	Therapeutic interventions often possible

Like Colles' fractures, on the other hand, incidence rates for some other disorders do not increase exponentially with aging (non-Gompertzian) as shown in Figure 5. These diseases, too, have common characteristics (Table I). Thus, Colles' fractures and postmenopausal vertebral crush fractures, which are most closely associated with Type I osteoporosis, are consistent with non-Gompertzian conditions that have relatively early onset and a variable clinical course often marked by remission. Such diseases affect a smaller proportion of the population, often have a specific etiology and may be more amenable to treatment.

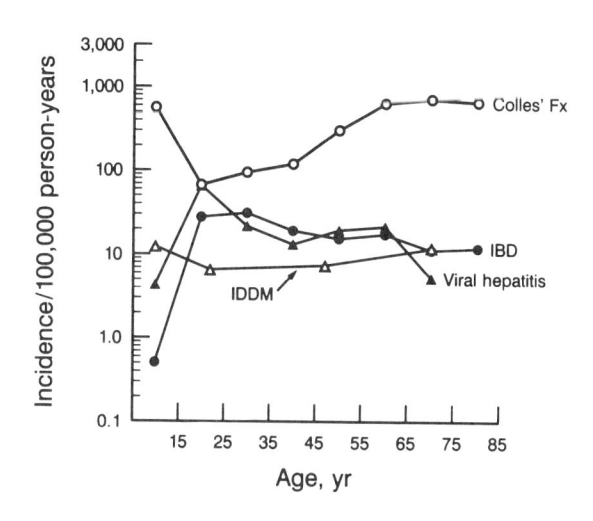

FIG. 5. Age-specific incidence of Colles' fracture, viral hepatitis, inflammatory bowel disease (IBD) and insulin-dependent diabetes mellitus (IDDM) among Rochester, Minnesota women.

These epidemiologic observations provide empirical support for the existence of two distinct syndromes of involutional osteoporosis. By this analysis, Type II osteoporosis (Gompertzian) and Type I osteoporosis (non-Gompertzian) are different diseases, even though they operate through the final common pathway of low bone mass and individual patients may be affected by both conditions. Hypotheses of pathophysiology are consistent with the Gompertzian model insofar as Type I osteoporosis is generally considered to be more closely linked with a specific factor, estrogen deficiency, which leads to increased bone turnover and accelerated bone loss, while the slower age-related bone loss of Type II osteoporosis is related to a complex set of age-related physiologic changes [26]. In any event, the Gompertzian analogy suggests that the search for etiologic explanations in Type I and Type II osteoporosis might be broadened to consider explanations for features held in common with other chronic diseases which share their epidemiologic patterns.

ACKNOWLEDGEMENTS

The author would like to thank Ms. Mary Roberts for help in preparing the manuscript. The work was supported in part by research grants AR-27065 and AR-30582 from the National Institutes of Health.

REFERENCES

1. W.M. Garraway, R.N. Stauffer, L.T. Kurland, and W.M. O'Fallon, Mayo Clin. Proc. 54, 701-707 (1979).
2. L.J. Melton in: Osteoporosis: Etiology, Diagnosis, and Management, B.L. Riggs and L.J. Melton, eds. (Raven Press, New York, 1988) pp. 133-154.
3. L.J. Melton, J.M. Sampson, B.F. Morrey, and D.M. Ilstrup, Clin. Orthop. 155, 43-47 (1981).
4. S.H. Rose, L.J. Melton, B.F. Morrey, D.M. Ilstrup, and B.L. Riggs, Clin. Orthop. 168, 24-30 (1982).
5. T.J. Arneson, L.J. Melton, D.G. Lewallen, and W.M. O'Fallon, Clin. Orthop. 234, 188-194 (1988).
6. R. Hedlund and U. Lindgren, Acta Orthop. Scand. 57, 423-427 (1986).
7. P.J. Daly, R.H. Fitzgerald, L.J. Melton, and D.M. Ilstrup, Acta Orthop. Scand. 58, 539-544 (1987).
8. M.J. Gibson, Danish Med. Bull. 34(Suppl. 4), 1-24 (1987).
9. L.J. Melton, S.H. Kan, H.W. Wahner, B.L. Riggs, J. Clin. Epidemiol. 41, 985-994 (1988).
10. L.J. Melton and B.L. Riggs, Clin. Geriatr. Med. 1, 525-539 (1985).
11. M.E. Tinetti and M. Speechley, N. Engl. J. Med. 320, 1055-1059 (1989).
12. B.L. Riggs, H.W. Wahner, E. Seeman, K.P. Offord, W.L. Dunn, R.B. Mazess, K.A. Johnson, and L.J. Melton, J. Clin. Invest. 70, 716-723 (1982).
13. L.J. Melton, E.Y.S. Chao, and J. Lane in: Osteoporosis: Etiology, Diagnosis, and Management, B.L. Riggs and L.J. Melton, eds. (Raven Press, New York 1988) pp. 111-131.
14. B.L. Riggs and L.J. Melton, N. Engl. J. Med. 314, 1676-1686 (1986).
15. L.J. Melton, H.W. Wahner, L.S. Richelson, W.M. O'Fallon, and B.L. Riggs, Am. J. Epidemiol. 125, 254-261 (1986).
16. S.L. Hui, C.S. Slemenda, and C.C. Johnston Jr, J. Clin. Invest. 81, 1804-1809 (1988).
17. R. Eastell, B.L. Riggs, H.W. Wahner, W.M. O'Fallon, P.C. Amadio, and L.J. Melton, J. Bone Min. Res. (in press).
18. P.D. Ross, R.D. Wasnich, and J.M. Vogel, J. Bone Min. Res. 3, 1-11 (1988).
19. L.J. Melton, H.W. Wahner, W.M. O'Fallon, and B.L. Riggs, Am. J. Epidemiol. 129, 1000-1011 (1989).
20. A.P. Iskrant and R.W. Smith Jr, Public Health Rep. 84, 33-38 (1969).
21. R.D. Wasnich, Osteoporosis Update 1987, H.K. Genant, ed. (Radiology Research and Education Foundation, San Francisco 1987) pp. 95-101.
22. S.L. Hui, C.W. Slemenda, and C.C. Johnston, Jr, Ann. Intern. Med. (in press).
23. L.J. Melton, S.R. Cummings, and C.C. Johnston, Bone Min. 2, 321-331 (1987).
24. L.J. Melton in: Proceedings of the International Symposium on Clinical Disorders of Bone and Mineral Metabolism (in press).
25. J.F. Fries in: Proceedings, Exploring New Frontiers of U.S. Health Policy, Graduate Program in Public Health, University of Medicine and Dentistry of New Jersey-Rutgers Medical School and Rutgers (The State University of New Jersey 1984).
26. B.L. Riggs and L.J. Melton, Am. J. Med. 75, 899-901 (1983).

Assessment and Modification of Hip Fracture Risk Predictions of a Stochastic Model

A. Horsman and M.N. Birchall

MRC Bone Mineralisation Group, Department of Medical Physics, The General Infirmary, Leeds, U.K.

ABSTRACT

By means of a stochastic model which simulates falls and bone loss from the proximal femur in an ageing female cohort, we have shown that in elderly women the risk of fracture of the hip following a fall increases exponentially with decreasing bone mineral density (BMD) in the femoral neck. Our model predicts that about 66% of all fractures occur in those 25% of women who at maturity had the lowest values of BMD, and that peak BMD value, rather than rate of decline of BMD in middle age, is the major determinant of lifetime risk of hip fracture.

Such risks could be modified by prolonged therapy which affected the course of age-related bone loss and possibly the risk of falls in individuals. The model has been used to calculate likely reductions in fracture incidence resulting from large-scale prophylaxis, taking into account potential effects on both factors. For different durations of prophylaxis, average numbers of patient years of treatment that must be administered to women selected at random in order to prevent one hip fracture have been calculated. The extent to which those numbers might be reduced by selectively treating only individuals with low values of BMD has also been estimated.

INTRODUCTION

Dual photon absorptiometry (DPA) of the proximal femur is now widely performed with the expectation that one of the resulting measurements, the bone mineral density (BMD) of the femoral neck in particular, predicts the risk that the person measured will later suffer an osteoporotic fracture of the hip [1]. Research effort and screening procedures based on this technique, using machines with either isotope or X-ray tube radiation sources, usually concentrate on postmenopausal women, who are collectively at much greater risk of hip fractures than young adults and elderly men [2]. The aim of screening is to identify those women most likely to benefit, in terms of reduced fracture risk, from prophylaxis given primarily to reduce subsequent bone loss from skeletal sites where fractures often occur [3,4].

We have previously examined some of the numerical consequences of the hypothesis that in women the amount of bone in the femoral neck is a determinant of the risk of hip fracture following a fall, using stochastic modelling techniques to implement two similar models of events occurring in an ageing female cohort [5,6]. Those two models, 'linear' and 'non-linear', are reviewed below. In the latter more realistic case, we were able to show that in elderly women the risk of fracture following a fall increases exponentially with decreasing BMD [6]. We also demonstrated that the mean bone mineral deficits in groups of elderly fracture cases (relative to age-matched non-fracture cases) predicted by the model were consistent with observed values [7].

In this paper, we explore in greater depth the predictions of a new variant of the non-linear model, including some situations in which model parameters were altered in order to simulate possible effects on fracture incidence of large-scale prophylaxis administered to an ageing cohort.

STOCHASTIC MODELS OF FEMORAL BONE LOSS, FALLS AND HIP FRACTURE RISK

Two similar stochastic models have been investigated previously [6], the non-linear model being an extension of the linear case and the more relevant to hip fracture risk assessment given currently available measurements on the femoral neck. Monte Carlo methods were applied in both models to simulate bone loss, falls and fractures in an ageing cohort, using techniques explained fully in a previous publication [5]. Fractures were assumed to occur only as a consequence of falling; hip fractures which are the cause of falls are rare. The frequency of falls, which increases with age, was described by the same function in both models.

The linear model was so-called because a linear function was used to describe age-related bone loss from the femoral neck. Denoting the risk that an individual will fracture following a fall by Q, and the bone measurement in the femoral neck at the time of the fall by BM then, by definition, $Q = F(BM)$ where $F(BM)$ was an unknown function to be determined. F was not a function of age.

In the later model, a non-linear function was used to describe the age-related decrease in bone mineral density of the femoral neck. An important difference between the non-linear model and the linear model was inclusion in the calculation of fracture risk of an extra age-dependent function, $S(a)$ (a denotes age), which was regarded as describing how the severity of falls increases with age; its inclusion was necessitated by the form used for the descriptor of age-related bone loss. For the non-linear model, by definition the risk $Q = S(a) \cdot G(BMD)$ where the fall occurs at age a and here BMD is the current bone mineral density. Initially, both $S(a)$ and $G(BMD)$ were unknown functions; they were ultimately determined in the course of the calculations.

CURRENT IMPLEMENTATION OF THE NON-LINEAR MODEL

An important feature of the current version of the non-linear model is the control exercised over the occurrence of multiple fractures (see below). This, and other less significant changes also introduced to make the current version more realistic, affected the ultimate values of some of the model parameters.

Overview

FIG. 1 outlines the approach we recently used to simulate events in a female cohort ageing from birth into extreme old age. Details are given in later sections.

1) Each individual was first allocated parameters describing her lifelong changes in BMD.

2) Each was then allocated falls on the basis of the known risk of falls as a function of age.
3) The function S(a) was set to 1 for all ages a.
4) Parameters determining the function Q = S(a).G(BMD), which reduces to Q = G(BMD) when S(a) is set to 1, were initially given arbitrary values.
5) For each individual, all falls were examined and a decision made whether or not to associate a fracture with each fall; BMD at the time of fall was computed and the risk of fracture, on which that decision was based, was usually interpolated from the function Q. However, if two fractures had already occurred in that individual, the risk was set to zero; in the simulations, no-one was allowed to have more than two hip fractures.
6) The predicted age-specific incidence of fractures was computed by counting the number of fractures occurring in 1 year intervals.
7) The predicted incidence was compared with the known true (idealised) incidence of hip fractures in women. Any mismatch was attributed to errors in the specification of the function Q.
8) Parameter values determining G(BMD) were adjusted in such a way as to improve the match between the predicted and true incidences in the lower age groups (in practice below age 70).
9) Steps 5) to 8) were repeated iteratively, as indicated by the dotted loop in FIG. 1, until a satisfactory match was obtained.
10) Values of the function S(a) were calculated for ages over 65 such that in the next step the predicted and true incidences would match at all ages up to 85. Above age 85, S(a) was linearly extrapolated.

Finally, steps 5) and 6) were repeated with a further refinement in step 5): that for every individual Q = S(a).G(BMD) described the risk of fracture only for falls up to and including that which resulted in the first fracture. For subsequent falls the multiplier S(a) was assumed to be 1 at all ages; this was done in order to constrain the frequency of second fractures to realistic levels.

Mortality

Simulations were carried out for the whole cohort ageing between 0 and 100 years. By not removing individuals (as a result of dying, in a real cohort), the simulation programs generated a database which contained an adequate pool of information about the very old. However, for certain calculations, a realistic representation of mortality within the model was essential; for that reason, each individual was assigned an age at death, and the fact that an individual had died was taken into account when necessary in answering certain queries posed to the database.

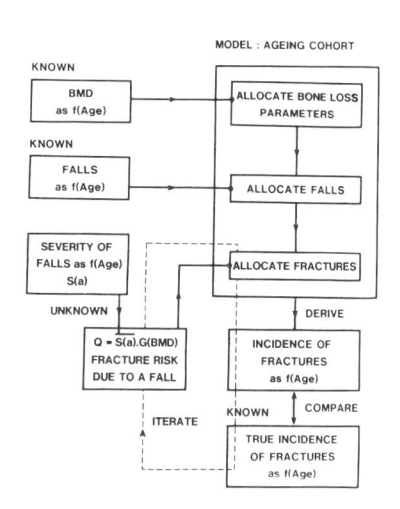

FIG. 1. Schematic diagram of the non-linear model.

Model parameters

Parameters describing how BMD changed with age in individuals are illustrated in FIG. 2. All variables were assumed to be Gaussianly distributed; standard deviations (SDs) are given below inside paretheses. Individual values were statistically independent of one-another. Units were arbitrarily chosen so that the mean value of BMD in young adults was approximately 90.

Growth occurred at mean rate R0=0.450(0.0405) until mean age of maturity A1=20(1). Thereafter the equilibrium phase (R1=0 in everyone) continued until mean age A2=35(2), when bone loss started with mean rate of change R2=-0.864(0.062). Later in life at mean age A3=60(2) bone loss slowed down to a mean rate of change R3=-0.27(0.027).

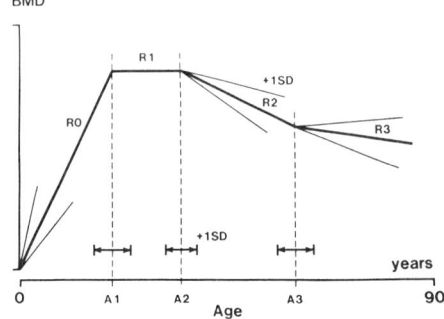

FIG. 2. Parameters of the non-linear model defining age-related changes in BMD.

The resulting mean values and SDs of BMD in those members of the ageing cohort who, up to any given age had not fractured, closely approximate published results of cross-sectional absorptiometric studies of the femoral neck in non-fracture cases [7]. Changes in BMD for the shrinking class of members of the cohort who remained free of fractures as age advanced are shown in relation to age by the curves in FIG. 3.

The age-related risk of falls in women was derived from two sources. Values in the range 50-70 years were taken from Aitken [8]; those from 60 onwards were obtained from a DHSS survey carried out in the UK (Cooper, personal communication). The period prevalence per week is a sigmoidal function of age [6]; it was represented as a unidimensional array of 100 elements in the simulation program. Element values at decade intervals from 50 onwards were 0.07, 0.35, 0.90, 1.35 and 1.48%.

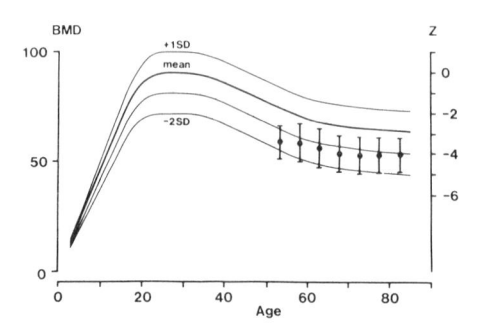

FIG. 3. Changes in BMD in the ageing cohort. Z is a linear transform of BMD. Points show mean values (1SD) in fracture cases.

Underlying the randomness of falls in the individual there might be systematic differences between individuals in the frequency of falling; each individual was therefore allocated a scaling factor for risk of falls that was applied in step 2) of the calculations. The factor had a mean of 1 and was arbitrarily assumed to have SD 0.3; the value of the SD did not affect conclusions drawn below.

The function S(a) was represented numerically, not analytically as before [6]; all 100 array elements were initialised to 1. The function G(BMD) was represented analytically as:

$$G(BMD) = \exp(k_1 - k_2 \cdot BMD)$$

with initial values of the two constants being 8 and 0.1. Those values changed in the course of iteration.

Because sets of real data on age-specific incidence of hip fracture vary due to sampling artefacts and systematic differences between populations studied, real data were idealised as an exponential rising to 50 cases/10,000/year at age 75 and doubling every 5 years. The idealised curve is shown in FIG. 4.

An age at death was allocated to each individual on the basis of death rates published for 5 year groups (DHSS statistics for England and Wales in 1985, using population structure based on 1981 census). In the simulations, nobody was allowed to survive beyond 100. Risk of death was such that the percentages of survivors at decade intervals from 50 onwards were 93%, 87%, 73%, 45% and 11%.

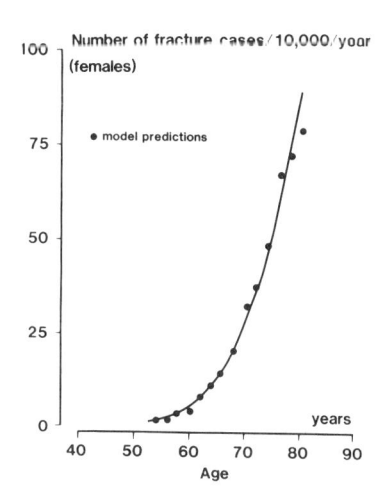

FIG. 4. Comparison of predicted (points) and idealised true hip fracture incidence (curve).

Practical implementation

Simulations were performed using a suite of programs written in compiled BASIC on an IBM compatible personal computer. Using a 30 megabyte hard disc to store the data for retrospective analysis, events in cohorts of 50,000 women were simulated without difficulty. A complete run of the programs took approximately 12 hours on a 20MHz machine with 80386 processor and 80387 math co-processor.

In many situations it was convenient to transform the scale on which BMD was expressed, the resulting variable being denoted by Z (a "Z score"). Z was a linear transformation of BMD such that Z=0 corresponded to the mean value of BMD in young women aged 25 years (say, B) and Z=-1 corresponded to a value of BMD 1SD below B (say, S). Small random variations in the computed values of B and S occurred between simulations.

PREDICTIONS OF THE NON-LINEAR MODEL

Values of B and S were about 90.1 and 9.29; the coefficient of variation of BMD in young adults was 11%. FIG. 4 shows the match achieved after 5 iterations between the age-specific incidence of fractures predicted by the non-linear model and the idealised incidence of hip fractures in women. Values of the previously unknown parameters k_1 and k_2 were 8.17 and

0.150 respectively. Values of S(a) from 65 to 85 at 5 year intervals were 1.00, 1.08, 1.40, 2.08 and 3.36.

What reductions in BMD are expected in hip fracture cases?

Predicted mean values of BMD or Z at the time of fracture in female hip fracture cases over 50 are shown with 1 SD limits in FIG. 3. Differences in the group means between fracture cases and controls were expressed as differences in Z, DZ. Values of DZ at mean ages 62.5 and 72.5 were -1.31 and -1.34 respectively. Those values are close to the observed differences [7]. In the older age groups, the magnitude of DZ diminished slightly.

What is the risk of a second fracture?

With the control mechanisms already described, the model generated a limited number of second fractures. The risk of second fracture was evaluated as a function of age. The annual risks at age 70 and 80 were 1.2% and 1.9% respectively. These values are of the same order as reported by Morgan [9] and attributed to Stewart [10].

What values of BMD did fracture cases have when they were young?

Results given in this and the next section apply to the ageing cohort diminishing in size as a result of mortality.

Because the young adult (peak) value of BMD for each individual was known, it was possible to allocate each member of the cohort in whom a fracture occurred into a category according to that value. It was found that 65.5% of all hip fractures occurred in women who when they were young were members of the lowest quartile of the BMD distribution. Corresponding figures for the lower middle, upper middle and highest quartiles were 22.1%, 9.3% and 3.1% respectively.

What values of rate of decrease of BMD did fracture cases have in middle age?

Following a similar approach, women with fractures were classified according to membership of quartiles of the distribution of rate of decrease of BMD during the first bone loss phase (see FIG. 2.) It was found that 31.1% of all fractures occurred in those who had been members of the quartile with the highest rates of loss. Corresponding figures for the other quartiles, in rank order, were 26.1%, 23.1%, and 19.7% respectively.

What is the lifetime risk of fracture in a woman for whom BMD is known?

The results given in TABLE I, again obtained by retrospective analysis of the database generated by the simulations, relate BMD expressed as a Z-score (Z(A)) measured in a woman of known age (A), to lifetime risk of hip fracture (R(S)), with survival time (S) as a parameter. For any age, the lifetime risk increases rapidly as Z(A) decreases.

What would be the effect on fracture incidence of delaying the onset of bone loss?

To answer questions of this kind, the simulation programs were re-run with different values for the parameters that define age-related bone loss. Delaying the onset of bone loss by T years in any individual was modelled by adding T to that individual's values of the breakpoints at ages A2 and A3 (see FIG. 2). T was the same for all women in whom bone loss was delayed ('treated' women). In the simplest case each and every woman was treated for T years from the age when bone loss would otherwise have first started in that woman; more complicated situations are discussed later. Simulations were carried out with T=10,15 and 20 years. (T=0 years corresponded to an untreated cohort, the results for which have already been presented above).

TABLE I. Lifetime risk of hip fracture in women. The BMD measurement obtained at age A years, expressed as a Z-score, is denoted by Z(A). R(S) is the percentage risk of fracture during the ensuing S years of survival. Values of Z(A) have been selected to cover the expected range of BMD at age A, with the centre value being equivalent to the mean, and values either side of that being displaced by multiples of one standard deviation.

Age A years	Z(A)	R(20)	R(30)	R(40)	R(50)
40	+1.56	-	-	-	0.7
	+0.55	-	0.2	0.6	2.4
	-0.47	-	0.6	2.6	11
	-1.49	-	2.1	10	38
	-2.50	-	9	36	83
50	+0.65	-	-	0.7	-
	-0.37	0.2	0.6	2.6	-
	-1.39	0.5	2.4	11	-
	-2.42	2.0	10	38	-
	-3.44	9	37	85	-
60	-0.17	0.2	0.7	-	-
	-1.21	0.5	2.5	-	-
	-2.24	2.3	10	-	-
	-3.27	9	37	-	-
	-4.30	33	82	-	-
70	-0.54	0.5	-	-	-
	-1.58	2.5	-	-	-
	-2.62	10	-	-	-
	-3.65	36	-	-	-
	-4.69	82	-	-	-

For each value of T, the total number of fractures occurring as the cohort aged from birth to death was counted and the number of fractures prevented by treatment calculated, using the expected number of fractures in the untreated cohort. The total number of patient-years of treatment administered to the ageing cohort was also computed; this was slightly less than T.N where N (=50,000) was the number of members of the cohort at birth, because some died before treatment could be administered, and others while it was being given. The number of patient years (py) of treatment invested in the cohort per fracture prevented could then be calculated. Results are summarised in TABLE II. Note the implicit assumptions that treatment had no effects on the risk of falling and/or mortality.

TABLE II. Predicted effect on fracture incidence of preventing bone loss for T years in all 50,000 women. When T=0 the expected number of fractures was 5368 as the cohort aged from birth to death. 'py' denotes patient years.

T years	Fractures occurring	Fractures prevented	% fractures prevented	py/fracture prevented
10	3853	1515	28	316
15	3168	2200	40	325
20	2425	2943	55	321

The magnitude of the figures for py/fracture prevented is surprising. The model predicts for example that on average about 22 women, selected at random, have each to be treated for 15 years to prevent one hip fracture.

Tests were also carried out to establish the likely magnitude of effects on fracture incidence produced by a treatment which not only prevented bone loss but also stabilised the risk of falling at the value it had in each individual at the start of the treatment period. For T=15 years, 1908 fractures occurred and 64% were prevented (compare with TABLE II.)

What would be gained by selecting women for treatment on the basis of BMD?

Special runs of the programs were carried out in which the aim was to examine the consequences of preventing bone loss for 15 years in all members of the cohort who satisfied the following criterion: that their young adult (peak) value of BMD, expressed as a Z-score, lay below a threshold value here denoted by ZT. In the particular case of ZT=+20, all women were selected for treatment; with ZT=0, approximately 50% (those below the mean) were selected.

TABLE III. Predicted effect on fracture incidence of preventing bone loss for 15 years in all women from a cohort of 50,000 who satisfied the criterion that their peak BMD value expressed as a Z score exceeded ZT. 'py' denotes patient years. Figures refer to the whole cohort.

ZT	%treated	Fractures occurring	% fractures prevented	py/fracture prevented
20	100	3168	40	325
0	50	3466	35	192
-1	16	4328	19	111
-2	2	5173	4	75

Results of runs with different ZT values are summarised in TABLE III above. As ZT was lowered the number of fractures prevented decreased. (The optimum treatment strategy if there were no limit to resources and no adverse health risks would be to treat everyone.) More important, the number of patient years of treatment administered per fracture prevented decreased quite rapidly as ZT decreased, with a factor of three between the values for ZT=20 (no selection) and ZT=-1 (treating the lowest 16%).

DISCUSSION

The aims of this work were twofold: to set up a mathematical framework, based on simple assumptions and a limited number of parameters, that would explain some of the facts known about female hip fracture cases; and having done so, to use the predictive power of the resulting model to answer questions which are currently of interest.

With regard to the first aim, we have illustrated how the model can generate an age-specific incidence of hip fractures which matches observations (see FIG. 4) and how the predicted reductions in BMD in fracture cases are then consistent with observation (see FIG. 3) [7]. In tailoring the model to make predictions and observations tally, we have found that in women up to age 70 or thereabouts, the risk of fracture following a fall can be described by an inverse exponential function of BMD in the femoral neck. That is not the only solution, but it is economical, involving only two parameters, and works well in practice. Results indicate that the risk of fracture following a fall increases by a factor of about 4.0 for each 1SD reduction in BMD; more exactly, the slope of $\ln [G(BMD)]$ against Z is -1.4 (and $\exp[1.4]=4.0$).

Our model provides indirect evidence that above age 70, an age-related factor other than (and independent of) BMD operates in determining the risk of fracture following a fall. We have regarded that factor, $S(a)$, as the severity of falls. However, $S(a)$ is better regarded as a function which ascribes to age those multiplicative risk factors which cannot be estimated from BMD at the time of the fall. Severity of falls may be relevant, as might other variables such as the number of microfractures per unit volume of the trabecular structure inside the proximal femur. It is also important to recognise that the final numerical values of $S(a)$ were dependent on three other functions: the idealised true age-specific incidence of fractures, which probably becomes increasingly unrealistic at ages over 80; the age-dependent frequency of falls, which might not be relevant to the population on whom BMD was measured; and the function describing how BMD changed with age in individuals (no data were available to verify some of the parameter values used). However in our view it is unlikely, even if all these limitations were overcome, that the function $S(a)$ would become redundant.

With regard to the second aim, we have used our model to answer queries which if posed as hypotheses to be tested in real life would involve prohibitively long and expensive experiments. Subject to the assumptions of the model and the validity of the parameter values we used, our results show that the majority (66%) of hip fractures occur in women whose peak BMD values, attained when young, were inside the lowest quartile of the distribution. Rate of bone loss in middle age, as measured by the decline in BMD, appears to be much less important; that conclusion might have to be modified if it is shown that in reality the variability between women in the rate of decrease of BMD in the femoral neck is greater than we have assumed. None the less, lifetime risk of fracture (for a given survival period) seems on present evidence to be dominated by the value of BMD attained in youth.

We have shown above how stochastic modelling techniques can be used to estimate numerical values of lifetime risks of hip fracture based on a measurement of the femoral neck at any age. This is a new application of the non-linear model which we have not previously explored. For the hip, as shown in TABLE I, lifetime risks rise rapidly with decreasing BMD, whatever the age and survival time; in practice, if an individual BMD value is to be translated into a lifetime risk, the most obvious choice of survival time is life expectancy.

Our approach has also allowed us to estimate the reduction in hip fracture incidence which might be brought about by long-term large scale prophylaxis against bone loss (see TABLE II). We have assumed the treatment to be 100% effective in stabilising BMD at the value it had at the start of treatment, and recognise that such an assumption may be too optimistic for such long treatment durations.

We have also used the model to estimate the economies likely to result from administering long-term prophylaxis selectively to those women with low BMD values; those economies have been evaluated solely in terms of the treatment investment necessary to prevent one fracture. Our results indicate that by using dual photon absorptiometry of the hip to measure BMD at that site the efficacy of treatment can be increased by as much as a factor of three (TABLE III). More sophisticated policies for the allocation of treatment on the basis of BMD observations are currently being explored within the model framework. The situation we have examined above, in which individuals below a prechosen threshold value are all treated for the same length of time, is not necessarily optimal in its use of resources. For example, even if a threshold criterion is applied to separate those who are to be treated from those who are not, it seems reasonable that amongst those treated the treatment duration should be longer in those with the lowest BMD values.

ACKNOWLEDGEMENTS

This work was carried out while the first author was supported by an MRC External Scientific Staff Programme Grant and the second by a Postgraduate Student Support Grant from the British American Tobacco Company Ltd.

REFERENCES

1. R.D. Wasnich, P.D. Ross, L.K. Heilbrun and J.M. Vogel, Am J Obstet Gynecol 153, 745-751 (1985).
2. J. Knowelden, A.J. Buhr and O. Dunbar, Brit J Prev Soc Med 18, 130-141 (1964).
3. B.E.C. Nordin, A. Horsman, D.H. Marshall, M. Simpson and G.M. Waterhouse, Clin Orthop Rel Res 140, 216-239 (1979).
4. A. Horsman, M. Jones, R. Francis and B.E.C. Nordin, New England Journal of Medicine 309, 1405-1407 (1983).
5. A. Horsman, D.H. Marshall and M. Peacock, Clin Orthop Rel Res 195, 207-215 (1985).
6. A. Horsman in: Proceedings of International Symposium 'Clinical Disorders of Bone and Mineral Metabolism' (Detroit, May 1988). In press (1989).
7. R.B. Mazess, H. Barden, M. Ettinger and E. Schultz E 1988, J Bone and Mineral Research 3, 13-18 (1988).
8. M. Aitken in: Osteoporosis in Clinical Practice (Wright, Bristol, 1984).
9. D.B. Morgan, Clinics in Endocrinology and Metabolism 2, 187-201 (1973).
10. I.M. Stewart, BMJ ii, 922-924 (1957).

Fracture Prediction

Charles W. Slemenda[*] and C. Conrad Johnston, Jr.[**]

[*]Regenstrief Health Institute, Indianapolis, Indiana
[**]Indiana University School of Medicine, Indianapolis, Indiana

ABSTRACT

The identification of women at high risk of fracture, particularly hip fracture, would have important public health implications. This paper reviews that data relevant to fracture prediction. Indirect evidence has been accumulated that shows bone strength is strongly related to bone mass. Bone mass is lower in fracture cases compared with controls, and prospective studies are uniform in their observations that bone mass predicts fracture incidence. These longitudinal studies are in agreement despite the fact that different techniques for bone mass measurements were used, and these studies usually did not have measurements at the site of fracture. Whether measurements at the skeletal site of interest would provide superior prediction remains to be answered, but for prediction of total fractures, measurements at peripheral sites do not seem to differ from measurements in the spine.

Fracture prediction might more precisely be referred to as the identification of those at the highest risk of future fractures. Hip fractures are probably the most serious result of osteoporosis. About one in every six women will suffer a fractured hip in her lifetime [1], and between 12 and 25% of the victims will die in the year following the fracture [2,3]. Of those who escape this fate about one-third will become totally dependent and almost all will be faced with a long and difficult rehabilitation. The public health costs associated with these fractures are in the billions of dollars each year. Importantly, the increasing age structure of most developed countries assures that the magnitude of this problem will increase in the years to come. The identification and successful treatment of those at greatest risk of hip fractures would have obvious benefits, both for individuals and for society.

Vertebral fractures, despite often being asymptomatic and requiring little or no treatment, are a problem for several reasons, including the concern created in patients with such fractures and the cumulative effects of multiple crush fractures. In addition, other osteoporotic fractures, including those of the distal radius, proximal humerus and pelvis produce pain and disability and generate considerable costs for medical care. Thus, the identification of those at the highest risk of all osteoporotic fractures would enable treatment for the prevention of bone loss to be applied more judiciously than is now possible; this is desirable, given the risks and costs involved with such therapy.

Although osteoporosis is defined as a loss of bone leading to greater susceptibility to fractures and low bone mass is almost certainly the primary cause of fractures in the elderly, there has been considerable debate regarding the clinical value of bone mass measurements. A number of authors have in the past concluded that such measurements should not be made in clinical situations, given their unproven ability to predict fractures [4,5]. However, a body of evidence has accumulated which now suggests that bone mass measurements may be clinically useful in the estimation of fracture risk, and in the decision to institute therapies to prevent bone loss.

In-vitro studies have shown that bone strength is strongly correlated with bone mass [6,7], and that approximately 80-90% of the ultimate strength of bone tissue may be accounted for by bone mass [8]. While these data do not address fracture prediction, they provide clear evidence that bone strength is strongly and directly related to bone mass.

Cross-sectional studies have shown that women with low bone mass have fracture histories which differ significantly from those with greater bone mass [9]. In this study of 557 women (mean age = 59), bone mass was significantly lower in those with any fractures since age 20 compared to those without a fracture in this time period. When stratified by age at time of fracture, the bone mass difference was diminished but consistent in direction.

Case-control studies comparing women with and without hip fractures have most often shown small differences in mean bone mass between these groups [1,10,11,12]. Many of the differences observed were significant, but the magnitude of these differences varied depending on the site measured. For example, many of the measurements of trabecular bone in the spine or iliac crest showed only small differences, while measurements of cortical bone in the radius or metacarpals consistently suggested that those with hip fractures had less bone, amounting to 10-15% in most cases, than their similarly-aged counterparts. Similarly, hip fracture patients have lower bone mass in the non-fractured hip compared with controls of similar ages [6,10,13,14]. In case-control studies of crush fractures, women with vertebral fractures have been shown to have less trabecular bone than similarly-aged comparison groups [10,15,16]. However, in almost all case-control studies the overlap between groups was considerable, generating some confusion regarding the differentiation between risk and diagnostic factors and the value of using risk factors for stratifying patients on the basis of fracture risk. Thus, just as serum cholesterol concentrations above 250 mg/ml are associated with an increased prevalence of myocardial infarction but most people with this risk factor have not suffered heart attacks, similarly women with mid-radius bone mass below 0.7 g/cm have an increased risk for fracture but most have not suffered osteoporotic fractures; the value of these measurements is determined by evaluating the predictive power of cholesterol or bone mass in assigning risk. In establishing absolute risk several elements are involved, including relative risk and the background incidence of the condition being studied. Case-control studies can establish an association between risk factors, such as bone mass, and events, such as fractures, but they cannot be used to determine the utility of the risk factor as a predictor.

For this purpose longitudinal studies are required. There have been prospective studies of osteoporotic fractures and bone mass for over 20 years. In 1969 Iskrant and Smith published the results of a longitudinal study of more than 2,000 women for whom baseline radiographic evaluation of spinal osteopenia was made [17]. In 8,000+ person-years of follow-up, a clear gradient of increasing fracture incidence with declining vertebral bone density was observed. In age-stratified analyses similar patterns were seen. Smith et al. [18] observed a higher prevalence of vertebral crush fractures in women with lower bone mass, and in a 1.7 year follow-up of 278 women found incident fractures to be more common in those with lower bone mass. No adjustment for age differences were made. This same group also studied 106 older women, and observed that 29 fractures occurred in the 2.5 years of follow-up [19]. Bone mass, but not the Singh index, predicted fracture incidence, but, again, age was not taken into account. Some of these earlier longitudinal studies were flawed, due either to problems with instrumentation and estimation of bone mass or failure to control for age [17,18,19], but each of these studies observed that lower bone mass was associated with an increased risk for fracture. None, however, studied hip fractures as separate entities (although hip fractures were included), and the follow-up in these three studies was relatively short (three years or less on average).

More recently, five prospective studies have further confirmed the results of the earlier work while controlling for the effects of age [20,21,22,23,24]. One of these studies has shown that a single bone mass measurement in the radius is predictive of time to first fracture, and importantly, time to first hip fracture [24]. Follow-up in this study ranged from 3 to 15 years and 89 of 532 subjects suffered 132 fractures, including 32 hip fractures. For each 0.1 g/cm decline in bone mass (one standard deviation = 0.12 g/cm) fracture risk increased 2.2 times. Others [20,21] have shown that bone mass measurements at various sites (including the radius, spine, and os calcis) predict total fractures, including and excluding spine fractures, and spine fractures alone. These authors have studied a population of Japanese-Americans and have estimated relative risk for incident spine fractures to be approximately 2.6 per standard deviation change in bone mass, similar to that for observed for non-spine fractures in Midwestern Caucasian women in the previously cited work. A third group [22] has obtained similar risk estimates in a 10-16 year follow-up of a mixed group of subjects which included referrals for suspected osteoporosis and fracture cases. The risk estimates obtained from all of these studies differ only slightly, with relative risks in the neighborhood of 2-3x per standard deviation change in bone mass. That is, a group of women with bone mass one standard deviation (about 0.12 g/cm in the radius or spine) below another group would be expected to have approximately twice as many fractures. The consistency of these predictions in three very different populations suggests that bone mass is a good predictor in a variety of circumstances, and across a number of age groups. Only Gardsell [22] failed to observe significant prediction in older women, and this may relate to the heterogeneity of his population or the sample size.

The mean period of follow-up in these studies was generally longer than that for the older work, ranging from slightly more than 3 years [20,21] to almost 13 years [22]. While these longer follow-ups greatly increase the strength of the work in this area, it remains to be shown that measurements around the time of menopause will predict fractures many years later. However, it is known that therapy around the time of menopause, specifically estrogen replacement, both reduces bone loss [25] and reduces fracture risk [26], both in the short term and many years later. Moreover, there is evidence that this protection extends to hip fracture risk, thereby increasing the potential importance of this approach in reducing the adverse public health impact of osteoporosis.

The question about which site to measure is unanswered at present. The studies with the longest follow-up [22,23,24] both employed single photon absorptiometry of the radius because this was the only technique available at the time of the initiation of these studies. However, both showed significant prediction of fractures, and one demonstrated significant prediction of hip fractures with this peripheral measurement [22]. The other studies of Japanese-Americans have utilized multiple measuring devices, but as yet have had too few hip fractures to analyze separately [20,21]. Moreover, they have had too few fractures of any type to have adequate statistical power to distinguish between the predictive power of different methods. Thus, while measurement at the site of interest would intuitively seem to offer the best hope for predicting fractures at this site, no direct data have yet been accumulated to support this concept.

Finally, there is reason to believe that modification of fracture risk is possible. Most recent studies suggest that estrogen therapy results in a small increase in bone mass, probably as a result of filling remodeling space as bone turnover is slowed. Calcitonin may have similar effects, although this remains to be established. Factors which may increase fracture risk include frequency of falling, reductions in muscle mass or adipose tissue, and behaviors which expose older people to environmental hazards. Information regarding any of these influences may at some time in the future allow more precise estimates of the critical importance of bone mass in the etiology of fractures.

REFERENCES

1. Cummings S, Kelsey J, Nevitt M, O'Dowd K. Epidemiology of osteoporosis and osteoporotic fractures. Epidemiol. Rev. 7, 178-208 (1985).
2. Gallagher J, Melton L, Riggs B, Bergstrath E. Epidemiology of fractures of the proximal femur in Rochester, Minnesota. Clin. Orthop. 150, 163-171 (1980).
3. Miller C. Survival and ambulation following hip fracture. J. Bone Joint Surg. (Am) 60A, 930-934 (1978).
4. Davis M. Screening for postmenopausal osteoporosis. Am. J. Obstet. Gynecol. 156, 1-5 (1987).
5. Cummings S, Black D. Should perimenopausal women be screened for osteoporosis? Ann. Intern. Med. 104, 817-823 (1986).
6. Mazess R. On aging bone loss. Clin. Orthop. 165, 239-252 (1982).
7. Hayes W, Gerhart T. Biomechanics of bone: Applications for assessment of bone strength. Chapter 9. In: Bone and Mineral Research/3, Peck W, ed. (Elsevier Science Publishers B.V., Amsterdam, 1985) pp. 259-284.
8. Melton L, Chao E, Lane J. Biomechanical aspects of fracture. Chapter 4. In: Osteoporosis: Etiology, Diagnosis, and Management. Riggs B, Melton L, eds. (Raven Press, New York 1988) pp. 133-154.
9. Nordin B, Chatterton B, Walker C, Wishart J. The relation of forearm mineral density to peripheral fractures in postmenopausal women. Med. J. Australia 146, 300-304 (1987).
10. Riggs B, Wahner H, Seeman E, Offord K, Dunn, W, Mazess R, Johnson K, Melton L. Changes in bone mineral density of the proximal femur and spine with aging: Differences between the postmenopausal and senile osteoporosis syndromes. J. Clin. Invest. 70, 716-723 (1982).
11. Krolner B, Pors Neilsen, S. Bone mineral content of the lumbar spine in normal and osteoporotic women: Cross sectional and longitudinal studies. Clin. Sci. 62, 329-336 (1982).
12. Aitken J. Relevance of osteoporsis in women with fractures of the femoral neck. Br. Med. J. 288, 597-601 (1984).
13. Horsman A, Nordin C, Simpson H, Speed R. Cortical and trabecular bone status in elderly women with femoral neck fracture. Clin. Orthop. 166, 143-151 (1982).
14. Bohr H, Schaadt O. Bone mineral content of femoral bone and the lumbar spine measured in women with fracture of femoral neck by dual photon absorptiometry. Clin. Orthop. 179, 240-245 (1983).
15. Firooznia H, Golimbu C, Rafii M, Schwartz M, Alterman E. Quantitative computed tomography assessment of spinal trabecular bone. II In osteoporotic women with and without vertebral fractures. CT: The Journal of Computed Tomography 8, 99-103 (1984).
16. Cann C, Genant H, Kolb F, et al. Quantitative computed tomography for prediction of vertebral fracture risk. Metab. Bone Dis. Relat. Res.

17. Iskrant A, Smith R. Osteoporosis in women 45 years and over related to subsequent fractures. Public Health Rep 84, 33-38 (1969).
5, 1-7 (1984).
18. Smith D, Khairi M, Johnston C. The loss of bone mineral with aging and its relationship to risk of fracture. J. Clin. Invest. 56, 311-318 (1975).
19. Khairi M, Cronin J, Robb J, Smith D, Yu P, Johnston C. Femoral trabecular pattern index and bone mineral content measurement by photon absorption in senile osteoporosis. J. Bone Joint Surg. 58A, 221-226 (1976).
20. Ross P, Wasnich R, Vogel J. Detection of prefracture spinal osteoporosis using bone mineral absorptiometry. J. Bone Min. Res. 3, 1-11 (1988).
21. Wasnich R, Ross P, Davis J, Vogel J. A comparison of single and multi-site BMC measurements for assessment of spine fracture probability. J. Nucl. Med. 1989 (in press).
22. Gardsell P, Johnell O, Nillson B. Predicting fractures in women by using forearm bone densitometry. Calcif. Tissue Int. 44, 235-242 (1989).
23. Hui S, Slemenda C, Johnston C. Age and bone mass as predictors of fracture in a prospective study. J. Clin. Invest. 81, 1804-1809 (1988).
24. Hui S, Slemenda C, Johnston C. Baseline bone mass measurements predict fracture incidence. Ann. Intern. Med. 1989 (in press).
25. Lindsay R, Aitken J, Anderson J, Hart, McDonald E, Clark A. Long-term prevention of postmenopausal osteoporosis by estrogen. Lancet 1, 1038-1041 (1976).
26. Kiel DP, Felson DT, Anderson JJ, Wilson PWF, Moskowitz MA. Hip fracture and the use of estrogens in postmenopausal women: The Framingham Study. N. Engl. J. Med. 317, 1169-1174 (1987).

METHODS OF ASSESSMENT

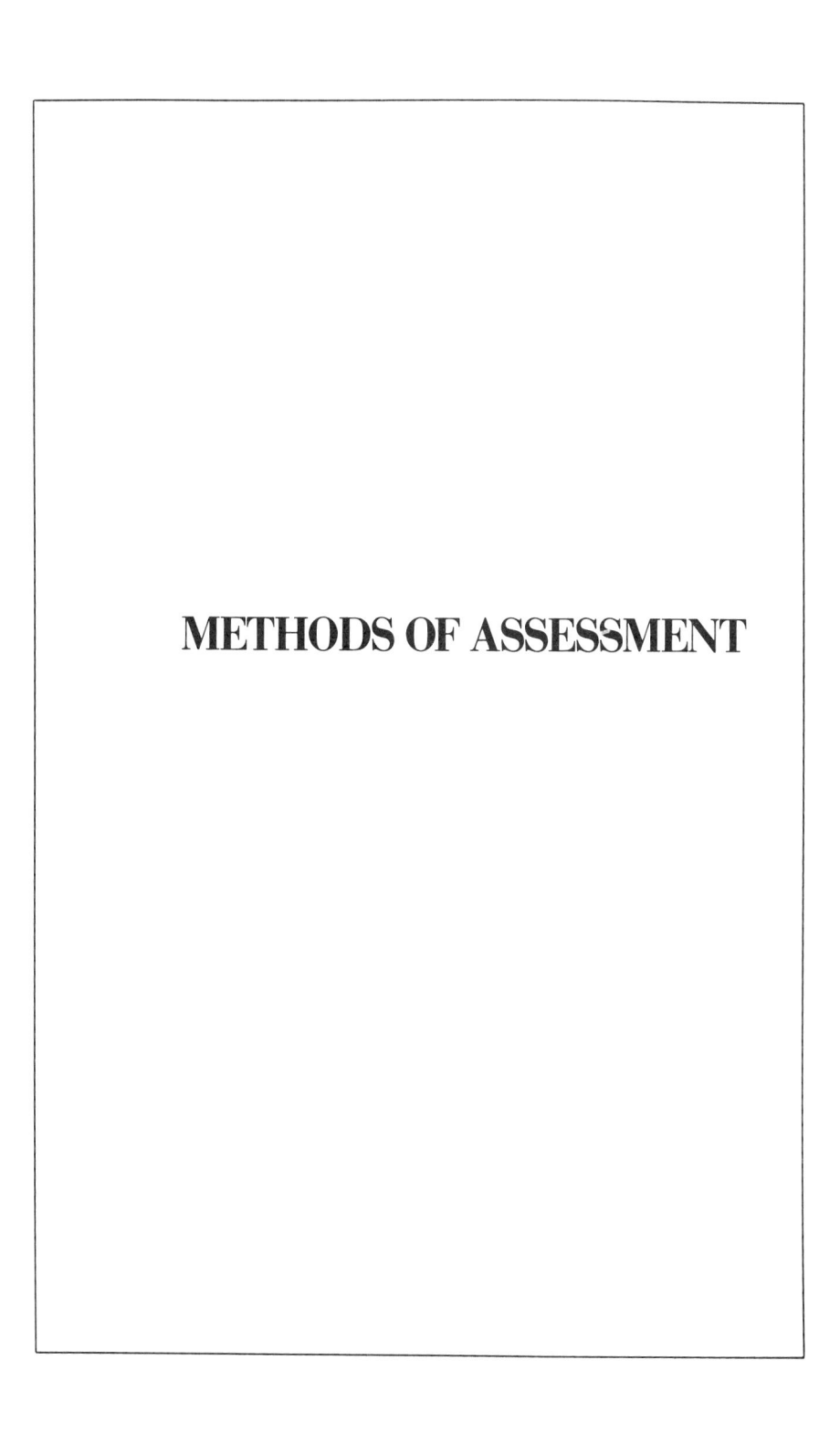

Bone Densitometry for Clinical Diagnosis and Monitoring

Richard B. Mazess

Department of Medical Physics, University of Wisconsin, and Lunar Radiation Corporation, Madison, Wisconsin

ABSTRACT

Bone densitometry increasingly is used for clinical diagnosis and monitoring, as well as for biomedical research. Studies *in vitro* have shown that bone mass and density account for 80-90% of the variance in strength independent of age. Epidemiologic studies have shown a steep gradient of increasing fracture risk with decreasing bone density. Site specificity is obvious.

A variety of methods for appendicular and axial measurement are available. Appendicular measurements are less sensitive for diagnosis, and inadequate for monitoring because appendicular bone, even purely trabecular bone of the distal radius or os calcis, is often unresponsive to therapies. Dual-photon absorptiometry provides low-dose (1 to 5 mrem) measurement of the total body, spine and proximal femur, with an average precision error *in vivo* of 1%, 2%, and 3% respectively. Dual-energy x-ray absorptiometry reduces scan times by a factor of 5, increases spatial resolution from 3 mm to 1.5 mm, and halves the precision error of DPA (2% to 1%). Lateral spine scans allow measurement of trabecular bone that hitherto was available only with quantitative computed tomography. The latter method typically has a high radiation dose (6 mrem/mas), accuracy errors due to fat and osteoid (20-25%), modest precision *in vivo* (3-8%), and limited applicability at sites other than the lumbar spine. The variety of methods available can greatly enhance patient management.

USE OF DENSITOMETRY

Bone densitometry is widely used today in over 1000 major medical centers for clinical management of metabolic bone disease [1-4]. Only a decade ago densitometry was used mainly for clinical research, but newer methods that measure the axial skeleton with good precision (1%) have made densitometry valuable for the individual patient [1-4]. There are two principal uses for densitometry. First, densitometry is used as an aid in the diagnosis of metabolic bone disease, in particular, for the ascertainment of the degree of osteopenia. In this regard densitometry provides an indication of future fracture *risk*, but is not diagnostic of existing fracture [5,6]. Radiographs are sensitive for the diagnosis for fracture, but are not sensitive to assess risk prior to fracture; densitometry indicates the potential for future fracture, as well as the seriousness of underlying bone loss in those who already have fractured. Second, changes over time are monitored either to assess the course of a disease, or its therapy. About 30-40% of osteoporosis in females, and 40-50% in males [7,8], is secondary to a primary medical condition (for example; renal calcium leak, malabsorption, Cushings disease), or iatrogenic (corticosteroids, neuroleptics, thyroxine, anticonvulsants). Effective patient management of secondary osteoporosis often involves monitoring. Monitoring also is considered essential by experts for effective therapeutic intervention in primary osteoporosis [9].

TABLE I. Indications for bone densitometry—Adapted from the Southern California Bone Club

A. Male hypogonadism
B. Premenopausal women with high risks including
   - surgical menopause
   - amenorrhea
   - anorexia nervosa
   - hyperprolactinemia; neuroleptic drugs
   - GnRH and LHRH agonists
C. Postmenopausal women with two or more major risk factors
   - positive family history
   - stature <160 cm, weight <50 kg
   - loss of >3 cm height
   - hypercalciuria, elevated GLA protein
D. Osteoporosis on radiograph
E. Fracture with minor trauma
F. Immobilization
G. Calcium deficiency for more than ten years and
   - hypercalciuria (24-hour, 4 mg/kg/day), kidney stones
   - gastrointestinal diseases
H. Rheumatoid arthritis over a five-year duration
I. Chronic corticosteroid excess, or methotrexate treatment
J. Anticonvulsant therapy over a five-year period
K. Kidney disease with a creatinine clearance of <50 ml/min, or renal tubular disorders
L. Osteomalacia, indicated by low serum calcium, and phosphorus Hyperparathyroidism (including mild cases to assess the need for therapy)
M. Thyroid replacement (over ten years)
N. Monitoring of treatment programs for osteoporosis
O. Immunosuppressant therapy (cyclosporine)

INDICATIONS FOR DENSITOMETRY

Some controversy about densitometry has arisen because of misunderstandings about the role of bone density in osteoporotic fractures [10]. Much of the controversy has been in reaction to claims that densitometry should be used for mass screening (for individuals without medical indications), rather than as a diagnostic aid for patients with indications. Some generally agreed upon indications for bone densitometry are given in Table I [11-13].

BONE DENSITY AND STRENGTH

Studies of bone strength *in vitro* [14-16] have demonstrated that the decrease of bone strength in both the spine and femur is directly proportional ($r = 0.9$) to bone mineral content (BMC) determined by dual-photon absorptiometry. The 35% and 45% decrease of BMC in the spine and hip respectively in fracture cases [17] decreases bone strength (ultimate load) of whole specimens by 45% and 55%, i.e., the strength decrease is only slightly greater than that of BMC, rather than 2-3X greater as might be expected based on isolated bone tissue (see Figure 1 & 2).

There have been far more equivocal results on the relation of quantitative computed tomography (QCT) to strength. The initial studies [18,19] showed that QCT density of the vertebral body was modestly correlated to strength; the predictive error was 20-30%. Later results have confirmed this [16, 20-21], but have shown that when the QCT density is multiplied by the area of the vertebra strength is better predicted. Of course, multiplying density by area, or volume, gives a value equivalent to the bone mass measured directly by DPA and DEXA.

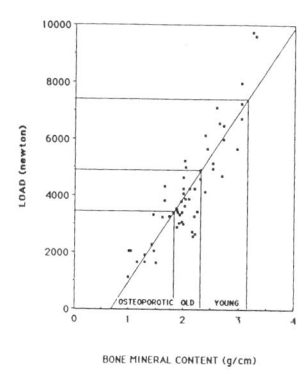

FIG 1. Relation between ultimate load and BMC of vertebral body adapted from Hansson et al [14]. Lines have been drawn to show average BMC, and load, for normal young (30 years), and older (70 years) females, and for osteoporotic women.

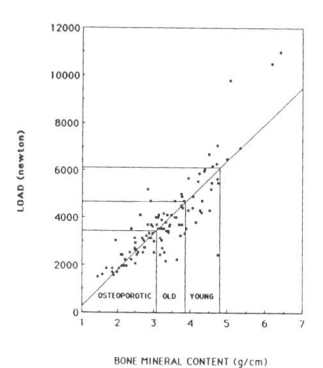

FIG. 2 Relation between ultimate load and BMC of femoral neck adapted from Dalen et al [15]. Lines have been drawn to show average BMC and load for normal young (30 years), and older (70 years) females, and for osteoporotic women.

Factors other than BMC and bone mineral density (BMD) may contribute to the decrease of strength, but it is unlikely that they have a substantial effect since the strength decrease is no greater than that due to the osteopenia itself. Porosity, trabecular anisotropy, and accumulation of microfractures may all contribute, but since these are correlated to BMC and BMD [22], they add little incremental information on strength. Studies using both DPA and QCT have shown that the basic regression relationship between mass or density, and load or load per unit area respectively, is *not* different for older or osteoporotic cases compared to normal young adults. All cases fall on a common regression line, with a variance that does not exceed that found in young normal subjects., This indicates that "structural factors" and "aging" probably have little effect on strength. With regard to hip fracture, the proclivity for falling, defective muscular buffering, and structural weakness of bone all seem to covary with lower bone mass and density. If age, or the factors contributing to strength other than bone mass that vary with age, were really important to bone strength, then we should find a different relationship between strength and bone mass in low density (older) bone than in high density (younger) bone. Since a single linear regression applies across the broad spectrum of bone mass, it is unlikely that fatigue, microfractures, anisotropy etc., impinge significantly on the mass-strength relationship. Secondly, if aging factors (susceptibility and severity of falls for example) were significant, we should find that older osteoporotics had higher BMD levels on the average, than younger patients. In fact, the values we observed for spine and femoral neck BMD in younger (50-69 years) and older (70-89) fracture patients were very similar (0.89 and 0.87 g/cm^2 for spine, and 0.63 and 0.59 g/cm^2 for femur). Moveover, ROC analysis showed that age, and age divided by body weight, accounted for a very small portion of the area under the ROC curve in spine fracture (~55%), and only a slightly higher percentage (~65%) in hip fracture (Table II). In contrast, BMD of the femur, and to a lesser extent that of the spine, accounted for larger portions of the ROC area. Femoral BMD was particularly important in hip fracture cases. In conclusion, bone densitometry appears to be an effective method for assessing fracture risk at axial fracture sites (spine and femur) because it indicates bone strength, and to a lesser extent because it reflects other degenerative aging changes.

TABLE II. Roc analysis (area under the ROC curve) of >400 normal women vs osteoporotics (age 50-89 years).

	Crush-Fracture (n=103) Area		Hip-Fracture (n=61) Area
Femur BMD	75%	Femur BMD	86%
Spine BMD	70%	Spine BMD	68%
Age	54%	Age	66%
Age/weight	57%	Age/weight	63%

BONE DENSITY AND FRACTURE

Epidemiological studies have shown a clear gradient of fracture risk related to BMD at each fracture site; individuals with low BMD have the greatest risk for fracture, while a high BMD, independent of age, confers protection [5,23-30]. This has been shown in numerous retrospective studies, and in at least three major prospective trials [23,27,28]. We investigated this gradient of risk for both spine and hip fractures in relation to BMD at fracture sites. BMD of the lumbar spine (L2-L4 region) and proximal femur (neck) were measured using DPA in 590 white women (ages 50-89 years; mean age 68 years); about 25% had spine (n = 105; mean age 68.5 years) or hip (n = 61; mean age 71 years) fractures. The increased prevalence of fracture was related directly to decreased BMD at each fracture site (Table III; Figures 3, 4, and 5).

TABLE III. Fracture prevalence [5] and relative risk (RR) related to BMD of the spine L2-L4 and femur neck.

		% WITH FRACTURE					
		Spine		Hip		Either/Both	
SPINE BMD (g/cm^2)	N	%	RR	%	RR	%	RR
>1.10	100	6.0	1.0	3.0	1.0	7.0	1.0
1.00-1.09	111	9.9	1.7	5.4	1.8	13.5	1.9
0.90-0.99	159	17.0	2.8	6.3	2.1	22.0	3.1
0.80-0.89	134	23.1	3.9	9.7	3.2	29.9	4.3
0.70-0.79	49	40.8	6.8	12.2	4.1	44.8	6.4
0.60-0.69	20	50.0	8.3	15.0	5.0	60.0	8.6
FEMUR BMD (g/cm^2)							
>.80	133	3.8	1.0	0.0	1.0	3.8	1.0
0.70-0.79	178	10.6	2.8	3.4	3.4	12.9	3.4
0.60-0.69	164	21.3	5.6	10.4	10.4	31.1	8.2
0.50-0.59	89	32.6	8.6	29.2	29.2	51.7	13.6
0.40-0.49	26	38.5	10.1	46.2	46.2	76.9	20.2

The mean BMD in women without fracture [31] was 1.00 g/cm^2 for the L2-L4 spine, and 0.75 g/cm^2 for femoral neck compared with 0.88 g/cm^2 and 0.57 g/cm^2 for women with mild spine osteoporosis and with femur fracture respectively. The relative risk (RR) of spine fracture increased about 1.5X for each 1 SD (0.1 g/cm^2 or 10%) decrease in either the spine or femoral neck BMD, and about 1.1X for a comparable change of radius BMD. The relative risk of femur fracture increased about 2.6X for every 1 SD (0.1 g/cm^2 or 10%) decrease in femur neck BMD, versus about 1.3X for the same decrease in spine BMD.

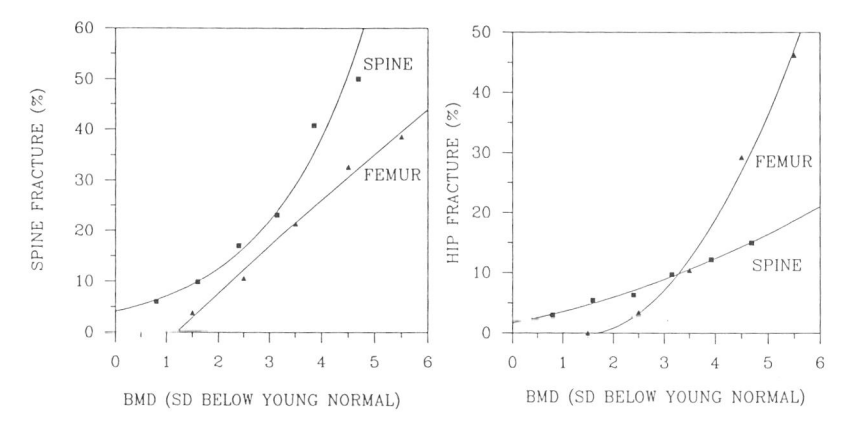

FIG 3. The prevalence of spine fracture in relation to BMD of the spine and femoral neck in white women >50 years.

FIG 4. The prevalence of femur fracture in relation to BMD of the spine and femoral neck in white women >50 years.

The risk of femur fracture for radius BMD change was similar to the spine BMD. Therefore femur BMD was twice as good an indicator of hip fracture as was either spine or radius BMD, and femur BMD indicated spine fracture as effectively as spine BMD. These data confirm that fracture risk increases greatly for even small decreases of BMD or strength, and suggest that the proximal femur should be the primary site for assessing the risk of osteoporotic fracture.

These data show that there is some gradient of risk for hip fracture using spine BMD, but it is much less than for femoral neck BMD. Several studies have shown that the spine BMD is not reduced in hip fracture patients, especially if there are not concomitant spine fractures (Table IV). The normal-abnormal difference divided by the intrapopulation variation (1 SD) is called the Z-score. In contrast, femoral neck BMD is much reduced (0.55 to 0.6 g/cm^2) in hip fracture patients, both male and female, compared to values in normal subjects without fracture (0.75 and 0.85 g/cm^2 in females and males respectively), or even in comparison to patients with fractures elsewhere (0.65 g/cm^2). The normal-abnormal difference is as great as or greater than for spine BMD in crush fracture cases [5,17,36] - see Figure 6. In terms of Z-score, the typical value is about 1.5 to 2.0 [17,36]. This is comparable to the Z-score observed for spine density in spinal osteoporosis of younger patients (Table V). In older patients (<70 years) similar in age to hip fracture patients, the Z-score is typically 1.0 to 1.5.

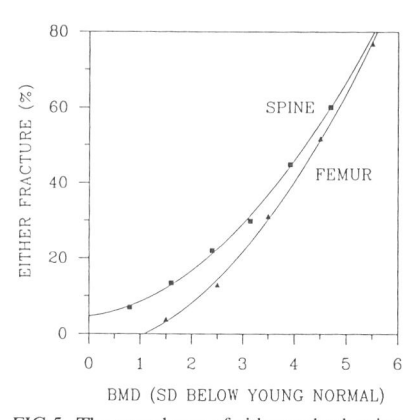

FIG 5. The prevalence of either or both spine and femur fracture in relation to BMD of the spine and femoral neck in white women >50 years.

TABLE IV. Spine density in hip fracture.

SOURCE	Z-SCORE	METHOD
Riggs et al 1982 [32]	+0.2	DPA
Bohr and Schaadt 1983 [33]	-0.3	DPA
Mazess et al 1987 [17]	-0.7	DPA
Harma et al 1985 [34]	-0.8	QCT
Firooznia et al 1986 [35]	-0.2^a	QCT
Firooznia et al 1986 [35]	-1.4^b	QCT

a. *hip FX alone*
b. *hip FX + spine FX*

TABLE V. Diagnostic sensitivity for spinal osteoporosis. Normal-abnormal differences (Z-score) for younger patients (<70 years). Variations among studies are due to measurement site and instrument. Z-score for spine BMD (using either QCT or DPA) averages twice as high as appendicular BMD (except with certain DPA/DEXA instruments).

SOURCE	SCANNER	Z-SCORE
Appendicular Bone (SPA)		
Ross et al 1988 [37]	Osteon	-0.6
Gotfredsen et al 1989 [38]	Nuclear Data	-0.8
Eastell et al 1989 [39]	Mayo	-0.8
Harma et al 1986 [34]	—	-0.8
Ott et al 1987 [40]	Norland	-0.9
Nuti et al 1988 [41]	Lunar	-1.0
Grubb et al 1986 [30]	Norland	-1.1
Spine (DPA/DEXA)		
Pacifici et al 1989 [42]	Hologic	-0.6
Ott et al 1987 [40]	Nuclear Data	-0.7
Reinbold et al 1987 [43]	Norland	-1.0
Gotfredsen et al 1988 [38]	Lunar	-1.0*
Krolner 1982 [43]	Novo	-1.3
Eastell et al 1989 [39]	Mayo	-1.6
Mautalen et al 1989 [44]	Lunar	-1.9
Pouilles et al 1988 [45]	Lunar	-2.0
Nuti et al 1987 [41]	Lunar	-2.0
Grubb et al 1986 [30]	Lunar	-2.2
Spine (QCT)		
Pacifici et al 1989 [42]	GE-9800	-0.9
Ott et al 1987 [40]	GE-8800/9800	-1.6
Harma et al 1986 [34]	—	-1.6
Reinbold et al 1987 [43]	GE-8800	-1.7

This system appears to have been defective, since a 4% precision error was reported, and the BMD values were deviant from other Lunar scanners.

Similarly, radius BMD is not especially reduced (usually within 1 SD of age-matched controls), in either hip or spine fracture cases [17,30]. We found the area under the ROC curve was 65% for radius BMD and 70% for spine BMD [46]. Total body BMD provides diagnostic sensitivity comparable to the spine or femur for spine and/or hip fractures [38,40,41]. More importantly, appendicular sites are poor indicators of early osteoporosis or osteopenia [47-49]. The advantage of spinal densitometry was demonstrated in our study of 1600 female patients [47]. We found there were 2-3X more osteopenic (>20% loss) cases using spine BMD than radius BMD between 40 and 60 years of age. Later in life appendicular loss caught up with axial loss, but the radius was still less sensitive than the spine. However, the ultradistal radius may prove to be a slightly better indicator for risk of Colles' fractures than other sites (Table VI).

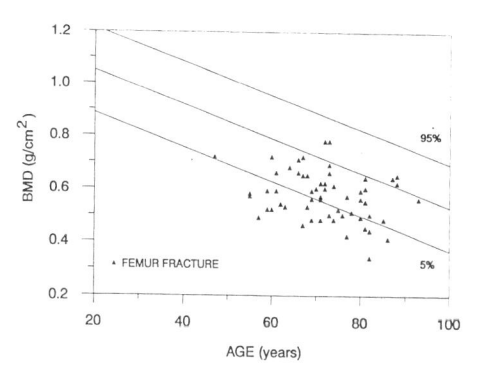

FIG. 6. The femoral neck BMD in 58 hip fracture patients plotted on the age regression for normals ($\pm$ 1 SEE).

Definite osteopenia is found in about 40% of all postmenopausal women; the critical levels are spine BMD <0.9 g/cm^2, or femoral neck BMD <0.7 g/cm^2 [53]. Severe osteoporosis occurs at BMD levels 0.1 g/cm^2 lower (i.e. 0.8 and 0.6 g/cm^2 for spine and femur respectively). About 70% of fractures occur with definite osteopenia, but even so, only about half of these osteopenic women as a group have a severe fracture, or multiple fractures. About 30% of fractures occur in women with mild or moderate osteopenia, and fractures do not occur at normal density levels unless there is severe trauma. The osteopenia that produces high fracture risk is not a "normal" consequence of aging in either males or females. Only a low peak bone mass, and/or accelerated and prolonged bone loss, causes osteopenia of 30 to 50% relative to young normals that characterizes the osteoporotic group. Normal women, for example, lose only 10-20% of their bone mass in the decade following the menopause, and no more than 15 to 25% by age 70 [31].

The strength of the relationship between fracture and BMD at appendicular sites is at least comparable to that between blood pressure and stroke, or cholesterol and coronary heart disease [23]. In fact, the attributable risk (excess risk/population risk) associated with BMD in fracture was 73% for the spine and 83% for the femur. This high figure may result because BMD possibly is a marker for frequency of falls, muscular strength, and how

TABLE VI. Bone density in Colles' fracture.

SITE	METHOD	Z-SCORE	SOURCE
Spine	DPA	0.55	Krolner et al 1982 [43]
Spine	DPA	0.58	Eastell et al 1989 [39]
Spine	QCT	0.70	Harma and Karjalainen 1986 [50]
Os Calcis	BUA	0.63	Johnson and Porter 1988 [51]
Radius	SPA	0.50	Harma and Karjalainen 1986 [50]
Radius	QCT	0.58	Hesp et al 1984 [52]
Radius	SPA	0.80	Eastell et al 1989 [39]

people fall, as well as bone strength. This compares to an attributable risk of 21% for cholesterol in heart disease in males, or of 78% for smoking and lung cancer [54]. Long-term prospective studies at appendicular sites have shown that for every 10% (1 SD) decrease in appendicular BMD, there is a 1.3X to 1.8X increase in risk for fracture [23,27,28]. Retrospective data like ours (Table III) show an increase of 2.5X of hip fracture for every 1 SD decrease of femoral neck BMD. Prospective studies currently underway are needed to confirm the greater predictive efficacy of axial bone densitometry for spine and femur fracture.

TYPE I AND TYPE II OSTEOPOROSIS?

Mayo Clinic researchers have elaborated Albrights' earlier speculations, and postulated that there are two types of osteoporosis [9,55]. The first (Type I) is presumed (a) to be due to estrogen deprivation, (b) affects trabecular bone, and (c) is responsible for crush and Colles' fractures. The type II, or senile, form is thought (a) to be associated with loss of both compact and trabecular bone, (b) causes wedge and hip fractures, and (c) has a multifactorial etiology. There is little hard evidence for this theoretical dichotomy in skeletal data. Trabecular bone loss from the axial skeleton appears prior to the menopause, and in fact occurs at similar rates in both males and females from the third decade of life onward [56]. Hip fracture, the hallmark of "senile" osteoporosis, is characterized by preferential femoral osteopenia in both older and younger patients [17,46]. As shown in Table IV, hip fracture is not accompanied by commensurate spinal osteopenia; the spinal BMD has about the same diagnostic sensitivity as age.

Most (70%) of osteoporosis is associated with low axial, but not appendicular, osteopenia in younger adults rather than with a high rate of postmenopausal bone loss [31,47,57,58]. The premenopausal children of osteoporotic patients have low axial density, but normal appendicular density [57,58]. The interaction of many factors (menopause, calcium utilization, bone turnover, inactivity) may exacerbate the underlying osteopenia and reduce bone levels at fracture sites. Spine fractures occur earlier than hip fractures because the former are associated with only 30-35% bone diminution in the spine, while the latter are associated with a 40-45% bone diminution in the femur. This implies that hip fractures would occur about a decade later than spine fractures on the average (assuming a 1% annual bone loss).

It may be more accurate and productive to consider osteoporosis as either (a) "generalized", affecting multiple skeletal areas, or (b) "focal", affecting specific areas such as the spine, femur/and humerus, and ultradistal radius, rather than as Type I and Type II.

MONITORING

Many therapies used today, with the notable exception of calcium, are effective for improving spine density, and arresting appendicular loss, but they do not work in all patients (Table VII). For example, about one-third of osteoporotic patients have high turnover and

TABLE VII. Nonresponders to therapy.

THERAPY	NON-RESPONDERS	(PREVALENCE)
Calcium	Intake >500 mg/day	(75%)
Vitamin D	Normal 1,25-D Levels	(40%)
Fluoride	Slow Responders	(30%)
Estrogen	Long term "Escape"	(20%)
Calcitonin	Normal Turnover	(20%)

respond well to calcitonin, but two-thirds have normal turnover. About one-third of these patients (20% of all the osteoporotic patients) did not respond with a lumbar spine increase [59]. There are other obvious examples. The response to vitamin D may depend on age, being low prior to age 60 when serum 1,25-D3 levels are normal, and high after age 70 when 1,25-D3 is low. Individual variability in response, and site differences within the skeleton (spine + +, femur +, radius $\pm$), mandates monitoring at several skeletal sites for clinical control. If only one site can be measured, the clinical consensus today is the spine. The decreases occurring in the spine at the menopause are twice as large as those in the peripheral skeleton [60], and the response of the spine to therapy is often several-fold greater than peripheral sites.

METHODS FOR DENSITOMETRY

Densitometric methods have been reviewed in several recent reports [61-63], and only major highlights, particularly on new developments, are detailed here.

SPA: Single-photon absorptiometry is a method developed 25 years ago for densitometry of the peripheral skeleton [64] that utilizes a single-energy radionuclide source, such as ^{125}I (28 keV). The source is coupled to a radiation detector, usually a sodium iodide crystal mounted on a photomultiplier tube. The narrow beam (1-3 mm) of radiation is passed across an area, usually the distal third of the radius shaft (compact bone), where anatomical uniformity allows precision of about 1% to 2%. The radiation dose is a few mrem. In the past decade SPA has used rectilinear scanners to measure an area several centimeters long on anatomically variable regions, such as the distal radius, or the os calcis, that have more trabecular bone [65,66]. Precision at these "irregular" sites is comparable to that on the radius shaft in research laboratories (1-2%), but the clinical precision is about 2% to 4%. BMD of the distal radius or os calcis is no more sensitive for spine or hip fractures than the radius shaft (see Table V and VI). On the other hand, the distal radius, particularly the "ultradistal" portion which is distal to the radius-ulna junction (trabecular bone 50%), may be more sensitive for Colles' fracture, while the os calcis is closely related to ankle and tibia fractures [27,66]. Peripheral trabecular bone, like compact bone, is not as responsive as axial bone to either aging decreases, or to therapeutic intervention [67-69]. It does not respond to fluoride, but it is stabilized by estrogen [70]. The radius shaft is particularly useful in hyperparathyroidism where compact bone seems more affected than trabecular bone [71,72].

EXPERIMENTAL METHODS: A variety of methods other than SPA have been used over the past 25 years to examine the peripheral skeleton. These include: peripheral QCT, ultrasound, compton scattering, neutron activation, radiogrammetry, radiographic photodensitometry. All suffer from limitations that restrict their application to research laboratories where technical expertise is sufficient to ensure precision. QCT of the peripheral skeleton is perhaps most promising as a clinical tool because of the excellent precision (< 1%) that is available on purely trabecular bone [73-75]. However, peripheral trabecular bone does not reflect that of the axial skeleton, and hence, measurements on the distal radius, the proximal tibia, or os calcis do *not* provide any better diagnostic sensitivity than is obtained on the radius shaft [27,48,66]. Moreover, trabecular bone of the peripheral skeleton is largely unresponsive to agents that cause osteopenia in the axial skeleton, such as corticosteroids, or to those that produce axial increases, such as fluoride. Still, such measurements could be of limited clinical value.

Most recently, ultrasound measurements have been advocated for measurement of appendicular bone. Ultrasound was first investigated over 20 years ago [76], but despite substantial efforts, the results have not been exceptional. There are two basic approaches, speed-of-sound [76,77] and broadband ultrasound attenuation [78,79]. The precision of both methods *in vivo* is worse than SPA, and the diagnostic sensitivity is unproven. There is *no* evidence that these methods provide an indication of bone strength or structural characteristics (Table VIII).

TABLE VIII. Measurements of bone using Speed-of-Sound (SOS) and Broadband Ultrasound Attenuation (BUA).

	SOS (m/sec)		BUA (dB/MHz)	
	Os Calcis [80]	Patella[77]	Os Calcis[79]	Os Calcis[80]
Normal	1500	1850	54.5	55
Osteoporosis	1480	1780	46.3	45
Difference	20	70	8.2	10
SD	20	90	12	13
Z-Score	1.0	0.8	0.8	0.8
Precision	6 (.4%)	40 (2%)	2 (4%)	3 (6%)

DPA: Dual-photon absorptiometry for spine and femur measurement is used in over 1,000 hospitals and clinics for the management of metabolic bone disease [1]. Most commonly, a rectilinear scanner is used to cover an area about 15x20 cm for regional scans [81]. The radioisotope source (153-Gd with emissions at 44 and 100 keV) is coupled to a scintillation detector, or detectors, on a rigid yoke. Scans of the total body, spine and femur have a precision error of < 1%, 2%, and 2% to 3%, respectively, with state-of-the-art equipment [2,82,83]. The total body scan takes 60-70 minutes [41,84-86], while spine and femur scans take about 15 to 20 minutes with standard scanners. Second-generation DPA scanners, with multiple scintillation detectors, provide scans of the spine and femur in about 10-minutes. This is also the case for gamma camera determinations [87]. In the latter case, a fixed 153-Gd source is used in a fixed geometry (magnification < 2X), and scattered radiation is minimized with focused grids. The basic DPA method has an accuracy error of < 3% and a radiation dose of about 1 to 5 mrem [82,83]. The accuracy is not influenced by overlying tissue or marrow fat [88,89].

The typical 1 Ci source of 153-Gd has a low output flux, so relatively large pixels (usually 2x3 mm) must be used to achieve reasonable data density. Also, the size of the source and beam limits the spatial resolution to about 3-4 mm. This resolution is adequate for scans of the femur or the spine of normal subjects. However, artifacts in the spine (osteophytes, endplate hypertrophy, disc degeneration, calcified aorta and fractures) occur in about 15%-20% of patients over age 65. These cause quantitative problems, and also make it difficult to identify a precise region-of-interest [90,91]. This, and the clinical import of the femur in the elderly, has lead to an increasing focus on the proximal femur in patients over age 65.

Some controversy regarding the diagnostic sensitivity of DPA has arisen in part because not all commercial DPA scanners provided measurements of spine BMD having a high diagnostic sensitivity for spine fracture. Scanners of a design similar to that used at the University of Wisconsin, showed a large normal-abnormal difference for spine BMD in women aged 50-65 years (Z-score 1.5 to 2.5 relative to age-matched) [17,45,47], but other scanners did not (Z-score < 1.0) [92,93]. Two adverse influences on sensitivity apparently are (a) use of a constant soft-tissue baseline for the entire spine region, and (b) inclusion of transverse processes. Similarly, only software patterned after that developed at the University of Wisconsin allowed discrimination of hip fracture cases using femoral neck

BMD [Z-score 1.5 to 2.0 in women aged 60-80 years [17,36]. Of course a complicating factor has been that investigators have sometimes mistakenly compared hip fracture cases to so-called "controls" who have fractures. Usually patients with crush fractures, or in fact fractures anywhere in the skeleton, will show osteopenia in the proximal femur [17,36].

DEXA: The new method of dual-energy x-ray absorptiometry [4,5] offers several advantages over DPA, including: improved spatial resolution (1-2 mm vs 4 mm), improved precision (1% vs 2%) and greatly decreased scan times (10 minutes for total body and around 5 minutes for spine or femur). One commercial system even provides 1-minute regional scans with precision comparable to DPA and even better images [94]. There is a high correlation (r > 0.95) between DEXA scans those using 153-Gd-DPA [94-98]. The long-term precision error for spine scans *in vitro* is about 0.4% while the precision *in vivo* is about 1% (Table IX).

TABLE IX. Relative precision *in vivo* (% error) with dual-energy x-ray absorptiometry for the lumbar spine (lateral and AP), femoral neck, and total body BMD.

Source		Scanner	Spine Lateral	AP	Femur Neck	Total Body
Ribot et al 1989	[99]	Lunar	—	0.8%	0.6%	—
Mazess et al 1989	[94]	Lunar	2.0%	0.9%	1.2%	0.7%
Kelly et al 1988	[98]	Hologic	—	1.0%	—	—
Slosman et al 1989	[100]	Hologic	6.3%	1.0%	1.8%	—
Wahner et al 1989	[95]	Hologic	—	1.3%	2.2%	—
Pacifici et al 1988	[97]	Hologic	—	1.0%	2.2%	—

There are two approaches to DEXA. First, a stable x-ray tube with constant voltage can be used with a K-edge filter to produce a dual-energy beam. The lower energy is quite invariant with this approach. One system (Lunar DPX) with a cerium filter has effective energies of 40 and 70 keV, while another system (Norland XR26) uses a samarium filter to give slightly higher energies (45 and 80 keV). In these systems, a NaI(T1) scintillation detector is used in pulse-counting mode. The effects of beam hardening and scattered radiation are corrected in software. Alternatively, the x-ray tube can be switched rapidly between high and low kVp settings, as was done with the first dual-energy x-ray systems 15 years ago [101], but this gives fluctuations in both output and effective energies. One system (Hologic QDR) compensates for the fluctuations on a pixel-by-pixel basis by placing a rotating wheel containing known reference materials in the beam [5,97,98]. The inherently stable K-edge approach provides a lower dose for any given precision (1 vs 3 mrem for regional scans) than the switched energy approach [102].

We tested the Lunar DPX densitometer that uses the K-edge approach [94]. The DPX system was stable for 85 sequential measurements of an annulus over a 7-hour period (CV = 0.4%). The output of the x-ray tube was constant over this period with the system running continuously, and over several months using the instrument intermittently. The densitometer performed spine and femur scans in about 5 minutes and 3 minutes respectively, with adequate resolution (1.2x1.2 mm). The dose was about 1 mrem. Total body scans require 10 minutes (or optionally 20 minutes); the radiation dose was < 0.05 mrem.

The high x-ray flux of DEXA scanners, coupled with better spatial resolution, gives a precision error that is half that of DPA systems using 153-Gd. A series of DPA measurements made on spine or femur phantoms of normal thickness (20 cm) usually shows a SD of 0.012 g/cm^2 (1.2%), while long-term measurements *in vivo* show an SD of about 0.02

g/cm² (2%); the SD of measurements on the same phantoms using DEXA was about 0.5% on the spine and about 0.8% on the femur. However, long-term precision on the spine or femur is dependent on technician skill. The correct sequence of vertebrae (L2-L4) can be confused (L1-L3 or L3-L5). Precision on the femur can be dependent on angulation of the leg and selection of the ROIs even with sophisticated software.

The long-term precision error with the DPX scanner was determined over 12 months by repeated measurements of a three-chamber calibration phantom (0.3%), and of a spine phantom consisting of three lumbar vertebrae embedded in an 18 cm block of tissue-equivalent (Figure 7). Precision error *in vivo* was about 0.6, 0.9 and 1.5% for spine scans (L2-L4) at slow, medium, and fast speeds respectively, in young subjects, while the error was 1.2 and 1.6% respectively, for femur scans at slow and medium speed (Table IX). Precision error in one male subject measured 50 times over one month was less than 1% for spine (0.62% for L1-L4 and 0.68% for L2-L4), and under 2% for the femur (1.6% for femoral neck and 1.2% for neck + trochanter).

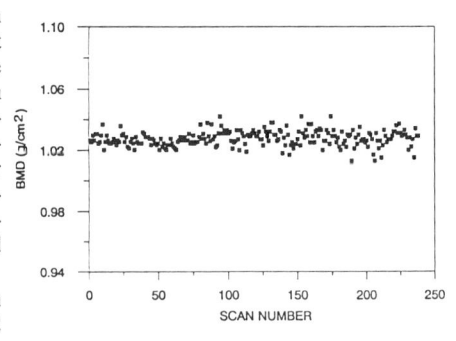

FIG 7. Precision of DEXA (Lunar DPX) over one-year on an 18-cm thick spine phantom was 0.47% (n=239) using a medium speed (4-minutes) and 0.45% (n=164) using a slow speed (8-minutes).

The precision error of total body scans on a skeleton over many scanners was 0.4% (n=34). The precision of total body BMD *in vivo* assessed over 4-7 days in 12 subjects was <0.6% at both the fast (10 minute), and medium (20 minute) speeds, and was 0.7% to 1.5% for major subregions (arms, legs, and trunk).

Some controversy has arisen with regard to calibration of DPA and DEXA instruments even though all instruments show a linear response to concentrations of calcium hydroxyapatite, and are relatively invariant to thickness or composition [94]. The DPX calibration provides accurate BMC measurements *in vivo* by making adjustment for marrow fat. All DPA and DEXA instruments necessarily show a small decrease of BMC with increasing fat. The DPX densitometer indicated accurately (within 1%) the actual amount of hydroxyapatite when the fat content was approximately twice that of the hydroxyapatite, the normal ratio of fat to bone *in vivo*. There was no significant effect of tissue thickness on mass, area or area density (BMD) between 10 and 24 cm of water [94]. Above 24 cm there can be changes that depend on composition. The effect of tissue increases above 24 cm must be determined using soft-tissue equivalent materials that correspond to those found *in vivo* (i.e. 15-40% fat).

Conventional DPA and DEXA scans are made in the AP projection. Scanning the spine in the lateral projection may minimize the effects of aortic calcification and posterior osteoarthritis, conditions of the elderly which can elevate BMD falsely. On the other hand, compression and wedge fractures, Schmorls nodes, and endplate hypertrophy can affect lateral scan results. Bone measurements have been done on the spine in lateral projection using radiographic photodensitometry by both U.S. and German investigators [103-107]. There was about a 1%/year loss of vertebral body density in both sexes. The U.S. studies showed this loss started in young adulthood, while the more extensive German studies showed loss beginning after attainment of peak mass at age 35-40 years. Thick tissue cover (30 cm) has complicated radiographic determinations because of: (a) scattered radiation, and (b) beam hardening.

Uebelhart et al [108] used an experimental DPA approach with 153-Gd to measure the spine in lateral projection. They found a larger aging decrease in the vertebral body (49%) than in the AP projection (27%). In that study, osteoporotics were 31% below controls in the lateral projection and 24% below controls in the AP projection. Mazess et al [109], using a DEXA scanner, confirmed the aging loss from the vertebral body in females was about double that from AP scans (45% vs 20%). The annual loss was actually identical (.01 g/cm^2), but was elevated as a percentage, because BMD in the lateral projection is half that in the AP projection. The larger relative decrease in the vertebral body may not increase diagnostic sensitivity because the within-population variance, at least as a percentage of the lower BMD, is increased by lateral scanning. The within-population SD in the AP projection is about 10%, while in the lateral projection the SD is 15-20%. For diagnostic sensitivity to be improved, the preferential decrease seen in lateral scans must exceed the increased variance associated with these scans.

The BMD of the vertebral body from lateral scans is correlated with that from the AP projection in excised bones and *in vivo* (r = 0.6 to 0.8), but the regression slope changes with age, sex and disease status [108-110]. Ouchi et al [110] used the DPX scanner to measure lateral BMD in males and females; both groups showed aging decreases that were more significant and larger than the decreases in the AP projection. The correlation of AP and lateral BMD values in younger subjects was greater than that in older subjects. Preferential loss from the body itself prevents prediction of lateral BMD from AP scans in elderly or osteoporotic patients.

Part of the reason for a relatively larger, within-population SD in lateral scans is associated with difficulties of measurement in this projection. Slight changes in positioning from time-to-time, or subject movement, can affect the results, since the projected area is sensitive to these factors. Measurement precision per unit time is lower in the lateral projection than in the AP because there is much greater attenuation due to thicker soft-tissue cover. As a consequence, scan times for a given radiation flux and precision level are greater in lateral determinations. Finally, there is a difficulty in precise location of a region-of-interest (ROI). Measurements *in vitro* and *in vivo* on excised vertebrae demonstrated a large regional variability of BMD. The ROI in the lateral projection may include the total vertebral body or the transverse processes can be excluded. The BMD of the body, with the transverse elements removed, is about 10% less than the BMD with the processes present. Manual adjustment of the ROI is associated with precision errors of >5%, but automatic algorithms give lower precision errors. Algorithms have been developed for automatic relocation of the ROI, including one for the anterior body that excluded the transverse processes [108,109]. The precision error for a ROI including the base of the neural arches, and for an ROI more anterior to the arches, was 2% and 3% respectively with the Lunar DPX scanner *in vivo* [109].

It is unclear if the diagnostic sensitivity of DEXA systems will be entirely comparable to that of DPA systems, but since the results from the two approaches are in general highly correlated (r > 0.95), there is reason to suppose that any DEXA system will provide diagnostic results similar to that demonstrated with DPA. However, one commercial scanner appears to provide spine BMD values having relatively poor sensitivity for crush fracture (Z-score of < 1.0 in women about 60 years old) [42] just as was the case with some DPA scanners [92,93].

QCT: Quantitative computed tomography (QCT) was developed by researchers at UCSF [111-114] for spinal measurement. A conventional x-ray tomographic scanner produces cross-sectional images of the 3 or 4 vertebrae. Since the x-ray output is variable, calibration standards must be measured together with the patient. Even with such calibration, however, density results may vary over time because of (a) machine drift, or (b) relocation of the vertebral region. The precision error in careful research laboratories is 5 mg/cm^3; this is 3% in normal young adults, but about 7-15% in an osteoporotic patient [115-118].

There are two approaches to QCT measurement. In order to get precision of 1%-3%, researchers use multiple contiguous transverse slices from each vertebra, in order to reconstruct a larger volume-of-interest for several vertebral bodies [119-121]. In contrast, the clinical approach uses only a small ROI (3 cm^3 or <5% of vertebral mass) from a single slice of each of 2 to 4 vertebrae. The latter approach is very dependent on (a) congruence of the lateral scout view and the tomographic slice, (b) angulation of each vertebra, and (c) selection of the region within the vertebra. A change of only 1 mm causes large changes [121]. New software programs for automatic localization reduces the large locational variation, and halves the precision error (Table X).

TABLE X. Precision of QCT (from references [115-118]).

	SD (mg/cm^3)	
	Manual	Auto
Single-Energy	5	—
Single-Energy	4	3
Dual-Energy	6	3

The results also vary ($\pm 7\%$) among different scanners [114]; direct comparability of results can be achieved on different scanners, or with change of an x-ray tube, only if extensive recalibration is done [122,123]. In research laboratories, these factors can be controlled [114], but in clinical settings the time required for system maintenance and quality control is often doubled. Given this variation, it is difficult to use published normal data from one scanner on another, particularly if the program for ROI location and kilovoltage, and the calibration standard differ. Results at 130 kVp on the same scanner will differ from those at 80 kVp.

The small ROI in the anterior vertebral body is not representative of the remainder of the body [21,122,125]. Typically, only 1 g of bone mineral is measured if 4 vertebrae are sampled, and this represents <5% of the trabecular mass of these same vertebrae. Furthermore, this ROI predicts vertebral strength with a 30% error [18-21] compared to larger regions which have a smaller error [16,122]. On the other hand, the anterior ROI often changes first with disease (oophorectomy, immobilization) or with treatment, perhaps because it is the least dense region. One remarkable finding has been that the density of purely trabecular bone in the spine is similar in males and females, and that the magnitude of aging bone loss is only 20% lower in males [124,126-128]. This is difficult to reconcile with the tenfold lower frequency of spine fracture syndrome (two or more fractures) in men. Kalender et al [128] have shown, however, that males lose little compact bone from the spine, but women lose as much compact bone as trabecular bone. The resistance of male vertebrae to fracture may be the result of the larger overall vertebral size, and to the disproportionate role of the compact outer shell to strength [129]. The anterior region of the body probably shows the greatest decreases with aging because it is the least critical to strength.

Radiologists often use standard imaging exposures for QCT, although a lower voltage (80 kVp) and exposure are recommended [111,113]. The radiation dose is relatively high in clinical practice; at 6 mrem per mass the usual dose is about 1000 mrem. The dose is as low as 200 mrem in research centers, but is substantially higher in most clinical settings (single-energy 700-1500 mrem; dual energy 1500-3500 mrem).

The high kVp usually used for QCT increases the inaccuracy associated with variable marrow fat and osteoid [130-147]. The normal fat content of vertebrae is 250 ± 100 mg/cm^3, but values can be as low as 100 mg/cm^3 in adolescents (or with fluoride therapy), or as high as 500 mg/cm^3 in elderly osteoporotics (or with corticosteroids). There is an error in apparent density of 10 to 13 mg/cm^3 for every 100 mg/cm^3 change of marrow fat. Given a conservative estimate for random variation of ±120 mg/cm^3 of marrow fat in patients, the uncertainty in ash density is ±12 to 20 mg/cm^3 (an accuracy error of 10% to 30% depending on age and density). This "fat error", results in (a) a systematic overestimation of aging decreases, (b) overestimation of the effects of estrogen withdrawal, (c) overestimation of corticosteriod effects, and (d) inaccurate assessment of fluoride effects. The menopausal decrease with QCT (5-10%/year) is about double the actual decrease. Both estrogen withdrawal and corticosteroids increase marrow fat and produce an apparent density decrease. The opposite is true of fluoride, which increases both osteoid and red marrow. Dual-energy QCT only partially corrects the problems due to variable marrow and osteoid. It does not increase the diagnostic sensitivity of the method, and it compromises both precision and dose [148]. Variation of erythropoietic activity (anemia, immunosuppressants) and matrix proliferation (fluoride therapy, renal disease) also lead to large uncertainties.

One major advance has been made recently. Boden et al [149] developed a method for precise (1% normal, 1-2% osteoporotic) QCT that uses tissue histogramming (paraspinal muscle and fat) for internal calibration instead of external standards. The location of external standards in the CT field in relation to the spine of the patient, was a source of variability, particularly with older liquid standards that were large, difficult to place, and occasionally unstable. By using internal calibration, the Boden method avoids the effects of (a) the air gap between the patient and standard, and (b) variable beam hardening due to patient size and composition. The method also avoids the large precision error associated with exact relocalization of the bone ROI by using a similar histogram approach. CT numbers appropriate for trabecular bone differ from those for compact bone, so the two can be isolated by providing a bone histogram for the vertebral body. Mispositioning the vertebral ROI up to 3.5 mm, which usually causes a 3-5% error in conventional QCT [116,122], did not affect the 1% precision. The new method correlated highly ($r=0.96$) with results on patients by the older UCSF method developed at UCSF. The well-documented error caused by variable fat and osteoid on single-energy QCT is unaffected by this approach.

QCT is used as an interim solution to meet bone densitometry needs in many institutions, but it cannot be a satisfactory solution until the errors are corrected, radiation dose lowered, and femur determinations are standardized. QCT has been used experimentally for examination of the proximal femur [150,151]; spinal QCT is of little value in relation to hip fracture [35]. Problems of CT scanner accessibility, and high costs, as well as reliability, limit the clinical usefulness of QCT although it remains important for biomedical research.

CLINICAL UTILITY: DIAGNOSTIC AND MONITORING RELIABILITY

The clinical utility of bone densitometry is not defined by the diagnostic sensitivity, or its precision alone, but rather by the reliability of the diagnostic assessment and the monitoring assessment. For example, the spinal density using single energy QCT is greatly diminished in osteoporotic patients compared to age-matched controls (65 vs 100 mg/cm^3); the difference is about 7 times the precision error of 5 mg/cm^3 (seen in the best laboratories), and 4 to 5 times the typical clinical precision error of 7-9 mg/cm^3. The normal-abnormal difference using DPA (or DEXA) (1.00 vs 0.85 g/cm^2) is also about 7 (or 14) times the typical precision error of .02 g/cm^2 (or .01 g/cm^2) respectively. It is this advantage for reliable assessment of skeletal status that makes DEXA superior to either DPA or QCT. The 1% precision that seems to be attained with the DEXA method, allows clinically meaningful changes to be evaluated with high confidence within 6 to 12 months of therapeutic intervention. A comparison of methods is given in Table XI.

TABLE XI. The normal-abnormal difference (Z-score) and precision (CV) appendicular and axial bone densitometry.

APPENDICULAR MEASUREMENTS

Method	Site	Z-Score	Diagnosis A	B	Monitoring C	Precision %
SPA	Radius	0.7	2	2	0.5	2
SPA	Os Calcis	0.7	2	2	0.5	2
SOS	Os Calcis	1.0	3	3	?	6
SOS	Patella	0.8	2	2	?	20
BUA	Os Calcis	0.8	3	6	?	4
QCT	Radius	0.8	13	13	2	1
QCT	Tibia	2.3	60	80	2	0.5

AXIAL MEASUREMENTS

Method	Site	Z-Score	Diagnosis A	B	Monitoring C	Precision %
QCT	Spine	1.3	7	5	2	5
DPA	Spine	1.2	7	7	2	2
DPA	Femur	1.2	8	5	0.5	2
DPA	Total	1.2	15	10	1	1
DEXA	Spine (AP)	1.1	14	14	4	1
DEXA	Spine (LAT)	1.3	13	12	4	2
DEXA	Femur	1.2	16	10	1	1
DEXA	Total	1.2	20	13	2	0.6

A. *(Normal-Abnormal)/Precision*
B. *(Within Populations SD)/precision*
C. *Annual Change/Precision*

CONCLUSION

Bone densitometry is essential to ascertain the risk of fracture, and for monitoring temporal changes. Multiple risk factors can isolate population segments at higher risk for fracture, but are not specific for individuals. Women who (a) are overweight, (b) have no family history of osteoporosis, (c) have a history of osteoarthritis, and (d) have no indications adversely affecting bone, will have only a slight risk of fracture (< 10%). Thin individuals with other risk factors can have 50-100% risk. Measurement methods for axial sites afford enhanced diagnostic sensitivity, particularly in younger patients when intervention options are greatest. The same methods provide a low precision error in the areas of clinical import (spine and femur) where therapeutic intervention must be monitored.

REFERENCES
1. H.S. Barden and R.B. Mazess. Bone densitometry of the appendicular and axial skeleton. Top Geriatr Rehabil 1989;4:1-12.
2. R.B. Mazess and H.S. Barden. Bone densitometry for diagnosis and monitoring osteoporosis. Proc Soc Exp Biol Med 1989;191:261-271.
3. D.J. Sartoris and D. Resnick. Osteoporosis: Update on densitometric techniques. J Musculoskel Med 1989;6:108-123.
4. D.J. Sartoris and D. Resnick. Dual-energy radiographic absorptiometry for bone densitometry: Current status and perspective. AJR 1989;152:241-246.
5. B.L. Riggs and L.J. Melton. Involutional osteoporosis. N Engl J Med 1986;314:1676-1686.
6. J.W. Davis, J.M. Vogel P.D. Ross and R.D. Wasnich. Disease versus etiology: The distinction should not be lost in the analysis. (Editorial). J Nucl Med 1989;30:1273-1276.
7. B.E. Johnson, B Lucasey, R.G. Robinson and B.P. Lukert. Contributing diagnosis in osteoporosis: The value of a complete medical evaluation. Arch Intern Med 1989;149:1069-1072.
8. E. Seeman, L.J. Melton, W.M. O'Fallon and B.L. Riggs. Risk factors for spinal osteoporosis in men. Am J Med 1983;75:977-983.
9. B.L. Riggs and L.J. Melton. Osteoporosis: Etiology, diagnosis, and management. Raven Press, New York, 1988.
10. S.R. Cummings and D. Black. Should perimenopausal women be screened for osteoporosis. Ann Intern Med 1986;104:817-823.
11. H.K. Genant, J.E. Block, P. Steiger, C.C Glueer, B. Ettinger and S.T. Harris. Appropriate use of bone densitometry. Radiology 1989;170:817-822.
12. W.A. Peck, B.L. Riggs and N.H. Bell. Physician's resource manual on osteoporosis: A decision-making guide. Washington, D.C., National Osteoporosis Foundation, 1987.
13. B.L. Riggs and H.W. Wahner. Bone densitometry and clinical decision-making in osteoporosis. Ann Intern Med 1988;108:293-295.
14. T. Hansson, B. Roos and A. Nachemson. The bone mineral content and ultimate compressive strength of lumbar vertebrae. Spine 1980;5:46-55.
15. N. Dalen, L.G. Hellstrom and B. Jacobson. Bone mineral content and mechanical strength of the femoral neck. Acta Orthop Scand 1976;47:503-508.
16. S.A. Ericksson, B.O. Isberg and J.U. Lindgren. Prediction of vertebral strength by dual photon absorptiometry and quantitative computed tomography. Calcif Tissue Int 1989;44:243-250.
17. R.B. Mazess, H.S. Barden, M. Ettinger and E. Schultz. Bone density of the radius, spine and proximal femur in osteoporosis. J Bone Min Res 1988;3:13-18.
18. R.J. McBroom, W.C. Hayes, W.T. Edwards, R.P. Goldberg and A.A. White. Prediction of vertebral body compressive fracture using quantitative computed tomography. J Bone Jt Surg 1985;67A:1206-1214.
19. F. Brassow, W. Crone-Munzebrock, L. Weh, R. Kranz and G. Eggers-Stroeder. Correlations between breaking load and CT absorption values of vertebral bodies. Europ J Radiol 1982;2:99-101.
20. M. Biggemann, D. Hilweg and P. Brinckmann. Prediction of the compressive strength of vertebral bodies of the lumbar spine by quantitative computed tomography. Skeletal Radiol 1988;17:264-269.
21. P. Brinkmann, M. Biggemann and D. Hillweg. Prediction of the compressive strength of human lumbar vertebrae. Spine 1989;14:606-610.
22. B. Vernon-Roberts and C.J. Pirie. Healing trabecular microfractures in the bodies of lumbar vertebrae. Ann Rheum Dis 1973;32:406-412.
23. S.L. Hui, C.W. Slemenda and C.C. Johnston. Age and bone mass as predictors of fracture in a prospective study. J Clin Invest 1988;81:1804-1809.
24. L.J. Melton, H.W. Wahner, L.S. Richelson, W.M. O'Fallon and B.L. Riggs. Osteoporosis and the risk of hip fracture. Am J Epidemiol 1986;124:254-261.

25. L.J. Melton, S.H. Kan, H.W. Wahner and B.L. Riggs. Lifetime fracture risk: An approach to hip fracture risk assessment based on bone mineral density and age. J Clin Epidemiol 1988;41:985-994.
26. B.E.C. Nordin, J.M. Wishart, M. Horowitz, M., A.G. Need, A. Bridges and M. Bellon. The relation between forearm and vertebral mineral density and fractures in post-menopausal women. Bone and Min 1988;5:21-33.
27. R.D. Wasnich, P.D. Ross, J.W. Davis and J.M. Vogel. A comparison of single and multi-site BMC measurements for assessment of spine fracture probability. J Nucl Med 1989;30:1166-1171.
28. P. Gardsell, O. Johnell and B.E. Nilsson. Predicting fractures in women by using forearm bone densitometry. Calcif Tissue Int 1989;44:235-242.
29. C.E. Cann, H.K. Genant, F.O. Kolb and B. Ettinger. Quantitative computed tomography for prediction of vertebral fracture risk. Bone 1985;6:1-7.
30. S.A. Grubb, P.C. Jacobson, B.J. Awbrey, W.H. McCartney, L.M. Vincent and R.V. Talmage. Bone density in osteopenic women: a modified distal radius density measurement procedure to develop an "at risk" value for use in screening women. J Orthop Res 1984;2:322-327.
31. R.B. Mazess, H.S. Barden, M. Ettinger, C.C. Johnston, B. Dawson-Hughes, D. Baran, M. Powell and M. Notelovitz. Spine and femur density using dual-photon absorptiometry in US white women. Bone and Min 1987;2:211-219.
32. B.L. Riggs, H.W. Wahner, E. Seeman, K.P. Offord, W.L. Dunn, R.B. Mazess, K.A. Johnson and L.J. Melton. Changes in bone mineral density of the proximal femur and spine with aging: differences between the postmenopausal and senile osteoporosis syndromes. J Clin Invest 1982;70:716-723
33. H. Bohr and O. Schaadt. Bone mineral content of femoral bone and the lumbar spine measured in women with fracture of the femoral neck by dual-photon absorptiometry. Clin Orthop 1983;197:240-245.
34. M. Harma, P. Karjalainen, V. Hoikka and E. Alhava. Bone density in women with spinal and hip fractures. Acta Orthop Scand 1985;56:380-385.
35. H. Firooznia, M, Rafii, C. Golimbu, M.S. Schwartz and P. Ort. Trabecular mineral content of the spine in women with hip fracture: CT measurement. Radiology 1986;159:737-740.
36. S. Ericksson and T.L. Widhe. Bone mass in women with hip fracture. Acta Orthop Scand 1988;59:19-23.
37. P.D. Ross, R.D. Wasnich and J.M. Vogel. Detection of prefracture spinal osteoporosis using bone mineral absorptiometry. J Bone Min Res 1988;3(1):1-11.
38. A. Gotfredsen, J. Podenphant, L. Nilas and C. Christiansen. Discriminative ability of total body bone-mineral measured by dual photon absorptiometry. Scand J Clin Lab Invest 1989;49:125-134.
39. R. Eastell, H.W. Wahner, W.M. O'Fallon, P.C. Amadio, L.J. Melton and B.L. Riggs. Unequal decrease in bone density of lumbar spine and ultradistal radius in colles' and vertebral fracture syndromes. J Clin Invest 1989;83:168-174
40. S.M. Ott, R.F. Kilcoyne and C.H. Chesnut III. Ability of four different techniques of measuring bone mass to diagnose vertebral fractures in postmenopausal women. J Bone Min Res 1987;2:201-210.
41. R. Nuti, G. Righi, G. Martini, V. Turchetti, C. Lepore and A. Caniggia. Methods and clinical applications of total body absorptiometry. J Nucl Med and Allied Sciences 1987;31:2;213-221.
42. R. Pacifici, M. Griffith, A. Chines, R. Rupich, N. Susman, and L.V. Avioli. Dual energy radiography (DER) versus quantitative computer tomography (QCT) for the diagnosis of osteoporosis. Endocrine Society of Seattle, June 1989 (abstract).
43. B. Krolner and S. Pors Nielsen. Bone mineral content of the lumbar spine in normal and osteoporotic women: Cross-sectional and longitudinal studies. Clinical Science 1982;62:329-336.
44. E. Vega, C. Mautalen, G. Ghiringhelli and G. Fromm. The bone mineral density in different types of osteoporotic females: (A) Generalized, (B) Femur specific. J Bone Min Res 1989;4(Supp):230 (abstract)

45. J.M. Pouilles, F. Tremollieres, J.P. Louvet, B. Fournie, G. Morlock and C. Ribot. Sensitivity of dual-photon absorptiometry in spinal osteoporosis. Calcif Tissue Int 1988;43:329-334.
46. R.B. Mazess and H.S. Barden. Discrimination of osteoporosis using a single-photon (SPA) and dual-photon absorptiometry (DPA). J. Dequeker, P. Geusens, and H.W. Wahner (eds.) Bone Mineral Measurements by Photon Absorptiometry: Methodological Problems. Leuven University Press, Belgium 1988. pp.109-115.
47. R.B. Mazess, H.S. Barden and M. Ettinger. Radial and spinal bone mineral density in a patient population. Arthritis Rheum 1988;31:891-897.
48. P. Schneider, W. Borner, R.B. Mazess and H.S. Barden. The relationship of peripheral to axial bone density. Bone Min 1988;4:279-287.
49. R.I. Price, M.P. Barnes, D.H. Gutteridge, M. Baron-Hay, R.L. Prince, R.W. Retallack and C. Hickling. Ultradistal and cortical forearm bone density in the assessment of postmenopausal bone loss and nonaxial fracture risk. J Bone Min Res 1989;4:149-155.
50. M. Harma and P. Karjalainen. Trabecular osteopenia in Colles' fracture. Acta Orthop Scand 1986;57:38-40.
51. K. Johnson and R.W. Porter. Broadband ultrasonic attenuation in patients with fracture of the distal radius Ultrasonic Studies of Bone. S.B. Palmer, C.M. Langton (eds.) Institute of Physics. No. 1987:65-66.
52. R. Hesp, L. Klenerman and L. Page. Decreased radial bone mass in Colles' fracture. Acta Orthop Scand 1984;55: 573-575.
53. R.B. Mazess. Bone density in diagnosis of osteoporosis: Thresholds and breakpoints. Calcif Tissue Int 1987;41:117-118.
54. W.S. Browner. Estimating the impact of risk factor modification programs. Am J Epidemiol 1986;123:143-153.
55. B.L. Riggs and L.J. Melton III. Evidence for two distinct syndromes of involutional osteoporosis. Am J Med 1983;75:899-901.
56. Mazess, R.B. On aging bone loss. Clin Orthop Rel Res 1982;162:239-252.
57. E. Seeman, J.L. Hopper, L.A. Bach, M.E. Cooper, E. Parkinson, J. McKay and G. Jerums. Reduced bone mass in daughters of women with osteoporosis. N Engl J Med 1989;320:554-558.
58. R.A. Evans, G.M. Marel, E.K. Lancaster, S. Kos, M. Evans and S.Y.P. Wong. Bone mass is low in relatives of osteoporotic patients. Ann Int Med 1988;109:870-873.
59. R. Civitelli, S. Gonnelli, F. Zacchei, S. Bigazzi, A. Vattimo, L.V. Avioli and C. Gennari. Bone turnover in postmenopausal osteoporosis: effect of calcitonin treatment. J Clin Invest 1988;82:1268-1274.
60. J.J. Stepan, J. Posciphal, J. Presl and V. Pacovsky. Bone loss and biochemical indices of bone remodeling in surgically induced postmenopausal women. Bone 1987;8:279-284.
61. J. Dequeker, P. Geusens and H.W. Wahner (eds.) Bone Mineral Measurements by Photon Absorptiometry: Methodological Problems. Leuven University Press, Belgium 1988.
62. P. Tothill. Methods of bone mineral measurement. Phys Med Biol 1989;34:543-572.
63. P.N. Goodwin. Methodologies for the measurement of bone density and their precision and accuracy. Seminars in Nucl Med 1987;17(4):293-304.
64. J.R. Cameron and J.A. Sorenson. Measurement of bone mineral in vivo: An improved method. Science 1963;142:230-232.
65. C. Christiansen and P. Robdro. Long-term reproducibility of bone mineral content measurements. Scand J Clin Lab Invest 1977;37:321-323.
66. J.M. Vogel, R.D. Wasnich and P.D. Ross. The clinical relevance of calcaneus bone mineral measurements: A review. Bone and Min 1988;5:35-58.
67. P. Ruegsegger, E. Ruegsegger, J. Ittner and M. Dambacher. Natural course of osteoporosis and fluoride therapy - a longitudinal study using quantitative computed tomography. J Comput Assist Tomogr 1985;9:626-627.
68. A.M. Parfitt, D. Sudhakar, J. Rao, A.R. Stanciu, M. Villanueva, M. Kleerekoper and B. Frame. Irreversible bone loss in osteomalacia. J Clin Invest 1985;76:2403-2412.
69. D. Briancon and P.J. Meunier. Treatment of osteoporosis with fluoride, calcium and vitamin D. Orthop Clinics N Am 1981;12:629-648.

70. C.J. Hosie, D.M. Hart, D.A.S. Smith and F. Al-Azzawi. Differential effect of long-term oestrogen therapy on trabecular and cortical bone. Maturitas 1989;11:137-145.
71. S.J. Silverberg, E. Shane, L. de la Cruz, D.W. Dempster, F. Feldman, D. Seldin, T.P. Jacobs, E.S. Siris, M. Cafferty, M.V. Parisien, R. Lindsay, T.L. Clemens and J.P. Bilezikian. Skeletal disease in primary hyperparathyroidism. J Bone Min Res 1989;4:283-291.
72. C. Mautalen, H.R. Reyes, G. Chiringhelli and G. Fromm. Cortical bone mineral content in primary hyperparathyroidism. Changes after parathyroidectomy. Acta Endocrinol 1986;111:494-497.
73. C.J. Hosie and D.A. Smith. Precision of measurement of bone density with a special purpose computed tomography scanner. Brit J RadioL 1986;59:345-350.
74. A. Mueller, E. Ruegsegger and P. Ruegsegger. Peripheral QCT: a low-risk procedure to identify women predisposed to osteoporosis. Phys Med Biol 1989;34:741-749.
75. T.N. Hangartner, T.N. Hangartner, J.J. Battista and T.R. Overton. Performance evaluation of density measurements of axial and peripheral bone with x-ray and gamma-ray computed tomography. Phys Med Biol 1987;32:1393-1405.
76. C. Rich, E. Klink, R. Smith, B. Graham and P. Ivanovich. Sonic measurement of bone mass. In: G.D. Whedon (ed.) Progress in the Development of Methods in Bone Densitometry National Aeronautics & Space Administration Publ. NASA SP-64, Washington, D.C., 1966.
77. R.P. Heaney, L.V. Avioli, C.H. Chesnut, J. Lappe, R.R. Recker and G.H. Brandenburger. Osteoporotic bone fragility. Detection by ultrasound transmission velocity. JAMA 1989;261:2986-2990.
78. S.B. Palmer and C.M. Langton (eds.) Ultrasonic Studies of Bone. Institute of Physics. 1987.
79. D.T. Baran, A.M. Kelly, A. Karellas, M. Gionet, M. Price, D. Leahey, S. Steuterman, B. McSherry and J. Roche. Ultrasound attenuation of the os calcis in women with osteoporosis and hip fractures. Calcif Tissue Int 1988;43:138-142.
80. R. Rossman, J. Zagzebski, C. Mesina, J. Sorenson and R.B. Mazess. Comparison of speed of sound and ultrasound attenuation in the os calcis to bone density of the radius, femur and lumbar spine. Clin Phys. (in press).
81. B. Krolner. Lumbar spine bone mineral content by photon beam absorptiometry. Dan Med Bull 1985;32:152-170.
82. O. Schaadt and H. Bohr. Bone mineral by dual photon absorptiometry. Accuracy-precision-sites of measurements. In: J. Dequeker, C.C. Johnston (eds.). Non-Invasive Bone Measurements 1982;59-72. IRL Press, Oxford.
83. R.B. Mazess, J.A. Hanson, J. Sorenson and H.S. Barden. Accuracy and precision of dual-photon absorptiometry. J. Dequeker, P. Geusens, and H.W. Wahner (eds.) Bone Mineral Measurements by Photon Absorptiometry: Methodological Problems. Leuven University Press, Belgium 1988. p157-164.
84. R.B. Mazess, W.W. Peppler, R.W., Chesney, T.W., Lange, U. Lindgren and E. Smith. Total body and regional bone mineral by dual-photon absorptiometry in metabolic bone disease. Calcif Tissue Int 1984;36:8-13.
85. J.C. Gallagher, D. Goldgar and A. Moy. Total bone calcium in normal women: Effect of age and menopause status. J Bone Min Res 1987;2:491-495.
86. J. Nijs, P. Geusens, J. Dequeker and A. Verstraeten. Reproducibility and intercorrelations of total bone mineral and dissected regional BMC measurements. J. Dequeker, P. Geusens, H.W. Wahner (eds.). Bone Mineral Measurements by Photon Absorptiometry: Methodological Problems. Leuven University Press, Belgium 1988. p.451-453.
87. S. Hoory, D. Bandyopadhyay and L.M. Levy. Use of a gamma camera to estimate bone mineral content based on the dual-photon technique. Phys Med Biol 1987;33:1377-1392.
88. S. Ericksson, B. Isberg and U. Lindgren. Vertebral bone mineral measurement using dual photon absorptiometry and computed tomography. Acta Radiol 1988;29:89-94.
89. H. Wahner, W. Dunn, R.B. Mazess, M. Towsley, R. Lindsay, L. Markhardt and D. Dempster. Dual-photon (153-Gd) absorptiometry of bone. Radiology 1985;156:203-206.
90. M.E. Stutzman, M.V. Yester and E.V. Dubovsky. Technical aspects of dual photon absorptiometry of the spine. J Nucl Med Tech 1987;15:177-181.
91. A. Hopkins, S. Zylstra and M. Hreshchyshyn. Normal and abnormal features of the lumbar spine observed in dual-photon absorptiometry scans. Clin Nucl Med 1988;14:410-414.

92. W.D. Reinbold, H.K. Genant, U.J. Reiser, S.T. Harris and B. Ettinger. Bone mineral content in early-postmenopausal and postmenopausal osteoporotic women: Comparison of measurement methods. Radiology 1986;160:469-478.
93. S.M. Ott, R.F. Kilcoyne and C.H. Chesnut. Comparisons among methods of measuring bone mass and relationship to severity of vertebral fractures in osteoporosis. J Clin Endocrinol Metab 1988;66:501-507.
94. R.B. Mazess, B. Collick, J. Trempe, H.S. Barden and J.A. Hanson. Performance evaluation of a dual-energy x-ray bone densitometer. Calcif Tissue Int 1989;44:228-232.
95. H.W. Wahner, W.L. Dunn, M.L., Brown, R. Morin and B.L. Riggs. Comparison of dual energy x-ray absorptiometry and dual photon absorptiometry for bone mineral measurements of the lumbar spine. Mayo Clinic Proc 1988;63:1075-1084.
96. J. Borders, E. Kerr, D.J. Sartoris, J.A. Stein, E. Ramos, A.A. Moscona and D. Resnick. Quantitative dual-energy radiographic absorptiometry of the lumbar spine: In vivo comparison with dual-photon absorptiometry. Radiology 1989;170:129-131.
97. R. Pacifici, R. Rupich, I. Vered, K.C. Fischer, M. Griffin, N. Susman and L.V. Avioli. Dual energy radiography (DER): A preliminary comparative study. Calcif Tissue Int 1988;43:189-191.
98. T.L. Kelly, D.M. Slovik, D.A. Schoenfeld and R.M. Neer. Quantitative digital radiography versus dual photon absorptiometry of the lumbar spine. J Clin Endocrinol Metab 1988;67:839-844.
99. C. Ribot, F. Tremollieres and J.M. Pouilles. Performance of an x-ray dual-photon scanner and comparison with conventional DPA. Proceedings of the Nineteenth Steenbock Symposium Osteoporosis H.F. DeLuca et al (eds.) Elsevier Science Publishers, New York. 1990. (in press).
100. D. Slosman, R. Rizzoli, A. Donath and J. Bonjour. Quantitative digital radiography and conventional dual-photon bone densitometry: study of precision at the levels of spine, femoral neck and shaft. J Bone Min Res 1989;4(Supp):394.
101. K.H. Reiss, K. Killig and W. Schuster. Dual-photon x-ray beam applications. In: R.B. Mazess (ed.) International Conference on Bone Mineral Measurement. Chicago, IL Oct. 12-13, 1973, 80-87.
102. J.A. Sorenson, P.R. Duke and, S.W. Smith. Simulation studies of dual-energy X-ray absorptiometry. Med Phys 1989;16:75-80.
103. G.P. Vose, S.A. Hoerster and P.B. Mack. New techniques for radiographic assessment of vertebral density. Am J Med Elect 1964;3:181-188.
104. D.J. Baylink, G.P. Vose, W.E. Dotter and L.M. Hurxthal. Two new methods for the study of osteoporosis and other metabolic bone diseases. II. Radiographic densitometry. Lahey Clin Bull 1964;13:217-227.
105. L.M. Hurxthal, G.P. Vose and W.E. Dotter. Densitometric and visual observations of spinal radiographs. Geriatrics 1969;24:93-106.
106. E. Krokowski. Calcium determination in the skeleton by means of x-ray beams of different energies. In: A.M. Jelliffe, B. Strickland (eds.). Symposium Ossium. E.S. Livinstone, Edinburgh, 1970.
107. H. Oeser and E. Krokowski. Quantitative analysis of inorganic substances in the body. A method using x-rays of different qualities. Brit J RadioL 1963;36:274-279.
108. D. Uebelhart, F. Duboeuf, P.J. Meunier and P.D. Delmas. Vertebral bone mineral density (BMD) measurement assessed by lateral dual-photon absorptiometry (DPA). Abstract: Europ Symp Calc Tissue, Jerusalem, 1989.
109. R.B. Mazess, J. Hanson, C. Gifford, J. Prete, and P. Peterson. Measurement of spinal density in the lateral projection. J Bone Min Res 1989;4(Supp):229 (abstract).
110. Y. Ouchi, A.C.A. de Souza, T. Nakamura, H. Orimo, J. Inoue and M. Shiraki. New method for the evaluation of lumbar vertebral body bone mineral density with dual energy x-ray absorptiometry. (abstract): Asia-Pacific Osteoporosis Conference, Honolulu, HI., March 1989.
111. C.E. Cann. Quantitative CT for determination of bone mineral density: a review. Radiology 1988;166:509-522.
112. H.K. Genant, P. Steiger, J.E. Block, C.C. Glueer, B. Ettinger, and S.T. Harris. Quantitative computed tomography: Update 1987. Calcif Tissue Int 1987;41:179-186.

113. C.E. Cann. Low-dose CT scanning for quantitative spinal mineral analysis. Radiology 1981;140:813-815.
114. C.E. Cann. Quantitative CT applications: comparison of current scanners. Radiology 1987;162:257-261.
115. O. Louis, R. Luypaert, W. Kalender and M. Osteaux. Reproducibility of CT bone densitometry: Operator versus automated ROI definition. Europ J Radiol 1988;8:82-84.
116. D.O. Rosenthal, M.A. Ganott, G. Wyshak, D.M. Slovik, S.H. Doppelt and R.M. Neer. Quantitative computed tomography for spinal density measurement factors affecting precision. Invest Radiol 1985;20:306-310.
117. W.A. Kalender, E. Klotz and C. Suess. Vertebral bone mineral analysis: An integrated approach with CT. Radiology 1987;164:419-423.
118. W.A. Kalender, H. Brestowsky and D.D. Felsenberg. Bone mineral measurement: Automated determination of mid-vertebral CT section. Radiology 1988;168:219-221.
119. L.M. Banks and J.C. Stevenson. Modified method of spinal computed tomography for trabecular bone mineral measurements. J Comput Assist Tomogr 1986;10:463-467.
120. C.E. Cann, M. Henzl, K. Burry, J. Andreyko, F. Hanson, G.D. Adamson, G. Trobough, L. Henrichs, and G. Stewart. In: Reversible bone loss is produced by the GnRH agonist nafarelin. D.V. Cohn, T.J. Martin, P.J. Meunier (eds.). Calc Regula and Bone Metab 1987;9:123-127.
121. E. Breatnach and P.J. Robinson. Repositioning errors in measurement of vertebral attenuation values by computed tomography. Brit J Radiol 1983;56:299-305.
122. R. Lambiase, D.J. Sartoris, L. Fellingham, M. Andre and D. Resnick. Vertebral mineral status: Assessment with single- versus multi-section CT1. Radiology 1987;164: 231-236.
123. H. Firooznia, C. Golimbu, M. Rafii, M.S. Schwartz and E.R. Alterman. Quantitative computed tomography assessment of spinal trabecular bone. II.In osteoporotic women with and without vertebral fractures. J Comput Tomogr 1984;8:99-103
124. H. Firooznia, C. Golimbu, M. Rafii, M.S. Schwartz and E.R. Alterman. Quantitative computed tomography assessment of spinal trabecular bone. I. Age-related regression in normal men and women. J Comput Tomogr 1984;8:91-97.
125. C.D. Jones, A.M. Laval-Jeantet, M.H. Laval-Jeantet and H.K. Genant. Importance of measurement of spongious vertebral bone mineral density in the assessment of osteoporosis. Bone 1987;8:201-206.
126. D.E. Meier, E.S. Orwoll and J.M. Jones. Marked disparity between trabecular and cortical bone loss with age in healthy men. Ann Int Med 1984;101:605-612.
127. D.E. Meier, E.S. Orwoll, E.J. Keenan and R.M. Fagerstrom. Marked decline in trabecular bone mineral content in healthy men with age: Lack of association with sex steroid levels. J Am Geriatr Soc 1987;35:189-197.
128. W.A. Kalender, D. Felsenberg, O. Louis, P. Lopez, E. Klotz, M. Osteaux and J. Fraga. Reference values for trabecular and cortical vertebral bone density in single and dual-energy quantitative computed tomography. Europ J Radiol 1989;9:75-80.
129. S.D. Rockoff, E. Sweet and J. Bluestein. The relative contribution of trabecular and cortical bone to the strength of human lumbar vertebrae. Calcif Tissue Res 1969;3:163-175.
130. J.E. Adams, S.Z. Chen, P.H. Adams and I. Isherwood. Measurement of trabecular bone mineral by dual energy computed tomography. J Comput Assist Tomogr 1982;6:601-607
131. J.G. Bradley, H.K. Huang and R.S. Ledleg. Evaluation of calcium concentration in bones from CT scans. Radiology 1978;128:103-107.
132. A.E. Burgess, B. Colborne and E. Zoffmann. Vertebral trabecular bone: comparison of single and dual-energy CT measurements with chemical analysis. J Comput Assist Tomogr 1987;11:506-515.
133. E.O. Crawley, W.D. Evans and G.M. Owen. A theoretical analysis of the accuracy of single-energy CT bone-mineral measurements. Phys Med Biol 1988;33-1113-1127.
134. M.M. Goodsitt, D.I. Rosenthal, W.R. Reinus and J. Coumas. Two post-processing CT techniques for determining the composition of trabecular bone. Invest Radiol 1987;22:209-215.
135. M.M. Goodsitt, R.F. Kilcoyne, R.A. Gutcheck, M.L. Richardson and D.I. Rosenthal. Effect of collagen on bone mineral analysis with CT. Radiology 1988;167:787-791.

136. D.J. Hawkes, D.F. Jackson and R.P. Parker. Tissue analysis by dual-energy computed tomography. Brit J Radiol 1986;59:537-542.
137. P.W. Henson and R.A. Fox. A relationship between the percentage of calcium by mass and the effective atomic number of regions containing bone. Phys Med Biol 1984;29:979-984.
138. A.M. Laval-Jeantet, B. Roger, S. Bouysse, C. Bergot and R.B. Mazess. Influence of vertebral fat content on quantitative CT density. Radiology 1986;159:463-466.
139. R.B. Mazess. Errors in measuring trabecular bone by computed tomography due to marrow and bone composition. Calcif Tissue Int 1983;35:148-152.
140. E.L. Nickoloff, F. Feldman and J.V. Atherton. Bone mineral assessment; New dual-energy CT approach. Radiology 1988;168:223-228.
141. G.U. Rao, I. Yaghmai, A.O. Wist and G. Arora. Systematic errors in bone-mineral measurements by quantitative computed tomography. Med Phys 1987;14:62-69.
142. R. Rohloff, H. Hitzler, W. Arndt, K.W. Frey and J. Lissner. Influence of fat content of bone marrow on bone mineral measurements by CT and photon-absorptiometry in trabecular bone. J Comput Assist Tomogr 1982;6:212-213.
143. M.A. Weissberger, R.G. Zamenhoff, S. Aronow and R.M. Neer. Computed tomography scanning for measurement of bone mineral in the human spine. J Comput Assist Tomogr 1978;2:253-262.
144. C.C. Glueer, U.J.. Reiser, C.A. Davis, B.K. Rutt and H.K. Genant. Vertebral mineral determination by quantitative computed tomography (QCT): Accuracy of single and dual energy measurements. J Comput Assist Tomogr 1988;12:242-258.
145. R.B. Mazess and J. Vetter. Comparison of dual-photon absorptiometry and dual-energy computed tomography for vertebral mineral. J Comput Assist Tomogr 1985;9:624-625.
146. R.B. Mazess and J. Vetter. The influence of marrow on measurement of trabecular bone using computed tomography. Bone 1985;6:349-351.
147. R.B. Mazess, J. Vetter and D.S. Weaver. Bone changes in oophorectomized monkeys: CT findings. J Comput Assist Tomogr 1987;11:302-305.
148. R. Pacifici, N. Susman, P.L. Carr, S.J. Birge and L.V. Avioli. Single and dual energy tomographic analysis of spinal trabecular bone: A comparative study in normal and osteoporotic women. J Clin Endocrinol and Metab 1987;64:209-214.
149. S.D. Boden, D.J. Goodenough, C.D. Stockham, E. Jacobs, T. Dina and R.M. Allman. Precision measurement of vertebral bone density using computed tomography without the use of an external reference phantom. J Digital Imag 1988;2:31-38
150. S. Bhasin, D.J. Sartoris, L. Fellingham, M.B. Zlatkin, M. Andre and D. Resnick. Three-dimensional quantitative CT of the proximal femur: Relationship to vertebral trabecular bone density in postmenopausal women. Radiology 1988;167: 145-149.
151. D.J. Sartoris, M. Andre, C. Resnick and D. Resnick. Trabecular bone density in the proximal femur: Quantitative CT assessment. Radiology 1986;160:707-712.

Quantitative Computed Tomography: Update 1989

Harry K. Genant, J.E. Block, P. Steiger, and C.C. Glueer

University of California, San Francisco, California

Quantitative computed tomography (QCT) is now a clinically established and widely applied method for noninvasive bone mineral assessment [1-56]. Currently, this technique has been implemented at over 1,000 sites (with approximately 10,000 advanced CT scanners worldwide) encompassing a wide geographic distribution and a wide array of commerical CT scanners. The usefulness of QCT for measurement of bone mineral lies in its ability to provide a quantitative image and, thereby, to measure trabecular, cortical or integral bone, centrally or peripherally. For measuring the spine, the potential strengths of QCT are its capability for precise three-dimensional anatomic localization, providing a direct density measurement, and its capability for spatial separation of highly responsive cancellous bone from less responsive compact bone.

Technical Considerations

QCT measurements of spinal trabecular bone are made on commerically available CT scanners using mineral reference standards for calibration, computed radiographs for localization, and either single or dual energy scanning techniques [7,19,22]. Representative volumes, (approximately 3 cc) of purely trabecular bone at the mid-plane of three to four lumbar vertebral bodies are quantified and averaged, and the results are expressed as mineral equivalents in mg/cc (Fig. 1). The examination requires approximately 10 minutes, and dedicated software reduces data analysis to several minutes. The cost for spinal CT measurement ranges from $100 to $250.

The absolute accuracy and longitudinal precision of QCT are influenced by a variety of technical (scanner drift, beam hardening, field non-uniformity, and scatter), operator (kVp, mAs, scout localization, and ROI selection), and patient (movement, size, and marrow composition) factors [6,7,22,25]. The performance characteristics, therefore, are highly machine, operator, and patient dependent. However, recent advances in CT instrumentation and software, and in quality assurance programs have improved the reliablity and the standardization of QCT results.

The long-term in vivo precision error for single energy (SE) QCT is 1-3% in normals and 2-5% in osteoporotics [2,7,14,19,22,40,41,48], and for dual energy (DE) QCT is approximately three-fold larger. As a reflection of accuracy spinal SEQCT density measurement in vitro correlates highly (r >.9) with vertebral ash determination (Fig. 2A) [6,25,36,47] and moderately well (r =.5-.8) with TBV by iliac histomorphometry [24,25]. The accuracy error for SEQCT is 5-10% in normals and 10-20% in osteoporotics, and for DEQCT is two-fold reduced (Figs. 2A&B) [1,6,25,30,33]. The fat-induced inaccuracy is machine and kVp dependent, ranging from -7 mg/cc (typical for GE 9800 at 80kVp) to -12 mg/cc (extreme) per 10% fat [6,25,33]. Extrapolating from reported data [25,33,58] on vertebral marrow fat content and applying the smaller error correction of -7 mg, then SEQCT measurement underestimates spinal mineral by about 20 mg/cc in the young and 30 mg/cc in the elderly with a residual uncertainty of about 5 mg/cc [20,25].

Copyright 1990 by Elsevier Science Publishing Co., Inc.
Osteoporosis: Physiological Basis, Assessment, and Treatment
Hector F. DeLuca and Richard Mazess, Editors

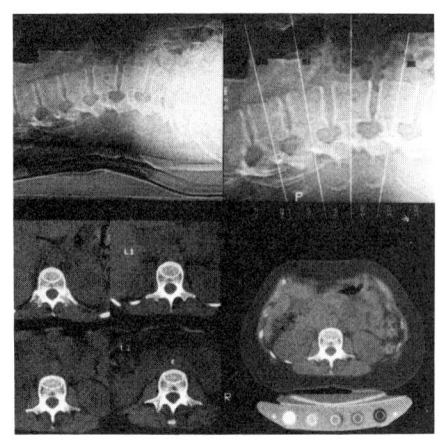

Fig. 1A&B   Lateral scout view provides rapid and simple localization approach in which the midplane of 4 vertebral bodies are defined on the video monitor and a single 10-mm thick section is obtained at each level. An oval region of interest, centered in the mid vertebral body, is used to determine cancellous bone mineral content (mg/cm3), while circular regions of interest are used to quantify the K2HPO4 solutions in the calibration phantom.

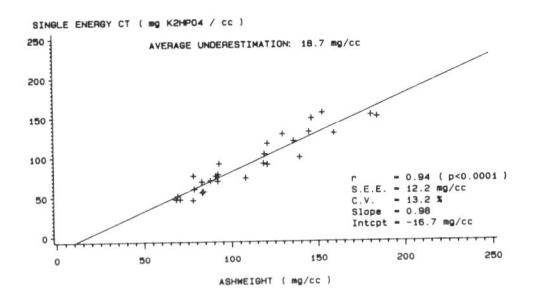

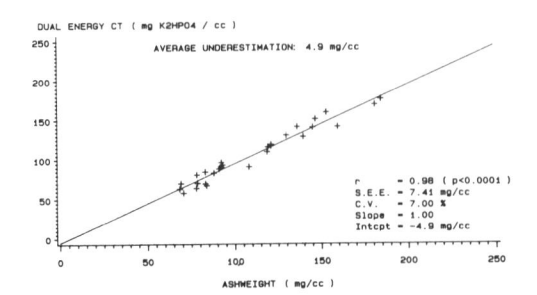

Fig. 2A&B   A) The accuracy [(25] of single energy QCT is shown for fresh vertebral specimen (derived from 62 samples) from 28 cadavers (20 males and 8 females with a mean age of 60). B) With dual energy QCT in the same specimen, the accuracy is improved two-fold.

The radiation exposure for SEQCT on most systems is 100-300 mrem (1/10 the normal imaging dose per slice, 1/10 the usual number of slices per study, and therefore, 1/100 the total integral dose of the routine abdominal imaging study) [8,10,22]. However, with certain systems on which the manufacturer has limited the capability for reducing kVp and mAs settings, the dose ranges as high as 500 to 1000 mrem [6,30]. The dose for DEQCT is generally two-fold higher than for SEQCT. Both the manufacturers and the users are taking steps to further reduce radiation dose for QCT studies.

Technical Advances in QCT

Important advances in QCT phantom design are being reported [15,22,30,43]. Aqueous dipotassium hydrogen phosphate solutions, used in the standard QCT phantom, have potentially limited long-term stability caused by gas bubbles, precipitation of the dissolved materials, and impurities. Because of these considerations, solid reference phantoms have been developed by Image Analysis, General Electric, Siemens and Chugai that are potentially more stable, sturdy, and resistant to damage. Reports [10,16,22,54] are appearing on the procedures necessary to provide cross-calibration among different calibration phantoms and among different QCT scanners. It is not yet clear which phantom material or design will prove most reliable.

Recent image-evaluation software, incorporating contour-tracking algorithms, allows for anatomically adapted and automatically placed regions of interest (ROIs) in the vertebrae and for automatic performance of calibration [22,30,53,54]. Automatic selection of the ROI eliminates operator influence and offers better reproducibility, especially if different operators are involved. In spinal studies, contour-tracking algorithms trace the cortical walls of the vertebral body, the spinal canal, and the posterior elements to select the optimum position and size of the ROI. Anterior or total trabecular density of the vertebral body, as well as total integral bone density (trabecular and cortical), can be automatically selected. Another new technique [31] automatically selects the mid-vertebral QCT slice on the lateral localization digital radiograph and promises faster studies and additional reductions in positioning errors due to operator influence.

Monitoring Bone Density Changes

Trabecular bone, constituting 20% of skeletal mass and 20-40% of vertebral mass [29,61], has nearly eight-fold greater turnover rate than that of cortical bone. As an index of sensitivity, the mean age-related trabecular bone loss in women from age 20-80 years is 1.2% annually, and the mean immediate postmenopausal bone loss is 5-7% annually, when measured by SEQCT [3,13,19,55]. These rates of spinal trabecular loss are approximately two- to three-fold larger than those observed by spinal integral BMC, and three- to five-fold larger than those by appendicular cortical BMC [13,19,57,62,63].

If two-point serial measurements are used [59], a QCT technique with a 2% precision error can detect changes in bone mass greater than 3.6% with 90% confidence (one-tailed analysis) [24]. Large annual losses of 5-20% from sites rich in trabecular bone can be observed and monitored in women undergoing surgical or natural menopause [13,19,55], and in patients initiating high-dose corticosteroid treatment [37]. Similarly, large annual gains of 5-15% are found in osteoporotic patients receiving investigational agents such as sodium fluoride [11], diphosphonates [23], or parathyroid hormone [52]. This ability to monitor changes in the individual patient by spinal QCT compares favorably with the abilities by spinal dual photon absorptiometry (DPA) or appendicular cortical single photon absorptiometry (SPA), in which slower rates of measured loss (assuming comparable precision) necessitate longer intervals and/or more measurements to reach similar levels of confidence (Fig. 3).

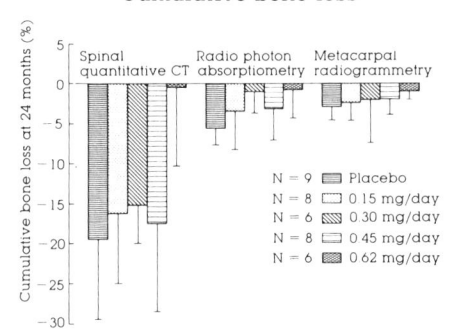

Cumulative bone loss

Fig. 3   Cumulative bone loss 24 months following oophorectomy in 37 women as a function of quantitative technique and estrogen therapy.

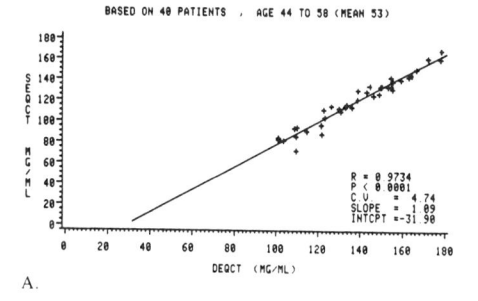

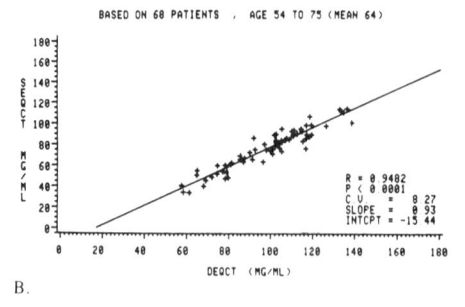

Fig. 4A&B   High correltion is shown for SEQCT versus DEQCT for (A) normal early postmenopausal women and (B) postmenopausal osteoporotic women, indicating a relatively small fat induced error with the GE 9800 CT scanner [42].

Correlations Between Measurements

In cross-sectional studies, SEQCT spinal measurements correlate highly (r >.95) with DEQCT spinal measurements (Figs.4A&B), moderately (r=.5-.8) with spinal integral BMC measurements by DPA (Figs.5A&B) and modestly (r=.2-.5) with appendicular cortical BMC measurements by SPA [21,45,48,50]. In longitudinal studies, the rates of change by SEQCT spinal measurement correlate only modestly (r=.4-.6) with spinal integral BMC changes and poorly (r=.2-.4) with appendicular cortical BMC changes [22]. Because of the large standard errors of the estimates, both cross-sectionally and longitudinally, measurement by one technique is a poor predictor of measurement by another technique for the individual patient. However for grouped patients, the correlations are significant, although the predictive values are low.

EARLY POSTMENOPAUSAL FEMALES: DPA VS. SEQCT
BASED ON 40 PATIENTS , AGE 44 TO 58 (MEAN 53)

A.

OSTEOPOROTIC FEMALES: DPA VS. SEQCT
BASED ON 68 PATIENTS , AGE 54 TO 75 (MEAN 64)

B.

Fig. 5A&B   A) Moderately good correlation is shown for DPA versus SEQCT for normal early postmenopausal women, while (B) for postmenopausal osteoporotic women, a modest correlation is shown for DPA versus SEQCT due to their respective sources of error in the elderly [42].

Spine Fracture Relationships

In vitro, spinal trabecular density by QCT or by ash determination correlates well (r=-.8) with vertebral fracture load [4,36]. In vivo, SEQCT measurement correlates well (r=-.6 to -.9) with spinal fracture severity (prevalence), compared with modest correlations (r=-.4 to -.6) by spinal integral BMC, and poor correlations (r=-.2 to .4) by appendicular cortical BMC [21,42,45], when assessed in the same populations (Figs. 6A&B). Data are not yet available on spinal QCT in relationship to spinal fracture incidence.

OSTEOPOROTIC FEMALES: FXI VS. SEQCT
BASED ON 68 PATIENTS , AGE 54 TO 75 (MEAN 64)

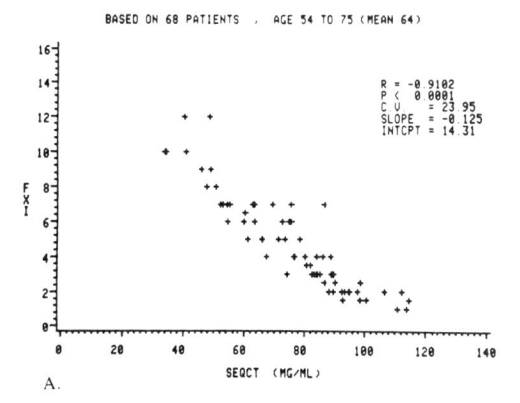

R = -0.9102
P < 0.0001
C.V. = 23.95
SLOPE = -0.125
INTCPT = 14.31

A.

OSTEOPOROTIC FEMALES: FXI VS. DPA
BASED ON 68 PATIENTS , AGE 54 TO 75 (MEAN 64)

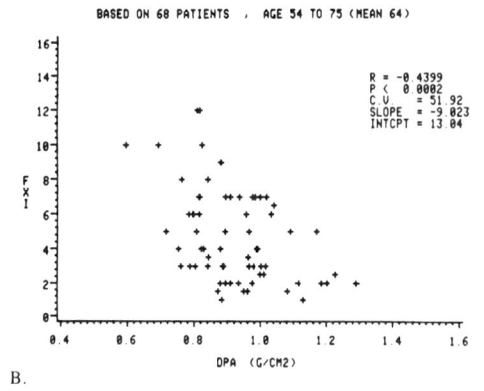

R = -0.4399
P < 0.0002
C.V. = 51.92
SLOPE = -9.023
INTCPT = 13.04

B.

Fig. 6A&B A) High correltion is shown for SEQCT versus spinal fracture index, while (B) modest correlation is shown for DPA versus spinal fracture index, in the same patients [42].

The decrement of spinal trabecular bone observed by SEQCT between young premenopausal women (165 ± 25 mg/cc) and elderly osteoporotic women (45 ± 25 mg/cc) is typically 120 ± 50mg/cc (50-90%) [14,21,40,42,45]. On the other hand, the decrement by QCT between early postmenopausal women and osteoporotic women is typically 25-65%, but compares favorably with the decrements of 15-25% by spinal integral BMC and 10-15% by appendicular cortical BMC when measured in the same populations. The overlap between spinal osteoporotic and age-matched controls, however, is substantial indicating that other factors are of importance [9,14,41]. Nevertheless, spinal QCT measurement appears to provide an index of relative risk for spinal fracture.

Hip Fracture Relationships

In vitro, femoral neck density by QCT correlates well (r=-.7 to -.8) with ash-weight, strength and fracture load [12]. In vivo, limited data have shown that spinal QCT measurements discriminate hip-fracture patients only weakly from age- and sex-matched controls [14,28]. While preliminary studies [26,43,51] show the feasibilty of direct femoral QCT measurements, clinical results have not yet been reported. However, the three-dimensional and high-resolution capabilities of QCT make this technology attractive for finite element analysis of strength and density relationships, for both the hip and the spine from an investigative and clinical perspective.

Osteoporosis/Fracture-Threshold Definitions

Recent studies [60,64] have addressed the inadequacies of defining osteoporosis by means of a dichotomous clinical variable, namely, fracture versus nonfracture, and have emphasized the role of bone densitometry, per se, in establishing this diagnosis or in assessing risk of its major complication, fracture. In the case of QCT, a consensus definition for osteoporosis has not been reached, with the issue complicated by variations across scanners, calibration standards and methodologies. Furthermore, QCT studies to date have been limited to analyses of fracture prevalence data.

SEQCT versus DEQCT

DEQCT generally improves the absolute accuracy of spinal measurement two-fold compared to SEQCT (r>.95 vs. r>.90, and SEE 3-7% vs. SEE 5-20% for in vitro studies) (see Figs. 2A&B), and has important research applications in which very high accuracy is required [6,25,30,33]. However, with typical CT scanners having -7 to -9 mg/cc per 10% fat errors [10,25], the use of DEQCT does not significantly reduce normal biological variation, improve fracture discrimination, or improve correlations with integral BMC measurements [20,42]. Furthermore, since DEQCT reduces precision three-fold, increases dose two-fold and is technically demanding, it is generally not recommended for clinical applications on most CT scanners.

Age-Related Bone Loss by QCT

QCT has been used to model patterns of vertebral bone diminution with aging [5,9,14,16,39,40,41]. New data [3] from the UCSF Osteoporosis Research Group on 538 healthy women between the ages of 20 and 80 indicate little skeletal involution of spinal trabecular bone prior to the onset of menopause. Various statistical regressions were performed for the entire population to describe the general pattern of bone loss from the spine; linear, quadratic, cubic and logarithmic models were found to be equally satisfactory in characterizing this pattern with R values of .65, .67, .68 and .67, respectively. QCT values were stratified into 5 and 10 year age brackets, and analyzed separately for pre- and postmenopausal women. The five and 10 year interval stratification revealed no identifiable bone mineral decrements prior to midlife; significant losses of bone mineral were noted to correspond with the usual time of menopause and to continue into old age. The statistical model of skeletal atrophy is best described as a two-phase regression, consisting of a pre-menopausal period of skeletal consolidation followed by a period of exponential postmenopausal involution (Fig. 7).

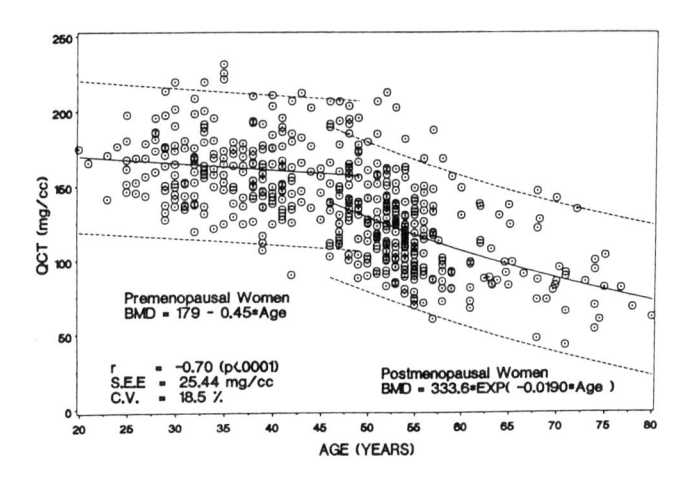

Fig. 7   Two-phase regression of bone density on age employing a premenopausal linear segment and a postmenopausal exponential segment.

Clinical Applications of QCT

QCT spinal measurement may be indicated as a diagnostic procedure in selected menopausal and osteoporotic women to determine current bone mass, as one of several osteoporotic risk factors, in making therapeutic decisions. Serial assessment by QCT measurement in certain postmenopausal women may be indicated to identify rapid bone losers or to document effectiveness of prophylaxis with low-dose estrogen replacement. Serial assessment may also be used in selected osteoporotic women to document effectiveness of osteotrophic therapy. Finally, QCT spinal measurement may be clinically indicated in a variety of metabolic bone disorders to assess the effects of the specific disorder on trabecular bone, and to determine the natural course of disease or response to therapy.

REFERENCES

1. Adams JE, Chen Sz, Adams PH, Isherwood I: Measurement of trabecular bone mineral by dual energy computed tomography. J Comput Assist Tomogr 1982;6:601-607.
2. Banks LM, Stevenson JC: Modified method of spinal computed tomography for trabecular bone mineral measurement. J Comput Assist Tomogr. 1986; 10(3):463-467.1. Genant HK, Boyd DP, Rosenthal D, Abols Y, Cann CE: Computed tomography. In: Cohn SH, ed. Noninvasive measurements of bone mass and their clinical application. Boca Raton, Fla.: CRC Press, 1981; 121-149.
3. Block JE, Smith R, Glueer CC, Steiger P, Ettinger B, Genant HK: Models of spinal trabecular bone loss as determined by quantitative computed tomography. J Bone Mineral Res 1989;4:249-257.
4. Brassow F, Crono Muenzebrock W, Weh L, Kranz R, Eggers-Stroeder G: Correlations with between breaking load and CT absorption values of vertebral bodies. Eur J Radiol 1982; 2:99-101.
5. Buchanan JR, Myers C, Lloyd T, Greer RB: Early vertebral trabecular bone loss in normal premenopausal women. J Bone Mineral Res 1988;3:583-587.
6. Burgess AE, Colborne B, Zoffmann E: Vertebral trabecular bone: Comparison of single and dual-energy CT measurements with chemical analysis. J Comput Assist Tomogr 1987;11:506-515.
7. Cann CE, Genant HK: Precise measurement of vertebral mineral content using computed tomography. J Comput Assist Tomogr 1980; 32:493-500.
8. Cann CE: Low dose CT scanning for quantitative spinal mineral analysis. Radiology 1981; 140:813-815.
9. Cann CE, Genant HK, Boyd DP, Kolb FO, Ettinger B: Quantitative computed tomography for prediction of vertebral fracture risk. Bone 1985; 6:1-7.
10. Cann CE: Quantitative CT applications: Comparison of current scanners. Radiology 1987; 162:257-261.
11. Duursma SA, Glerum JH, Van Dijk A, Bosch R, Kerkhoff H, Van Putten J, Raymakers, JA: Responders and non-responders after fluoride therapy in osteoporosis. Bone 1987;8:131-136.
12. Esses SI, Hayes WC, Goldberg RP: Fracture risk of the proximal femur by quantitative computed tomography. 32nd Annual Orthopaedic Research Society, New Orleans, Louisiana, Feb. 17-20, 1986.
13. Ettinger B, Genant HK, Cann CE: Postmenopausal bone loss is prevented by low-dosage estrogen with calcium. Ann Intern Med 1987; 106:40-45.
14. Firoozina H, Rafii M, Golimbu C, Schwartz MS, Ort P: Trabecular mineral content of the spine in women with hip fracture: CT measurement. Radiology 1986; 159:737-740.
15. Fujii Y, Tsunenari T, Tsutsumi M et al. Quantitative computed tomography: Comparison of two calibration phantom. JBMM 1988;6:17-20.
16. Fujii Y, Tsutsumi M, Tsunenari T, Fukase M, Yoshimoto Y, Fujita T, Genant HK: Quantitative computed tomography of lumbar vertebrae in Japanese patients with osteoporosis. Bone Mineral 1989;6:87-94.
17. Genant HK, Boyd DP: Quantitative bone mineral analysis using dual energy computed tomography. Invest. Radiology 1977; 12:545-551.
18. Genant HK, Boyd DP, Rosenthal D, Abols Y, Cann CE: Computed tomography. In, Cohn SH (ed). Noninvasive measurements of bone mass and their clinical application. Boca Raton, Fl, CRC Press, 1981, pp 121-149.
19. Genant HK, Cann CE, Ettinger B, Gordan GS: Quantitative computed tomography of vertebral spongiosa: a sensitive method for detecting early bone loss after oophorectomy. Ann Intern Med 1982; 97:699-705.

20. Genant HK, Cann CE, Boyd DP, Kolb FO, Ettinger B, Gordan GS: Quantitative computed tomography for vertebral mineral determination. In: Frame B, Potts JT, eds. Clinical Disorders of Bone and Mineral Metabolism. Amsterdam: Excerpta Medica, 1983; 40-47.
21. Genant HK, Powell MR, Cann CE, et al: Comparison of methods for in vivo spinal mineral measurement. In: Christiansen C, Arnaud CD, Nordin BEC, et al, eds. Osteoporosis. Denmark: Aalborg Stiftsbogtrykkeri, 1984, 97-102.
22. Genant HK (ed): Osteoporosis Update 1987, University of California Press, Berkeley, CA, 1987.
23. Genant HK, Harris ST, Steiger P, Davey PF, Block JE: The effect of etidronate therapy in postmenopausal womenh: Preliminary results. In, Christiansen C, Johansen JS, Riis BJ (eds). Osteoporosis 1987. September 27-October 2, Denmark, Copenhagen:Osteopress ApS 1987:2:1177-1181.
24. Genant HK, Block JE, Steiger P, Glueer CC, Ettinger B, Harris ST: Appropriate use of bone densitometry. Radiology 1989;170:817-822.
25. Glueer CC, Reiser UJ, Davis CA, Rutt BK, Genant HK: Vertebral mineral determination by quantitative computed tomography (QCT): Accuracy of single and dual energy measurements. J Comput Assist Tomogr 1988;12:242-258.
26. Glueer CC, Genant HK: Quantitative computed tomography of the hip. In, Genant HK (ed): Osteoporosis Update 1987. University of California Press, Berkeley, CA 1987.
27. Hangartner TN, Overton TR: The Alberta gamma CT system. J Comput Assist Tomogr 1983; 6:1156.
28. Harma M, Karjalainen P, Hoikka V, Alhava E: Bone density in women with spinal and hip fractures. Acta Orthop Scand 1985; 56:380-385.
29. Jones CD, Laval-Jeantet AM, Genant HK: Importance of measurement of spongious vertebral bone mineral density in the assessment of osteoporosis. Bone, 1987;8:201-206.
30. Kalender WA, Klotz E, Suess C: Vertebral bone mineral analysis: an integrated approach to CT. Radiology 1987;164:419-423.
31. Kalender WA, Brestowsky H, Felsenberg D; Bone mineral measurements: Automated determination of the midvertebral CT section. Radiology 1988;168:219-221.
32. Kleeman BC, Edwards WT, Hayes WC, Zamenhof RG, Sarno RC, Nachemson AL, White AA III: Prediction of vertebral fracture risk using quantitative computed tomography in vivo. 33rd Annual Meeting, Orthopaedic Research Society, January 19-22, 1987, San Francisco, CA.
33. Laval-Jeantet AM, Roger B, Bouysse S, Bergot C, Mazess RB: Influence of vertebral fat content on quantitative CT density. Radiology 1986; 159:463-466.
34. Mazess RB: Errors in measuring trabecular bone by computed tomography due to marrow and bone composition. Calcif Tissue Int 1983; 35:148-152.
35. Mazess RB, Vetter J: Comparison of dual photon absorptiometry and dual energy computed tomography for vertebral mineral. J Comput Assist Tomogr 1985; 9:624-625.
36. McBroom RJ, Hayes WC, Edwards WT, Goldbert RP, White AA: Prediction of vertebral body compressive fracture using quantitative computed tomography. J Bone Joint Surg 1985; 67:1206-1214.
37. Montag M, Belter SV, Meyer-Galander HM, Peters PE; BMC of the spongiosa in lumbar spine, measured by QCT: follow-up study in patients suffering from pemphigus and treated with high doses of cortisone (Abstract). Sixth International Workshop on Bone and Soft Tissue Densitometry, Buxton, England, Sept. 22-25, 1987.
38. Montag M, Peters PE: Computertomographisch bestimmter Mineralgehalt in det LWS-Spongiosa. Radiologe 1988;28:161-165.

39. Nilsson M, Johnell O, Jonsson K, Redlund-Johnell I: Quantitative computed tomography in measurement of vertebral trabecular bone mass. Acta Radiol 1988;29:719-725.
40. Odvina CV, Wergedal JE, Libanati CR, Schulz EE, Baylink DJ: Relationship between trabecular vertebral body density and fractures: A quantitative definition of spinal osteoporosis. Metabolism 1988;37:221-228.
41. Pacifici R, Susman N, Carr S, Birgo S, Avioli L: Single and dual energy tomographic analysis of spinal trabecular bone: A comparative study of normal and osteoporotic women. J Clin Endocrinol Metab 1987, 64:209.
42. Reinbold WD, Genant HK, Reiser UJ, Harris ST, Ettinger B: Bone mineral content in early-postmenopausal and postmenopausal osteoporotic women: Comparison of measurement methods. Radiology 1986; 160:469-478.
43. Reiser U, Genant HK: Determination of bone mineral content in the femoral neck by quantitative computed tomography (Abst). 70th Assembly and Annual Meeting of the Radiological Society of North America. Washington, DC, November 26-30, 1984.
44. Reiser U, Genant HK: New water and bone equivalent solid phantom materials used for calibration in quantitative CT. 70th Scientific Assembly of the Radiological Society of North America, Washington, DC, Nov. 26-30, 1984.
45. Richardson ML, Genant HK, Cann CE, Ettinger B, Gordan GS, Kolb FO, Reiser U: Assessment of metabolic bone diseases by quantitative computed tomography. Clin Orthop 1985; 195:224-238.
46. Richardson ML, Pozzi-Mucelli RS, Kanter AS, Kolb FO, Ettinger B, Genant HK: Bone mineral changes in primary hyperparathyroidism. Skeletal Radiology 1985;15:85-95.
47. Rohloff VR, Hitzler H, Arndt W, et al: Vergleichende Messungen des Kalk salzgenhaltes spongioser Knochen mittels Computer tomographie und I-125 Photonen Absorptions-methode. In: Lissener J, Doppman J (eds): CT '82 Internalationales Computertomographie symposium. Konstanz, Schnetztor-Verlag, 1982, 126-130.
48. Rosenthal D, Ganott M, Wyshak G, Slovik DM, Spooelt SH, Neer RM: Quantitative computed tomography for spinal density measurement-factors affecting precision. Intern Med 1982; 20:306-310.
49. Ruegsegger P, Elsasser U, Anliker M, et al: Quantification of bone mineralization using computed tomography. Radiology 1976; 121:93-87.
50. Sambrook PN, Bartlett C, Evans R, Hesp R, Katz D, Reeve J: Measurement of lumbar spine mineral: a comparison of dual photon absorptiometry and computed tomography. Br J Radiol 1985; 58:621-624.
51. Sartoris DJ, Andre M, Resnick C, Resnick D: Trabecular bone density in the proximal femur: Quantitative CT assessment. Radiology 1986; 160:707-712.
52. Slovik DM, Rosenthal DI, Doppelt SH, Potts JT, Daly MA, Campbell JA, Neer RM: Resoration of spinal bone in osteoporotic men by treatment with human parathyroid hormone (1-34) and 1,25-Dihydroxyvitamin D. J Bone Mineral Res 1986; 1:377-381.
53. Steiger P, Steiger S, Block JE, Glueer CC, Genant HK: Bone mineral density of different vertebral compartments in pre-, early post-, and postmenopausal women. J Bone Mineral Res 1988;3(suppl):S124.
54. Steiger P, Glueer CC, Genant HK: Simultaneous calibration in QCT: A comparison of commercial calibration phantoms. Calcif Tiss 1989;44:146.
55. Stevenson JC, Banks LM, Spinks TJ, Freemantle C, McIntyre I, Hesp R, Lane G, Endacott JA, Padwick M, Whitehead MI: Regional and total skeletal measurements in the early postmenopausal. J Clin Invest 1987; 80:258-262.

56. Torres A, Lorenzo V, Gonzales-Posada JM: Comparison of histomorphometry and computerized tomography of the spine in quantitating trabecular bone in renal osteodystrophy. Nephron 1986; 40:282-287.
57. Awbrey BJ, Jacobson PC, Grubb SA, McCartney WH, Vincent LM, Talmage RV: Bone density in women: A modified procedure for measurement of distal radial density. J Orth Res 1984; 1:314-321.
58. Dunnill MS, Anderson JA, Whitehead R: Quantitative histological studies on age changes in bone. J Pathol Bacteriol 1967; 94:275-291.
59. Heaney RP: En recherche de la difference ($p < 0.05$). Bone and Mineral 1986; 1:99-114.
60. Melton LJ, Kan SH, Wahner HW, Riggs BL: Lifetime fracture risk: An approach to hip fracture risk assessment based on bone mineral density and age. J Clin Epidemiol 1988;41:985-994.
61. Nottestad SY, Baumel JJ, Kimmel DB, Recker RR: The proportion of trabecular bone in human vertebrae. J Bone Mineral Res. In press.
62. Riggs BL, Wahner HW, Melton LJ, Richelson LS, Judd HL, Offord KP: Rates of bone loss in the appendicular and axial skeletons of women. J Clin Invest 1986; 77:1487-1491.
63. Riis B, Thomsen K, Christiansen C: Does calcium supplementation prevent postmenopausal bone loss? N Engl J Med 1987; 316:173-177.
64. Ross PD, Wasnich RD, Heilbrun LK, Vogel JM: Definition of a spine fracture threshold based upon prospective fracture risk. Bone 1987;8:271-278.

Bone Histomorphometry

F. Melsen, E.F. Eriksen, Le. Mosekilde, Li. Mosekilde, T. Steiniche, and A. Vesterby

University of Aarhus, Denmark

INTRODUCTION

Bone histomorphometry is a method for quantitative estimation of the skeletal constituents providing a description of the amount, structure and quality of bone by which microanatomical deviations in calcium metabolic disorders may be classified. This has for the last two to three decades been based upon the ideas of Frost [1] of a "basic multicellular unit" (BMU) (Fig. 1) by which the internal reorganization of bone takes place at localized sites through a sequential coupling between activation (A), resorption (R), and subsequent formation (F). Further, within the last few years, the quantum concept and the introduction of time^{-1}, obtained by

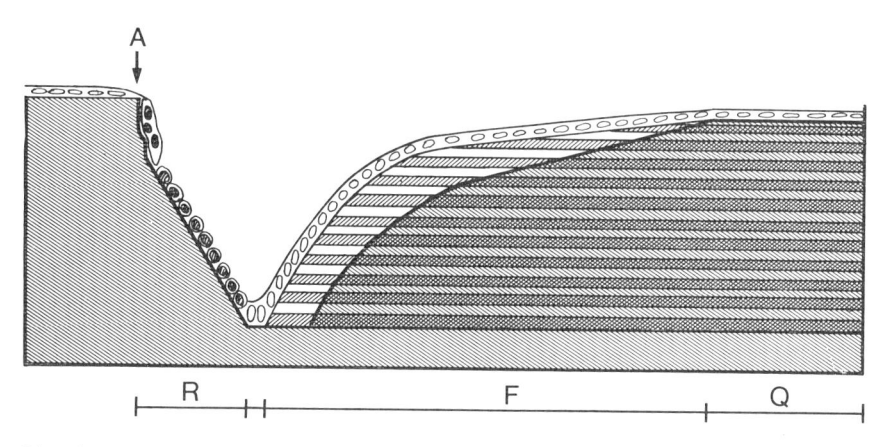

Fig. 1. Complete remodeling sequence in trabecular bone. A: activation frequency; R: resorption period; F: formation period; Q: quiescent phase

tetracycline double labeling [2,3] has played a very important role. The quantum concept which is of great importance for the prediction of bone mass is based upon determination of bone removed during resorption and formed during formation and the calculation of the balance between resorption and formation per modeling cycle. The tetracycline double labeling is a necessity for the estimation of bone formation rates and calculation of resorption rate. Based upon these dynamic estimates the life spans of resorptive and formative periods, as well as the activation frequency, the frequency by which new modeling sites per unit bone are initiated, can be calculated. All this leads to a combination of parameters among which resorption depth, balance per modeling unit, activation frequency and the life spans of resorptive and formative phases are the only determinants for amount and structure of bone. The biomechanical competence, a very important property of bone, is, of course, proportional to the amount and structure of the bony elements. These are, on the other hand, not the only determinants for the strength of the bone since bone quality may interfere. Altered quality of bone may occur when the mechanism of bone formation is disturbed. This may lead to accumulation of wide osteoid seams (see below under osteomalacia) hypomineralized bone with reduced strength or to the formation of non lamellar bone as seen in certain high turnover conditions, during fluoride treatment and in certain congenital bone disorders. A third factor that may interfere with the biomechanical properties is the degree of mineralization of the formed structural units of bone or rather the fraction of newly formed primary mineralized structures which is proportional to the activation frequency. Newly-formed less-mineralized structures are supposed to be strong and elastic and the older ones to be less strong due to stiffness and fragility.

Remodeling

Activation of a certain site of a bone surface is the mechanism by which osteoclasts are recruited for bone resorption [1]. This occurs with a certain frequency given by the number of newly created resorptive sites per unit time per unit bone or by which a given site on the bone surface undergoes remodeling. The activation frequency therefore is one of the two main determinants for the number of resorptive and later formative sites.

After recruitment of the multinuclear osteoclasts they remove bone to a certain depth at which resorption partly is taken over by mononuclear cells [4] until a final depth of resorption is reached. This depth of resorption is in normal approximately 60-70 μm when evaluated by new unbiased techniques [4]. Coupled to the resorption [5] a subsequent formation takes place. This is initiated by recruitment of preosteoblasts that will differentiate into osteoblasts. The osteoblasts start laying down matrix, in most cases with lamellar structure, until it reaches a certain thickness or age (the initial mineralization lag time). Then mineralization starts and the following osteoid formation and mineralization more or less completely refills the resorption cavity. The duration of resorptive and formative phases in normal adult trabecular bone is approximately 40 and 150 days [4].

The activation frequency and the coupling between the duration of the resorptive and formative phases are the determinants of the fractional occurrence of resorptive and formative sites on the bone surface. An isolated increase in activation frequency will after a certain period lead to a proportional increase in number or extent of resorptive and formative sites. This alteration cannot be separated by static histomorphometry from an isolated prolongation of the remodeling sequences stressing the importance of dynamic measurements and calculations of the activation frequency and life spans of the remodeling phases. Isolated alterations in the activation frequency thus will lead to proportional deviations in both resorptive and formative sites. On the other hand, many deviations in the life span, either the resorptive or formative, lead to deviations in the proportion of resorption to formation. This has by some investigators been regarded as uncoupling, which it is not. Uncoupling only occurs when resorption is not followed by formation or when formation occurs without preceeding resorption as seen in the process of modeling.

Amount and Structure of Bone

After the growing phase of life the trabecular bone is continuously internal reorganized. This remodeling of trabecular bone determines its amount and structure. The amount is under influence of two factors, the remodeling space, and balance between resorption and formation in the remodeling cycle. An increase in the remodeling space, which may be due to increased activation frequency and/or prolongation of the life spans of the remodeling phases, will lead to a decrease in amount of bone simply due to an increased porosity following the increased number of resorption cavities and the increased fraction of osteoid due to more formative sites. A decrease in activation frequency, and/or shortening of the remodeling phases, will lead to the opposite situation. These deviations on bone mass are to be regarded as reversible as bone mass returns to normal (or almost to normal) when normal activation frequency and/or life spans are reestablished.

An irreversible alteration in trabecular bone mass may be due to two isolated or combined factors, namely the balance between resorption and formation in the remodeling cycle, and the occurrence of trabecular perforations.

An imbalance between bone resorbed and formed will create an irreversible loss or gain in bone mass. Since a small amount of bone is either lost or gained per remodeling cycle, this effect on the amount of bone may be accelerated or reduced by an increase or a decrease respectively in the activation frequency.

Trabecular perforations by osteoclasts is another mechanism for irreversible bone loss. If the depth of resorption lacune or the depth of two lacunes on each site of a trabecula exceeds the thickness of the trabecula, a perforation occurs. This may create a true uncoupling at the structural basis for the bone formation is lost [6]. This disintegration of the trabecula network, which is proportional to the activation frequency, is probably of greatest importance for the bone strength.

Bone Biopsy

For the quantitative study of metabolic bone diseases the iliac crest is the preferred sampling site by most investigators. This is due to (a) the very easy approach to the region, (b) no difference in amount and remodeling of bone between right and left site allowing repeated biopsies [7], and (c) a usually sufficient representation of cortical and trabecular bone for histomorphometric analysis. Further, the iliac crest biopsy procedure is a safe procedure with very few complications [8]. A precondition for the study of bone remodeling is preparation of undecalcified histologic sections. This is necessary not only for the discrimination between mineralized and unmineralized matrix, but for the evaluation of tetracycline labelings and thereby the bone dynamics as well. Various plastic embedding compounds have been suggested for biopsy embedding purpose among which methylmethacrylate is the most commonly used. This allows cutting of undecalcified sections on special microtomes and will to a great extent prevent shrinkage of the specimen and distortion of the sections. In our laboratory 7 μm thick sections stained with Massontrichrome and Goldner-trichorme are used for estimation of the static parameters. For the estimation of bone dynamic variables, 10 or 20 μm thick unstained sections may be used to identify tetracycline double labelings in fluorescent microscope.

Measuring Principles

Measurements of the various variables can be carried out either according to a random sampling of structure interfaces using microscopic grids and point counting or by using computerized digitizing devices for tracing complete tissue structures. The manual grid method is, at least in our hands, the most convenient, precise and reliable and should be recommended except for two point discrimination (measuring of distances in width determinations) where recording of data is facilitated by the use of computerized devices.

Traditional bone histomorphometry, whether point counting or computerized methods are used, has suffered from the lack of suitable stereological parameters related to the structure of the bone. Further bone histomorphometrists seem to have overlooked the fact that bone structure is anisotropic. Consequently parameters related to structures have been biased to an uncertain degree. Recently the introduction of anisotropic, transiliac crest sections, the so-called vertical sections, has, however, made it possible to obtain unbiased stereological estimates. The vertical section technique which must be combined with a special cyloid grid is probably the most recommendable manual histomorphometric method (for more information see Vesterby et al. [9]).

Using the above mentioned histomorphometric methods, the static remodeling parameters can be estimated: fractional extent of resorptive surfaces, and extent, width and amount of osteoid. Further, the amount and structure of trabecular bone can be estimated. Using a new and unbiased technique [4] the final resorption depth and the man width of the structural units can be measured and the balance per remodeling cycle calculated.

If tetracycline is given in two separated doses with an interval of i.e., 10 days prior to biopsy and dynamics in bone remodeling can be measured: bone formation rate at cellular, BMU and tissue levels and mineralization lag time. From these measurements, and the static parameters of bone remodeling, life spans of bone formation, resorption and quescent periods can be calculated. Finally a complete reconstruction of BMU and the activation frequency may be estimated.

Relation Between Iliac Crest Trabecular Bone Volume and Skeletal Strength

The representativity of the iliac crest trabecular bone volume (TBV) for trabecular bone in other parts of the skeleton is critical for its clinical applicability. Assessment of mass and mechanical competence of vertebral trabecular bone or whole vertebral bodies is of importance in order to evaluate patients at risk for spinal osteoporosis with spontaneous fractures [10].

It has previously been demonstrated [11,12] that the maximum compressive strength of vertebral trabecular bone as well as whole vertebral bodies correlates to the compressive strength of horizontal iliac crest trabecular bone cylinders in normal individuals. However, in most clinical situations equipment for mechanical testing of bone biopsies is not available and the biopsies are subjected to histomorphometric examination which include determination of trabecular bone volume (TBV) [13,14]. Although the average trabecular bone volume in the iliac crest is higher than in the vertebral bodies, a strong correlation has been demonstrated between the two volumetric measurements (Table I) [15-17]. This

TABLE I. Predictive value of iliac crest trabecular bone volume (TBV) for (a) vertebral trabecular bone volume, (b) ash density, (c) trabecular stress, (d) total vertebral body stress, and (e) strength in normal individuals aged 15 - 87 years [17]
SEE: Standard error of estimate of vertebral quantity from iliac crest trabecular bone volume

Vertebral variable	n	r	p	SEE
Trabecular bone volume, %	25	0.81	<0.001	1.96
Ash density, g/cm^3	24	0.61	<0.01	0.033
Trabecular bone stress, MPA	24	0.65	<0.001	0.99
Total vertebral body stress, MPA	22	0.69	<0.001	1.24
Total vertebral body strength, N	22	0.59	<0.01	1524

correlation, however, may not indicate that iliac crest trabecular bone volume can predict the mechanical competence of weightbearing vertebral trabecular bone [18]. The mechanical competence is related not only to bone mass but also to the architecture of the trabecular lattice [19-22]. Furthermore, iliac crest trabecular bone is nearly isotropic in all age groups [23], whereas vertebral trabecular bone has anisotropic properties that increase with age [11,24,25]. However, a recent study [17] has demonstrated significant positive correlation between iliac crest trabecular bone volume and vertebral bone mass as well as biomechanical competence in normal individuals (Table I). As expected, vertebral trabecular bone stress showed a weaker correlation to iliac crest than to vertebral trabecular bone volume. Of the variation in vertebral trabecular bone strength only 40% could be explained by variation in vertebral trabecular bone volume.

Table II compares the predictive value of invasive and noninvasive clinical methods for estimating whole vertebral body compressive strength

TABLE II. Efficacy of estimating whole vertebral body compressive strength (MPa) in normal individuals from invasive measurements on the iliac crest and noninvasive densitometric measurements on the spine [12,17]
SEE: Standard error of estimate of vertebral body compressive strength

	r	SEE MPa	age range years
Iliac crest			
Travecular bone volume, %	0.69	1.24	15-87
Compressive strength, MPa	0.78	0.92	15-87
Spine			
Dual photon absorptiometry, g/cm^3	0.47	0.75	43-95

in normal individuals. It appears that mechanical testing on the iliac crest gives a better estimate of vertebral body strength than iliac crest trabecular bone volume. Furthermore, dual photon absorptiometry (DPA) estimates vertebral body compressive strength with a smaller standard error of estimate than the invasive measurements on the iliac crest.

From a clinical point of view, the whole vertebral body load (N), is probably the most important measurement. This quantity was not well estimated (Table I), and only 35% of the variation in this parameter could be explained from variations in iliac trabecular bone volume. Furthermore, by multiple correlation analysis vertebral trabecular bone strength showed no partial correlation to iliac trabecular bone volume when age was also considered but a significant inverse relation to age when bone volume was taken into account [17]. This indicates that the observed correlation between vertebral trabecular bone strength and iliac trabecular bone volume is mainly created by an age-induced covariation between the two indices and that individual estimation of iliac trabecular bone volume in normal individuals adds no further information on vertebral trabecular bone strength than age itself. Such age-adjusted analyses have not been reported for the noninvasive measurements based on dual photon absorptiometry, quantitative digital radiography or quantitative computerized tomography.

Relation Between Histomorphometric Estimates of Bone Turnover and Biochemistry

It is well established that histomorphometric estimates of bone remodeling are changes in a variety of clinical states with abnormal bone and calcium metabolism [8,26]. However, in well defined clinical situations it has been difficult to establish significant relations between histomorphometric variables of bone remodeling and disease activity or biochemical bone markers. This difficulty, which may be related to the small sample size and the fact that only trabecular bone is investigated has been used to incriminate the histomorphometric technique for being insufficient for clinical and scientific purposes. Relations between histomorphometric and other variables, however, depend not only on the method error and representatively of trabecular bone quantitative histomorphometry but also on the accuracy and sensitivity of the biochemical variables and the range of the disease activity.

In hyperthyroid patients with a wide scatter of disease activity significant positive correlations have been found between free thyroxine index and trabeculat osteoclastic resorption surfaces, Haversian canals with active resorptioin and cortical porosity [27] indicating that an increase in thyroid activity enhance osteoclastic resorption in the endosteal as well as intracortical envelope leading to a reversible bone loss with increased cortical porosity (Table III). The extent of labeled surfaces was inversely related to thyroid activity indicating a suppression of bone formation with increasing hyperthyroidism [27]. These observations are in accordance with latter results based on a complete reconstruction of the remodeling cycle in hyperthyroidism [4], which demonstrate an increase in activation frequency with a defect in bone formation compared to bone resorption.

Furthermore, positive correlations have been found in hyperthyroidism between cortical osteoclastic resorption, cortical porosity and serum levels and renal excretions of calcium and phosphorus [27] (Table IV)

TABLE III. Correlation between thyroid function (free thyroxine index) and histomorphmetric indices of bone resorption, bone formation and cortical porosity in patients with hyperthyroidism [27]

	n	r	p
Trabecular bone			
Resorptive surfaces, %	37	0.38	<0.05
Labeled surfaces, %	26	-0.51	<0.01
Cortical bone			
Canals with resorption, %	37	0.52	<0.001
Cortical porosity, %	37	0.69	<0.001

indicating that enhanced cortical osteoclastic activity in hypertyroidism is followed by cortical bone loss and mobilization of bone mineral.

TABLE IV. Correlation Between Cortical Osteoclastic Resorption, Cortical Porosity and Biochemical Variables Related to Bone Mineral Mobilization in Hyperthyroidism [27]
Urinary calcium and phosphorus are expressed per mol creatinine.

	Cortical osteoclastic resorption		
	N	r	p
Bone mass			
Cortical porosity, %	38	0.71	<0.001
Mineral mobilization			
serum calcium, mmol/l	38	0.55	<0.001
serum phosphorus, mmol/l	37	0.43	<0.01
urinary calcium	37	0.53	<0.001
urinary phosphorus	37	0.45	<0.01

These results demonstrate that histomorphometric values describing bone remodeling are related to disease activity and calcium homeostases in well defined patient materials. This is further corroborated by the finding that medical treatment in hyperthyroidism and surgical treatment in primary hyperparathyroidism are followed by qualitatively identical changes in histomorphometric and biochemical parameters of bone turnover [28-30]. Furthermore, estrogen treatment in postmenopausal spinal crush fracture osteoporosis indicates a decrease in trabecular bone activation frequency with a reduction in trabecular bone resorption and formation followed by identical changes in urinary hydroxyproline excretion and serum alkaline phosphatase [31].

The Bone Biopsy As A Diagnostic Tool

Bone histomorphometric techniques are best suited for the characterization of basic mechanisms of disease in grouped materials. The method error associated with most pertinent histomorphometric indices (wall thickness (W.Th), osteoid thickness (O.TH), mineral appositional rate (MAR), resorption depth (Rs.De) is in the order of other techniques of biomedical research (e.g., RIA), i.e., between 5 and 15% [4]. For some secondary derived indices, like formation period (FP), erosion rate (ER) and bone balance (delta BV), the method error approaches 20-30%, but these higher values have to be viewed in the context of the changes in these indices observed in metabolic bone disease, changes that may amount to several hundred percent [4]. In this relative sense, the method error on the volume-based bone balance of trabecular bone, which lies around 30% is much lower than the value obtained from calcium balance studies, which amounts to 70%.

In the single individual, the relatively high intra-bone variance (i.e., the variance of bone histomorphometric indices between different compartments of bone in the same individual when subjected to repeat biopsies) [7], and the overlap with normal remodeling, preclude a firm diagnosis in most cases. In atyical cases of suspected thyrotoxicosis, myxedema, primary hyperparathyroidism or osteoporosis, the bone biopsy may be a valuable adjuvant to other clinical tests, but none of the histomorphometric changes are pathognomonic [4,13,19]. When it comes to one group of diseases, however, bone biopsy is still an important tool, namely when oteomalacia is suspected. In a recent study of osteomalacia after gastrectomy [31] we found that out of 8 patients who fulfilled the criteria for severe osteomalacia only 3 revealed abnormalities in S-AP, S-25 (OH)D_3 or S-Ca. The remaining patients exhibited serum values within the 95% confidence interval. These data suggest that the diagnosis of osteomalacia may be missed if based on screening blood tests alone. Therefore, a bone biopsy should be performed in all cases where the clinical picture leads to the suspicion of osteomalacia.

The diagnosis of osteomalacia is based on two criteria: (a) increased mineralization lag time and (b) increased osteoid seam thickness [32,33]. Both criteria have to be met, otherwise inclusion of low turnover bone disease (e.g., myxedema) may occur. The presence of increased osteoid surface (OS) has often been taken as a sign of osteomalacia. Increased OS may, however, occur in low as well as high turnover bone disease without any sign of mineralization defect, and is therefore less well suited as a criterion for osteomlacia. Increased osteoid width alone is also an insufficient criterion. A lot of high turnover states (e.g., hyperthyroidism and PHP) may lead to increased O.Th due to presence of early osteoid seams with osteoid thickness in the range of 10-20 μm [4]. The mineralization lag time, will, however, be normal in these conditions.

The Use of Bone Biopsies for Monitoring Effects of Treatment

Most techniques used in calcium metabolic research (e.g., calcium kinetics, assays of bone markers in serum, photon absorptiometry) measure changes in whole skeletal turnover. These changes constitute the sum of changes in individual cell activity at the level of the individual Basic Multicellular Unit (BMU) and the number of BMU's currently active. Consequently, a detailed analysis of osteoclastic and osteoblastic activity and changes in the birth rate of new BMU's is impossible with these techniques.

Any change in the birth rate of new BMU's will lead to changes in apparent bone mass, as measured with photon absorptiometry, due to expansion or reduction of the remodeling space (i.e., the volume of bone currently being turned over in the remodeling process) [4,20]. The studies currently available on effects of estrogen on bone [34] suggest that reductions in activation frequency are the main determinants for the increases in bone mass observed with photon absorptiometry in women treated with these compounds. The amount of bone marker (e.g., BGP) liberated to serum from bone will depend on the number of remodeling sites currently engaged in osteoblastic bone formation and the individual activity of osteoblasts at these sites. Thus, serum levels of bone markers as well as calcium kinetics indices and photon absorptiometric readings depend on a variety of factors that have to be elucidated in order to evaluate the changes observed.

Bone histomorphometry is the only method that allows the investigator to discriminate between changes in activation frequency and alterations of cellular activity. Thus, bone histomorphometric evaluation of bone biopsies constitute a "sine qua non," when it comes to evaluating effects of new treatment regimens in metabolic bone disease.

REFERENCES

1. H.M. Frost, Calcif. Tissue Res. 3, 211 (1969).
2. H.M. Frost in: Mathematical Elements of Lamellar Bone Remodeling (Charles C. Thomas, Springfield 1964)
3. H.M. Frost in: Bone Biodynamics, H.M. Frost, ed. (Little Brown & Co., Boston 1964)
4. E.F. Eriksen, Endocrine Rev. 7, 379 (1986).
5. A.M. Parfitt, Metab. Bone Dis. Rel. Res. 4, 1 (1982).
6. A.M. Parfitt, Calcif. Tiss. Int. 36S, 123-128 (1984).
7. F. Melsen, Histomorphometric analysis of iliac bone in normal and pathologic conditions, Ph.D. thesis, University of Aarhus, Aarhus, Denmark (1978).
8. F. Melsen and L. Mosekilde, Orthop. Clin. North AM 12, 571 (1981).
9. A. Vesterby, J. Kragstrup, H.J.G. Gundersen, and F. Melsen, Bone 8, 13 (1987).
10. J.K. Weaver and J. Chalmers, J. Bone Joint Surg. 48A, 289-298 (1966).
11. Li Mosekilde, A. Viidik, and Le Mosekilde, Bone 6, 291-295 (1985).
12. Li Mosekilde and Le Mosekilde, Bone 7, 207-212 (1986).
13. F. Melsen, B. Melsen, Le. Mosekilde, and S. Bergmann, Acta. Pathol. Microbiol. Scand. 86, 70-81 (1978a).
14. F. Melsen, B. Melsen, and Le Mosekilde, Acta Pathol. Microbiol. Scand. 86, 63-69 (1978a).
15. P. Meunier, P. Courpron, C. Edouard, J. Bernard, J. Bringuier, and G. Vignon, Clin. Endocrinol. Metab. 2, 239-256 (1973).
16. J.M. Giroux, P. Courpron, and P. Meunier, Histomorphometrie de l'osteonenie physiologique senile, Thesis, Lyon, France (1975).
17. Li Mosekilde and Le Mosekilde, Bone 9, 195 (1988).
18. R.B. Mazess, Clin. Orthop. 165, 239-252 (1982).
19. G.H. Bell, O. Dunbar, J.S. Beck, and A. Gibb, Calc. Tiss. Res. 1, 75-86 (1967).
20. A.M. Parfitt, H.E. Mathews, A.R. Villanueva, M. Kleerekoper, B. Frame, and D.S. Rao, J. Clin. Invest. 4, 1396-1409 (1983).
21. M. Kleerekoper, A.R. Villanueva, J. Stanciu, R.A. Sudhaker, and A.M. Parfitt, Calcif. Tissue. Int. 37, 594-597 (1985).
22. Li Mosekilde, Le Mosekilde, and C.C. Danielsen, Bone 8, 79-85 (1987).
23. W.J. Whitehouse, Calc. Tiss. Tes. 23, 67-76 (1977).
24. J.S. Arnold, M.H. Bartley, S.A. Tont, and D.P. Jenkins, Clin. Orthop. 49, 17-38 (1966).
25. P.J. Atkinson, Calc. Tiss. Res. 1, 24-32 (1967).

26. F. Melsen, L. Mosekilde, and J. Kragstrup in: Bone Histomorphometry, Techniques and Interpretation, R. R. Recker, ed. (CRC Press Inc, Boca Raton 1983) pp. 109-142.
27. L. Mosekilde, Effects of thyroid hormones on bone remodeling, bone mass and calcium homeostasis in man, Ph.D. thesis, University of Aarhus, Aarhus, Denmark (1978).
28. L. Mosekilde, M.S. Christensen, F. Melsen, and N.S. Sorensen, Acta Endocrinol. (Kbh.) 87, 743 (1978).
29. L. Moseskilde and F. Melsen, Acta Med. Scand. 204, 97 (1978).
30. L. Mosekilde and F. Melsen, Acta Endocrinol. (Kbh.) 87, 751 (1978).
31. S. Bisballe, Forstyrrelser i kalkmetabolismen med affektion af knoglesystemet efter gastrektomi. Privopgavebesvarelse ved Aarhus Universitet (1984).
32. F. Melsen and L. Mosekilde, Acta Pathol. Microbiol. Scand (A) 88, 83 (1980).
33. A.M. Parfitt, D.S. Rao, J. Stanciu, A.R. Villanueva, M. Kleerekoper, and B. Frame, J. Clin. Invest. 76, 2403 (1985).
34. T. Steiniche, C. Hasling, E.F. Ericksen, F. Melsen, and L. Mosekilde, In: Proceeding Fifth International Congress on Bone Morphometry, Niigata, Japan, abst. 59.

Biochemical Assessment of Bone Turnover in Osteoporosis

P.D. Delmas

INSERM Unit 234 and University C. Bernard, Hôpital E. Herriot, Lyon, France

ABSTRACT

Considerable efforts have been made in the past few years to develop new circulating markers of bone turnover. Among other markers of bone formation, serum bone gla protein (osteocalcin) has been shown to be a sensitive index of osteoblastic activity in patients with osteoporosis. In addition to the well known urinary excretion of hydroxyproline and to the plasma levels of tartrate-resistant acid phosphatase, the urinary excretion of the pyridinoline crosslinks of collagen is a new promising marker of bone resorption. The use of several markers reflecting specific aspects of osteoblast and osteoclast metabolism should enlighten our understanding of the complex and subtle abnormalities of bone turnover in osteoporotic patients and should be useful to analyze the mechanisms by which specific treatments act in vivo.

INTRODUCTION

In contrast to metabolic bone diseases such as Paget's disease of bone or renal osteodystrophy characterized by dramatic changes of bone turnover, osteoporosis is a condition where subtle modifications of the bone remodeling activity can lead to a substantial loss of bone mass after a long period of time. This explains why most conventional markers are normal in a patient with osteoporosis and why there is a need for sensitive biochemical markers of bone turnover.

The rate of formation or degradation of the bone matrix can be assessed either by measuring a prominent enzymatic activity of the bone forming or resorbing cells -such as alkaline and acid phosphatase activity- or by measuring bone matrix components released into the circulation during formation or resorption (Table I). As discussed below, these markers are of unequal specificity and sensitivity, and some of them have not been yet fully investigated. In addition, because circulating levels of these markers can be influenced by factors other than bone turnover such as their metabolic clearance, their clinical significance should be validated by comparison with the direct assessment of bone formation and resorption by iliac crest histomorphometry.

BIOCHEMICAL MARKERS OF BONE FORMATION

Serum alkaline phosphatase

Serum alkaline phosphatase activity is the most commonly used marker of bone formation but its lacks sensitivity and specificity (1). Nevertheless,

Table I. Biochemical markers of bone turnover.

Formation	Resorption
Serum - Total and bone specific alkaline phosphatase - Bone gla-protein (BGP, osteocalcin) - Procollagen I extension peptides - Other non collagenous bone proteins (?)	Plasma - Tartrate-resistant acid phosphatase - Free gamma-carboxyglutamic acid - Fragments of non collagenous proteins (?)
Urine - Non dialyzable hydroxyproline (?)	Urine - Total and dialyzable hydroxyproline - Hydroxylysine glycosides - Pyridinoline crosslinks (HP and LP)

several studies have shown that its activity increases with aging in adults, especially in women after menopause. In patients with vertebral osteoporosis, values are either normal or slightly elevated and poorly correlated with bone formation determined by iliac crest histomorphometry (2, 3). Also, a moderate increase of serum alkaline phosphatase is ambiguous as it may reflect a mineralization defect in elderly patients, or the effect of one of the numerous medications which have been shown to increase the hepatic isoenzyme of alkaline phosphatase. In an attempt to improve the specificity and the sensitivity of serum alkaline phosphatase measurement, techniques have been developed to differentiate the bone and the liver isoenzymes which only differ by posttranslational modifications as they are coded by a single gene. These techniques rely on the use of differentially effective activators and inhibitors (heat, phenylalanine and urea), separation by electrophoresis and separation by specific antibodies (4-6). In general, these assays have slightly enhanced the sensitivy of this marker, but most of them are indirect and/or technically cumbersome. A real improvement should be obtained by using a monoclonal antibody recognizing the bone but not the liver and kidney isoenzyme, a reagent likely to be available in a near future.

Serum bone gla-protein (BGP)

BGP, also called osteocalcin, is a small non collagenous protein specific for bone tissue and dentin, the precise function of which remains unknown (7). BGP is predominantly synthesized by the osteoblasts and incorporated into the extracellular matrix of bone but a fraction of neosynthesized BGP is released into the circulation where it can be measured by radioimmunoassay (8-10). Because antibodies directed against bovine BGP cross react with human BGP, most systems have been developed with bovine BGP as a tracer, standard and immunogen. Depending on the epitopes recognized by the antibody, some antisera may see -in addition to the intact molecule- fragments of BGP released during bone resorption in a high turnover state (11). In our experience, most polyclonal antibodies raised against the intact molecule do not recognize significant amounts of BGP fragments in serum (Figure 1). This pattern implies that such assays are specific markers of bone formation whenever formation and resorption are uncoupled, such as in multiple myeloma, but also in patients with vertebral osteoporosis (2, 12-14).

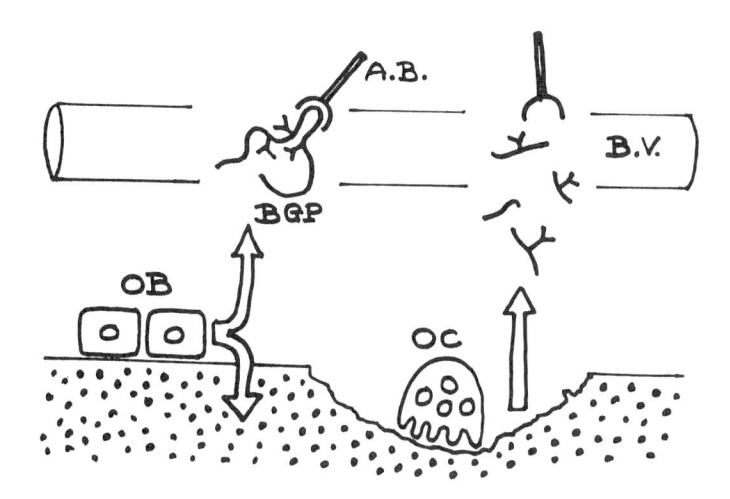

FIG. 1. Anti BGP antiserum which binds to the fraction of neosynthesized intact BGP released into the circulation but not to fragments of BGP released during osteoclastic bone resorption.
A.B. : anti-BGP antibody ; B.V. : blood vessel ; O.B. : osteoblast ;
O.C. : osteoclast

Serum BGP and aging.

In women, serum BGP increases gradually from the fourth to the tenth decade, along with a smaller but significant increase of serum alkaline phosphatase and urinary hydroxyproline (15). These increments reflect an age-related increase of bone turnover as recently demonstrated (16) by direct measurement on iliac crest biopsy from young normal women and from healthy elderly women who had passed their menopause 17 years ago (Table II). Superimposed on this age-related pattern, the menopause induces a

Table II. Bone turnover in young and healthy elderly women. From Eastell et al. (16)

	Younger women	Older women	P
N	12	11	
Age (yr)	36±3	66±1.3	
Serum BGP (ng/ml)	6.7±2.0	9.9±1.3	<0.01
Serum bone alkaline phosphatase	223±22	388±42	<0.01
Urinary hydroxyproline (mmol/dl GFR)	109±28	148±27	<0.005
Histomorphometry :			
- Bone Formation Rate (%/yr)	15.1±2.7	31.1±4.9	<0.01
- Active eroded surfaces (%)	1.84±0.95	2.89±0.95	<0.05

marked and transient acceleration of bone turnover with a two fold increase of serum BGP which can be reduced to premenopausal levels by estrogen therapy (17) (Table III). Two independent studies have shown that in untreated

Table III. Effect of estrogens (oestradiol valerate, 2 mg/day) on plasma BGP in early postmenopausal women (50±2.4 yr old). In 39 premenopausal women of the same age (49.7±2.6 yr), plasma BGP was 5.7±2.8 ng/ml.
From J.S. Johansen et al. (17)

	Plasma BGP (ng/ml)			
Group (n)	before	3 months	12 months	24 months
Estrogen (32)	10.5±3.4[a]	6.7±3.4[b]	5.3±2.7[b]	4.7±2.2[b]
Placebo (33)	12.0±6.6[a]	12.0±6.5[a]	12.9±6.3[a]	12.0±6.5[a]

[a] $p < 0.001$ vs premenopausal values [b] $p < 0.05-0.001$ vs initial values

post-menopausal women followed for 2 to 4 years, serum BGP is the best single biochemical marker reflecting the spontaneous rate of bone loss assessed by repeated measurements of the bone mineral content of the radius and of the spine (17, 18). Whether slow losers and fast losers of bone do so for a prolonged period of time after the menopause is debated, but the combination of bone mass measurement and assessment of bone turnover by a battery of specific markers is likely to be helpful in the future for the screening of patients at risk for osteoporosis who should be treated.

Serum BGP in vertebral osteoporosis

In patients with untreated vertebral osteoporosis, there is a wide scatter of individual values beyond the normal range reflecting the histological heterogeneity of the disease. Serum BGP is in the lower range of normals in patients with a low osteoblastic activity and significantly increased in the one third of patients having a high bone turnover. When serum BGP is compared with the bone remodeling activity measured on undecalcified iliac crest biopsy, there is a significant correlation with histological parameters reflecting bone formation but not with those reflecting resorption, both at the trabecular and the cortico-endosteal envelope (2, 19). Recognizing this variable level of bone turnover might be important for choosing the optimal therapy. Indeed, a recent study has shown that the subgroup of osteoporotic patients with high turnover -characterized by an increased whole body retention of Technetium-labelled diphosphonates and by increased serum BGP and urinary hydroxyproline- showed a significant increase of spinal bone mineral density after one year of calcitonine therapy. In contrast, those with low turnover had no increase of bone mass despite the same therapy (20). In patients treated with fluoride, the increase in serum BGP parallels the increase in bone mineral density of the spine (21). Finally, long-term corticosteroid treatment results in a marked inhibition of osteoblastic activity which is reflected by subnormal levels of serum BGP (22). The decrease of serum BGP is dependent on the daily dose of prednisone, can be observed even after a short term treatment and is not prevented by an exercise program (23). In those patients who had vertebral osteoporosis, we have found the same correlations with histological parameters as in primary osteoporosis, i.e. with formation and not resorption (12).

Procollagen I extension peptides.

During the extracellular processing of collagen I, there is a cleavage of the aminoterminal (p coll-I-N) and carboxyterminal (p coll-I-C) extension peptides prior to the fibril formation. These peptides circulate in blood where they might represent useful markers of bone formation, as collagen is by far the most abundant organic component of bone matrix. Using a radioimmunoassay for p coll-I-C, Simon et al. have shown that a single dose of 30 mg of prednisone suppresses serum p coll-I-C without decreasing urinary hydrxyproline suggesting that, indeed, circulating p coll-I-C reflects bone formation (24). In patients with vertebral osteoporosis serum p coll-I-C was found to be weakly correlated with histological bone formation, with r values ranging from 0.36 to 0.50 (25). An assay for p coll-I-N using a synthetic peptide as an immunogen has been recently reported (26) but data in osteoporosis are not yet available. It should be noted that, in contrast to what was initially believed, a fraction of p coll-I-N is incorporated into the bone matrix where it has been identified as the 24 K phosphoprotein of bone (27). Therefore, the release of fragments of p coll-I-N during resorption might be a source of serum immunoreactivity of p coll-I-N according to the epitope seen by a given antiserum. Clinical studies are necessary to assess the potential utility of procollagen I extension peptides in osteoporosis.

Other bone proteins.

Because of its hydroxyapatite and collagen-binding properties, and because its concentration is decreased in the bone of patients affected with a variety of osteogenesis imperfecta (28), osteonectin was regarded as an interesting potential marker of bone metabolism in osteoporosis. Osteonectin circulates in blood where it can be measured by radioimmunoassay (29). Unfortunately, platelets contain significant amounts of osteonectin that are secreted during thrombin stimulation, thus contributing largely to the levels detected in serum (30). The use of a monoclonal antibody recognizing osteonectin from bone but not from platelet origin might be useful and needs further investigation (31). Finally, there are other major bone related proteins, such as the sialoprotein I (osteopontin) and II which represent potential markers of osteoblastic activity.

BIOCHEMICAL MARKERS OF BONE RESORPTION.

Urinary hydroxyproline

Because free hydroxyproline released during degradation of collagen cannot be reutilized in collagen synthesis, its urinary excretion reflects the resorption of bone matrix which contains half of human collagen. As previously mentioned, urinary hydroxyproline increases with aging in normal women, if corrected by the glomerular filtration rate (15). Given the parallel decrease of bone mass, it implies a significant increase of the fraction of bone matrix which is resorbed with aging. This pattern is difficult to demonstrate by histomorphometry due to the limitation of histological methods assessing resorption rate but still can be shown if appropriate normal women are selected (Table II). In patients with vertebral osteoporosis, the mean value of urinary hydroxyproline is normal or slightly increased, but analysis of individual values show that up to 30% of patients have values above the normal range. Urinary hydroxyproline is poorly correlated with bone resorption assessed by calcium kinetics or bone histomorphometry, and there is an obvious need for a more sensitive marker of bone resorption.

Urinary hydroxylysine glycosides.

Like hydroxyproline, released hydroxylysine cannot be reutilized as it results from a posttranslational modification of lysine residues in collagen. The relative proportion and total content of galactosyl hydroxylysine and glucosyl-galactosyl hydroxylysine varies in bone and soft tissues which suggests that their urinary excretion might be a more sensitive marker of bone resorption than urinary hydroxyproline. Urinary galactosyl hydroxylysine increases with aging (32) and might be a useful marker in patients with osteoporosis (33).

Plasma tartrate-resistant acid phosphatase.

Tartrate-resistant acid phosphatase (TRAP) is abundant in osteoclasts and released into the circulation in which it corresponds to plasma isoenzyme 5. Plasma TRAP is increased in a variety of metabolic bone disorders with increased bone turnover (34) but its clinical utility in osteoporosis remains to be investigated. TRAP is a labile enzyme which can be decreased in stored frozen plasma samples and which can originate from blood cells, and these limitations should be kept in mind when analyzing the data obtained with this assay. The development of radioimmunoassay using monoclonal antibodies specifically directed against the bone isoenzyme should be valuable to assess the ability of plasma TRAP to predict osteoclastic bone resorption in osteoporotic patients.

Serum gamma-carboxyglutamic acid.

Gamma-carboxyglutamic acid (GLA) results from the vitamin K-dependent posttranslational modification of some glutamic acid residues in at least two bone proteins (BGP and matrix gla-protein), in some coagulation factors (factors II, VII, IX, X) and in plasma proteins C, S and Z. Increased levels of urinary GLA have been reported in patients with osteoporosis, but its significance has not been fully investigated (35). Using an original assay involving O-phthalaldehyde derivatization of plasma, reversed-phase high pressure liquid chromatography (HPLC) and detection of the GLA peak by fluorimetry, we have shown that free gla circulates in blood with a mean level in adults of 167±46 pmol/ml (36). Serum free gla is increased in patients with primary hyperparathyroidism and Paget's disease of bone. We have shown that serum free gla originates both from the metabolism of the vitamin K-dependent clotting factors and from bone metabolism (36) and that the fraction derived from bone is related to bone resorption and not to formation (unpublished data). However, because of its mixed origin, serum free gla is probably not sensitive enough to assess the subtle changes of bone resorption occuring in osteoporosis.

Urinary excretion of the collagen pyridinium crosslink.

Hydroxylysylpyridinoline (HP) and lysylpyridinoline (LP) are the two non reducible pyridinium crosslinks present in the mature form of collagen. This posttranslational covalent cross-linking generated from lysine and hydroxylysine residues is unique to collagen and elastin molecules. It creates interchain bonds which stabilize the molecule. The concentration of HP and LP in connective tissues is very low and varies dramatically with tissue type. HP is widely distributed in the type I collagen of bone and in the type II collagen of cartilage but is absent in skin collagen. Most interestingly, the LP form has only been found in the type I collagen of bone, at a concentration of 0.1-0.2 mol/mol of collagen, and not in cartilage, tendon, skin or cornea (37). We have purified HP and LP from human bone and developed an assay for total (free and peptide-bound) HP and LP in urine derived from previously published methods (37, 38). Because HP and LP are naturally fluorescent, they can be measured after reversed-phase HPLC of a cellulose-bound extract of hydrolyzed urine. With this assay, we have shown that urinary HP and LP represent a more sensitive marker of bone resorption than hydroxyproline in Paget's disease of bone and primary hyperparathyroidism (39). Some preliminary cross-sectional data indicate that there is a two fold increase of HP and LP at the menopause, contrasting with a milder increase of urinary hydroxyproline (Table IV).

Table IV. Urinary excretion of HP and LP pyridinium crosslinks and of hydroxyproline (OHP) in healthy young and postmenopausal women (w.)

groups	n	Age	OHP (mg/g creat)	HP (pmol/μmol creat)	LP
Young w.	12	29±4	37±14*	16±12	3.4±2.7
Postmenopausal. w.	9	55±3	58±16**	37±8***	8.2±2.4***

* mean ± 1 SD   ** $p < 0.01$ and   *** $p < 0.001$ vs young w.

CONCLUSION

There is not yet an ideal marker of bone formation but circulating BGP is the most satisfactory at the present time. New developments include the use of sheep BGP (40) and human BGP (41) as an immunogen, and monoclonal antibodies which may recognize fragments of BGP released during resorption (42). Unresolved questions include the volume of distribution of BGP, its metabolic clearance in human and the relative fraction of newly synthesized BGP incorporated into the matrix and released into the circulation which may vary in some diseases. The specific measurement of bone alkaline phosphatase, the assay of procollagen fragments and of other non collagenous bone-related proteins will allow in the future a more precise assessment of the complex osteoblastic functions in normal and pathological conditions. Finding a sensitive and specific marker of resorption is a challenge because all constituents of bone matrix are likely to be degraded into minute peptides during osteoclastic bone resorption. The measurement of pyridinium crosslinks and of TRAP by a bone-specific monoclonal antibody are the most tangible improvements in this area. These markers need to be validated by comparison with data obtained with direct measurement of bone turnover on iliac crest biopsy. It should be remembered, however, that circulating markers reflect the cellular activity of the whole skeleton, including cortical and trabecular bone and depend both on the number and on the activity of bone cells. Conversely, bone histomorphometry is limited to a small area of the trabecular envelope but allows to detect a specific defect at the cellular level. These differences should be kept in mind, as there is growing evidence that bone mass and bone turnover of osteoporotic patients before and during treatment varies in different appendicular/axial and cortical/trabecular compartments.

ACKNOWLEDGMENTS.

I am grateful to Dr B. Demiaux, B. Fournier, L. Malaval, and D. Uebelhart for their contribution, to E. Gineyts and B. Merle for excellent technical assistance. I thank Dr P.J. Meunier for his longstanding support and advice.

REFERENCES

1. P.D. Delmas in: Osteoporosis, B.L. Riggs and L.J. Melton, eds. (Raven Press, New York ,1988) pp. 297-316.
2. J.P. Brown, P.D. Delmas, L. Malaval, C. Edouard, M.C. Chapuy, and P.J. Meunier, Lancet i. 1091-1093 (1984).
3. J. Podenphant, J.S. Johansen, K. Thomsen, B.J. Riis, A. Leth, and C. Christiansen, J. Bone Min. Res. 2, 497-503 (1987).
4. D.W. Moss, Clin. Chem. 28, 2007-2016 (1982).
5. J.R. Farley, C.J. Chesnut, and D.J. Baylink, Clin. Chem. 27, 2002-2007 (1981).

6. R.J. Duda, J.F. O'Brien, J.A. Katzmann, J.M. Peterson, K.G. Mann and B.L. Riggs, J. Clin. Endocrinol. Metab. 66, 951-957 (1988).
7. P.A. Price in: Calcium Regulation and Bone Metabolism. Basic and Clinical Aspects, D.V. Cohn, T.J. Martin, and P.J. Meunier, eds. (Elsevier Science Publishers BV, 1987) vol. 9, pp. 419-426.
8. P.A. Price, M.K. Williamson, and J.W. Lothringer, J. Biol. Chem. 256, 12760-12766 (1981).
9. P.A. Price, J.G. Parthemore, and L.J. Deftos, J. Clin. Invest. 66, 878-883 (1980).
10. J.B. Lian, and C.M. Gundberg, Clin. Orthop. Rel. Res. 226, 267-291 (1988).
11. C. Gundberg, and R.S. Weinstein, J. Clin. Invest. 77, 1762-1767 (1986).
12. P.D. Delmas, L. Malaval, M.E. Arlot, and P.J. Meunier, Bone 6, 339-341 (1985).
13. P.D. Delmas, B. Demiaux, L. Malaval, M.C. Chapuy, C. Edouard, and P.J. Meunier, J. Clin. Invest. 77, 985-991 (1986).
14. R. Bataille, P. Delmas, and J. Sany, Cancer 59, 329-334 (1987).
15. P.D. Delmas, D. Stenner, H.W. Wahner, K.G. Mann, and B.L. Riggs, J. Clin. Invest., 71, 1316-1321 (1983).
16. R. Eastell, P.D. Delmas, S.F. Hodgson, E.F. Eriksen, K.G. Mann and B.L. Riggs, J. Clin. Endocrinol. metab. 67, 741-748 (1988).
17. J.S. Johansen, B.J. Riis, P.D. Delmas, and C. Christiansen, Eur. J. Clin. Invest. 18, 191-195 (1988).
18. C. Slemenda, S.L. Hui, C. Longcope and C.C. Johnston, J. Clin. Invest. 80, 1261-1269 (1987).
19. J.P. Brown, P.D. Delmas, M. Arlot, and P.J. Meunier, J. Clin. Endocrinol. Metab. 64, 954-959 (1987).
20. R. Civitelli, S. Gonnelli, F. Zacchei, S. Bigazzi, A. Vattimo, L.V. Avioli, and C. Gennari, J. Clin. Invest. 82, 1268-1274 (1988).
21. C.Y.C. Pak, K. Sakhaee, J.E. Zerwekh, C. Parcel, R. Peterson, and K. Johnson, J. Clin. Endocrinol. metab. 68, 150-159 (1989).
22. I.R. Reid, G.E. Chapman, T.R.C. Fraser, A.D. Davies, A.S. Surus, J. Meyer, N.L. Huq and H.K. Ibbertson, J. Clin. Endocrinol. Metab. 62, 376-383 (1986).
23. D.R. Garrel, P.D. Delmas, C. Welsh, M.J. Arnaud, S.E. Hamilton, and M.M. Pugeat, Metabolism 37, 257-262 (1988).
24. L.S. Simon, and S.M. Krane in: Clinical Disorders of Bone and Mineral Metabolism, B. Frame and J.T. Potts Jr., eds. (Excerpta Medica, Amsterdam 1983) pp. 108-111.
25. A.M. Parfitt, L.S. Simon, A.R. Villanueva, and S.M. Krane, J. Bone Min. Res. 2, 427-436 (1987).
26. M.E. Kraenzlin, S. Mohan, and D.J. Baylink, Europ. J. Clin. Invest. 19, A86 (1989).
27. L.W. Fisher, P.G. Robey, N. Tuross, A.S. Otsuka, D.A. Tepen, F.S. Esch, and S. Shimasaki, J. Biol. Chem. 262, 13457-13463 (1987).
28. L.W. Fisher, M.A. Drum, P.G. Robey, K.M. Conn, and J.D. Termine, Calcif. Tissue Int., 40, 260-264 (1987).
29. L. Malaval, B. Fournier, and P.D. Delmas, J. Bone Min. Res. 2, 457-465 (1987).
30. D.D. Stenner, P.T. Russel, B.L. Riggs, and K.G. Mann, Proc. Natl. Acad. Sci. 83, 6892-6896 (1986).
31. L. Malaval, B. Darbouret, C. Preaudat, J.P. Jolu and P.D. Delmas, J. Bone Min. Res. 3, S208 (1988).
32. L. Moro, R.S.P. Mucelli, C. Gazzarrini, C. Modricky, F. Marotti, and B. de Bernard, Calcif. Tissue Int. 42, 87-90 (1988).

33. L. Moro, C. Modricky, L. Rovis, and B. de Bernard, Bone Min. 3, 271-276 (1988).
34. J.J. Stepan, E. Silinkova-Malkova, T. Havrenek, J. Formankova, M. Zichova, J. Lachmanova, M. Strakova, P. Broulik, and V. Pacovsky, Clinica Chimica Acta 133, 189-200, (1983).
35. C.M. Gundberg, J.M. Lian, P.M. Gallop, and J.J. Steinberg, J. Clin. Endocrinol. Metab. 57, 1221-1225 (1983).
36. B. Fournier, E. Gineyts, and P.D. Delmas, Clinica Chemica Acta (in press).
37. D. Eyre in: Methods in Enzymology 144, 115-139 (1987).
38. D. Black, A. Duncan, and S.P. Robins, Anal. Biochem. 169, 197-203 (1988).
39. D. Uebelhart, E. Gineyts and P.D. Delmas, ASBMR-ICCRH meeting, Montreal, September 9-14 (1989).
40. P. Pastoureau, and P.D. Delmas, Calcif. Tissue Int. 44, S-85 (1989).
41. A.K. Taylor, S.G. Linkhart, S. Mohan, and D.J. Baylink, Metabolism 37, 872-877 (1988).
42. R.P. Tracy, M.L. Lamphere, B.L. Riggs and K.G. Mann in: Osteoporosis II, C. Christiansen, J.S. Johansen and B.J. Riss, eds. (Osteopress Aps, Kobenhaun, Denmark 1987) pp. 688-690.

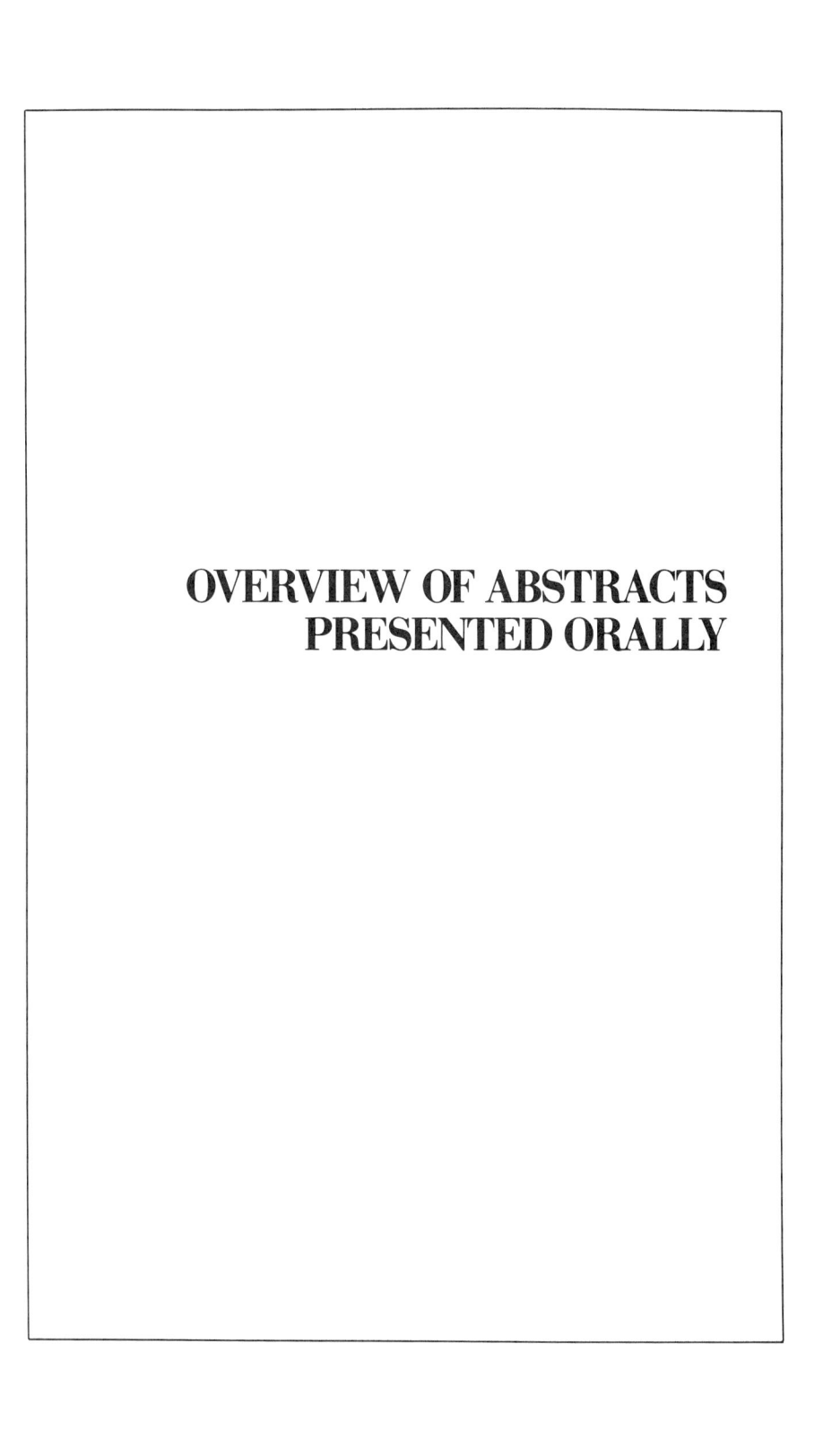

OVERVIEW OF ABSTRACTS PRESENTED ORALLY

Overview of Abstracts Presented at the Steenbock Symposium on Osteoporosis: Series 1—8:30 to 10:00—Tuesday, June 6, 1989

Lawrence G. Raisz

University of Connecticut Health Center, Farmington, Connecticut

In this session the selected papers were largely concerned with the role of sex hormones and vitamin D in the pathogenesis and treatment of osteoporosis. A clinical analysis of an unusual group of patients with acromegaly and varying degrees of hypogonadism was presented (Diamond, Neri and Posen, Abstract D04). These patients were used to assess the relative effects of growth hormone and its mediator, insulin-like growth factor (IGF-1), and sex hormones on bone. In acromegalics with high growth hormone and/or IGF-1 levels, forearm bone density was generally increased. However, in those subjects who are hypogonadal, bone density in the spine was decreased whether or not the growth hormone and IGF-1 levels were elevated. The fact that forearm and spinal bone density changed in opposite directions has important implications for the pathogenesis and treatment of osteoporosis. Presumably, the maintenance of trabecular bone requires gonadal steroids. Why high GH and IGF-1 levels did not oppose this effect remains to be determined, but suggests that if GH and IGF-1 are to be used to increase trabecular bone, this may require the presence of adequate levels of gonadal steroids.

The importance of sex hormones was further emphasized by a study comparing bone mass in young athletes with and without oligomenorrhea and in normal women who were being treated with oral contraceptives (Lloyd, Abstract L02). In the former group, as has been demonstrated previously, bone mass was lower in the oligomenorrheic than the eumenorrheic group and lowest in those who had had the fewest periods since menarche. In contrast, despite their low endogenous estrogen levels, women on oral contraceptives had normal bone mass. Presumably, this was due to an effect of the exogenous estrogen in these patients, since they received a dose of mestranol which was similar to that used previously to prevent bone loss after oophorectomy.

In two studies animal models of ovariectomy were used to assess the potential role of calcitriol and related compounds in preventing bone loss. In the dog, indirect evidence using bone biopsies showed that the initial bone loss after ovariectomy must have been due, at least in part, to increased bone resorption, but that this loss was maintained by decreased osteoblast function (Malluche et al., Abstract M02). Treatment with 1,25-dihydroxyvitamin D could reverse the bone loss, but after several months osteoblastic activity decreased, perhaps because of decreased activation of new bone remodeling units. In the rat, a novel vitamin D metabolite, 2β (3-hydroxypropoxy) calcitriol, was also shown to prevent the bone loss after ovariectomy and to be more potent than calcitriol (Takita et al., Abstract T01). This analog also appeared to mobilize calcium *in vivo* as well or better than calcitriol, although it was less effective *in vitro*. Clearly further studies of the possible selective effects of this and other vitamin D analogs on bone mass represent a fruitful approach for potential pharmacologic intervention in osteoporosis.

Another agent which has been widely studied in osteoporosis is calcitonin. Its use has been limited by the necessity for subcutaneous injection, so that the development of a form suitable for intranasal administration would represent an important advance. However, based on its effects on serum calcium, salmon calcitonin administered by the nasal route is substantially less potent than after parenteral administration (Vega et al., Abstract V01). Since the amounts of calcitonin required for effective treatment of osteoporosis have not been determined, it is possible that the lower levels and perhaps more prolonged presence of calcitonin after nasal administration could be adequate for prevention of bone loss in osteoporotic patients.

Another quite different but important clinical aspect of osteoporosis was examined in an epidemiologic study of hip fracture and falls (Hayes et al., Abstract H05). It was found that subjects who fell on the hip or side of the leg were most likely to fall, and that the average potential energy available in falls from a standing height is substantially more than the amount required to fracture a cadaveric hip in the biomechanics laboratory. This type of fall may be a substantially more significant component of hip fracture risk than has been presumed previously. Studies such as this, which identify some of the risk factors for falling and the types of falls which are most likely to cause hip fracture, can be used to develop preventive strategies which might help us to reduce the frequency of hip fracture which now results in substantial morbidity and mortality and represents a large health care cost. Further studies are needed to determine the relative contribution of age-related bone loss to fracturing in individuals who have "high risk" falls and assess the relative effectiveness of efforts to minimize such bone loss, as compared to efforts to reduce the frequency and severity of falls. It is possible that the exercise programs which were discussed elsewhere at the Steenbock Symposium could accomplish both goals by improving agility and balance as well as bone strength in the hip.

Overview of Abstracts Presented at the Steenbock Symposium on Osteoporosis: Series 2—8:30 to 10:00—Wednesday, June 7, 1989

Charles H. Chesnut III

University of Washington, Seattle, Washington

The second morning abstract session provided a number of interesting and occasionally controversial papers.

Dr. C. Marx described a retrospective, clinic-based controlled study assessing the effects of fluoride and estrogen in 92 postmenopausal osteoporotic women over 6 to 41 months, with assessment of bone mass by DPA. This interesting study concluded that estrogen increased spinal bone mineral density at a rate of 5.3%/year, with the benefit predominantly in the first 18 months of treatment. Most importantly, such beneficial effects of estrogen on bone mass were noted in women over age 65 (7.7%/year increase in BMD), roughly equivalent to the beneficial effect of estrogen in younger women. Further documentation of this potentially positive therapeutic information for elderly women is needed.

Dr. M. Tilyard then described a family practice-oriented clinical trial of the effects of calcitriol vs. calcium alone in 626 postmenopausal osteoporotic women. The primary efficacy endpoint in this ongoing study is vertebral fracture rate, or loss of anterior vertebral height. Preliminary assessment of the data indicated a preservation of anterior height in the calcitriol group, although no difference in recurrent vertebral fracture was noted between the two groups. Side effects of a dosage of .5 mcg per day of calcitriol were minimal. The study, indicating potential benefit of calcitriol without significant side effects, needs to be compared with other studies that failed to show efficacy at lower doses and others showing efficacy at higher dosages. Quite obviously, more information is needed on calcitriol's effects on bone mass of osteoporotic women.

Dr. M. Parfitt then presented a somewhat disturbing paper on the effects of sodium fluoride on vertebral fracture rate in 21 postmenopausal osteoporotic women, followed prospectively in an uncontrolled clinical trial. Intermittent sodium fluoride plus calcium therapy was not associated with a decrease in vertebral fractures. Most worrisome, and the true "pearl" of the study, was the fact that BMC by DPA improved during this study, but as noted, was not associated with a decrease in fracture rate, implying that assessment of bone mass quantity alone cannot be used to assess such therapies as sodium fluoride which may affect not only quantity but quality of bone.

Dr. T. Fujita then described a clinical trial of a new calcium preparation from Japan, oyster shell electrolysate, demonstrating the beneficial effect of this agent in a controlled study over 12 months. An improvement of radial cortical bone mass of 7% and of spinal trabecular bone mass (QCT-determined) of 6% after 12 months was noted, compared to losses in the control group. Such a study confirms other currently available information, demonstrating a stabilizing effect of increased calcium intake on bone mass in elderly osteoporotic women.

The actions of exogenous parenteral parathyroid hormone (synthetic 1-38 fragment) in osteoporotic patients was then described by Dr. A. Hodsman. In this study, significant increases in serum $1,25(OH)_2D$ and GI calcium absorption were noted, as well as expected increases in serum calcium, urinary phosphate, urinary cyclic AMP, urinary hydroxyproline, and serum alkaline phosphatase, and decreases in serum phosphate. Assessment by the authors of the latter changes were felt to reflect changes in bone resorption and formation, rather than changes responding to the increases in GI calcium absorption. As parenterally administered PTH has a therapeutic role in some osteoporotic patients, the above information regarding renal and skeletal responses to its usage is of value.

Lastly, Dr. G. Dalsky provided a "change of pace" from the previous abstracts, which had dealt primarily with treatment of osteoporosis. Dr. Dalsky noted that axial and total body bone mineral density were determined (predicted) more by fat-free (muscle) mass and specific muscular strength parameters than by aerobic power or body mass index. The study was performed on male runners and power-lifters. Such data provide further information on the relationships between muscle strength, bone mass, exercise intensity, etc.; relationships which have obvious effects upon clinical osteoporosis.

ESTROGEN

Estrogens in Prevention and Treatment of Osteoporosis

Robert Lindsay[*†] and Jack Tohme[†]

[*]*Helen Hayes Hospital, Regional Bone Center, West Haverstraw, New York*
[*†]*Department of Medicine, Columbia University, College of Physicians and Surgeons, New York, New York*

ABSTRACT

Numerous studies using a variety of techniques have demonstrated that failure of ovarian function increases skeletal remodeling, which results in acceleration of bone loss. Usually these phenomena follow menopause and oophorectomy, but occur also in other situations such as hypothalamic amenorrhea. There is general acceptance that estrogen therapy specifically prevents bone loss in this situation. The minimum effective dose is conjugated equine estrogen (as Premarin) 0.625mg/day or equivalent. The route of administration appears not to be important so long as serum 17 beta-estradiol levels in the mid-follicular range are achieved. The effects persist for as long as therapy is provided (at least 10 years), and result in reduction in fracture risk of about 50% for fractures of the hip and distal radius to perhaps as much as 90% for vertebral crush fractures. The addition of a progestogen does not appear to significantly affect the response of the skeleton to estrogen. Estrogens may also be successfully used in the treatment of established osteoporosis where prevention of further bone loss can be achieved with often small but significant increases in bone mass. Estrogen remains the single most potent agent for prevention and treatment of postmenopausal osteoporosis, although other agents such as calcitonin and diphosphonates are alternates for those who cannot or will not take estrogen therapy.

INTRODUCTION

Albright's original observations on osteoporosis first highlighted the importance of loss of ovarian steroids in the pathogenesis of osteoporosis (1). He also suggested more than 40 years ago that estrogens could be used therapeutically for this disorder (2). Although considerable data have been accumulated and published since then, there is still some confusion about the relationship between sex hormones and estrogen in particular and the skeleton. The evidence presented here will highlight the importance of estrogen loss in the pathogenesis of osteoporosis and the efficacy of these hormones in prevention and treatment of bone loss among the aging female population.

Copyright 1990 by Elsevier Science Publishing Co., Inc.
Osteoporosis: Physiological Basis, Assessment, and Treatment
Hector F. DeLuca and Richard Mazess, Editors

The Effects of Estrogen Deprivation

Many studies have demonstrated that bone mass among females is fairly constant at most skeletal sites until the 5th decade and then begins to decline at all skeletal sites. This fall coincides with the gradual onset of ovarian failure and declining estrogen production (3). Recent studies have demonstrated that there is gradual reduction in bone mass that accompanies the decline in estrogen production by the ovary, prior to the overt menopause (4). In our early studies, designed to examine the relative importance of loss of ovarian function, we were able to demonstrate reduced bone mass within three years of oophorectomy, with no equivalent loss in hysterectomized women with intact ovarian function (Figure 1,

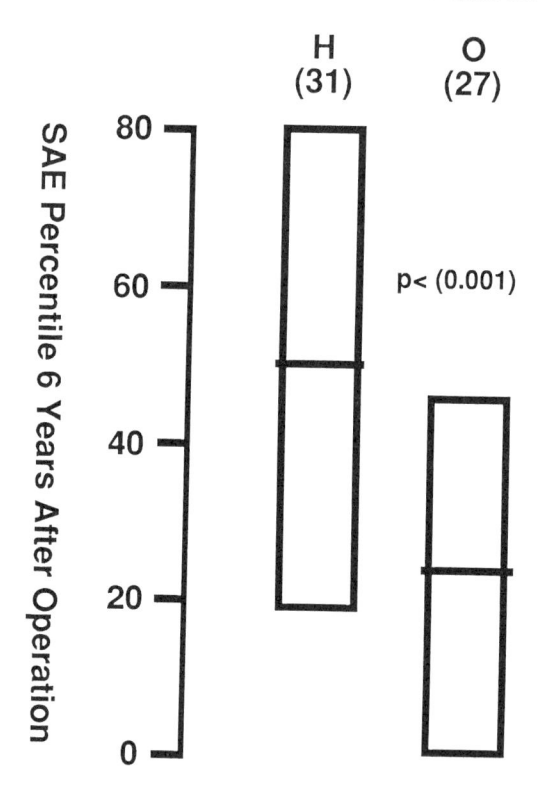

1. Bone loss in women after oophorectomy. The left hand panel demonstrates bone mass in hysterectomized oophorectomized women compared with hysterectomized women whose ovarian function was conserved 3 years after surgery.

ref 5). In a differently designed but some what similar study the Mayo Clinic group examined the reduction in bone mass in women 20 years after oophorectomy and demonstrated that bone mass in that group was equivalent to bone mass in 70 year old women, even though the mean age of the oophorectomized group was only 50 years (6). Thus loss of ovarian function appears more important a determinant of bone loss than age.

Prospective studies also suggest that bone loss accelerates after ovarian failure, the period of increased bone loss being 2-10 years depending on the individual and the bone that is measured. However, although bone loss slows, it remains sensitive to estrogen intervention demonstrating the dependence of rate of loss on remaining estrogen status (7). Bone mass at the time of menopause can now be demonstrated to be an important determinant of bone mass in later life, which in turn is the major determinant of fracture risk (8). Thus, those individuals with lowest bone mass at the time of ovarian failure may also be those most at risk of fracture in later life.

The changes in bone mass that occur across menopause are accompanied by alterations in calcium homeostasis (9-11). The efficiency of calcium absorption across the intestine declines. Urinary calcium rises, and net calcium loss from the body is increased (12). Indicators of bone turnover in serum and urine, alkaline phosphatase, osteocalcin, and hydroxyproline are also increased. These changes suggest that the primary effects of estrogen deficiency occur within the skeleton, and the alterations in calcium homeostasis are secondary to an intrinsic change in skeletal metabolism.

Bone loss appears to accompany estrogen deficiency at any point in life. Thus situations which create reduced hypothalamic-pituitary-ovarian function appear also to predispose to osteoporosis. Included in this category are exercise induced amenorrhea (13-15), hyperprolactinemia when accompanied by reduced ovarian function (16), and the amenorrhea of weight loss as in Anorexia Nervosa or Bulimia. Turner's Syndrome with congenital absence of functional ovarian tissue is also associated with osteoporosis at a young age, although in part the problem appears prior to the normal age of menarche and may be part of the congenital syndrome as well as consequent upon the failure to produce estrogen (17-18). In males the presence of Klinefelter's syndrome or loss of testicular function appears to increase the risk of osteoporosis (19), and thus sex hormones in general may play an important role in determining the status of the skeleton. The role of androgens in the female has not been evaluated although progestogens may be important.

The rate of bone loss in the postmenopausal female is dependent on the supply of endogenous estrogen. We demonstrated this biochemically several years ago (20) and more recently confirming data on bone mass have been published (28). The estrogen levels that are associated with virtual elimination of bone loss are within the physiological premenopausal range probably lying close to 40-100pg/ml, for 17 beta-estradiol. The precise level at which bone loss is completely inhibited may vary both with individuals and with skeletal site.

The Effect of Estrogen

The introduction of estrogen replacement therapy has been shown in a variety of studies to prevent the loss of bone that follows menopause. In our long term controlled studies (21-25), initially double-blind, we have demonstrated that prevention of bone loss lasts for as long as estrogens are provided, at least ten years (Figure 2), and that inhibition of loss occurs at all skeletal sites (Figure 3). It is clear that bone loss is prevented at sites (25) at which osteoporotic fracture occur especially the spine and femoral neck. Preservation of total body bone mass has also been demonstrated in the elegant studies from Christiansen's group, using a variety of estrogen preparations and routes of administration (26,27).

The skeleton appears, perhaps not surprisingly, to be extremely sensitive to exogenous estrogen therapy. The minimum effective dose (24) is 0.625mg/day conjugated equine estrogen (as Premarin). It appears as though, if sufficient estrogen can be supplied to provide circulating 17beta-estradiol levels equivalent to those obtained in the mid to late follicular phase of the regular cycle, then the method by which that estrogen is delivered is inconsequential.

The proof of the importance of estrogen was confirmed by our demonstration that cessation of therapy results in restoration of bone loss (28). Epidemiological data have demonstrated that estrogen therapy reduces the risk of fractures of the femoral neck and distal radius (29-32). The majority of the data suggest that there will be a risk reduction of at least 50%, provided estrogen treatment is initiated within a short period after menopause and continued for at least 5 years. Delaying bone loss it can be suggested will delay the rise in hip fracture risk beyond current life expectancy. Estrogen treatment in our prospective studies also reduced vertebral deformities assessed by lateral radiographs, by about 90%. Thus estrogen remains the best documented agent for prevention of postmenopausal osteoporosis.

The introduction of estrogen reduces bone turnover and inhibits bone resorption. Since these effects can be seen in any population of postmenopausal women at least up to the age of seventy years, estrogen therapy can be used as treatment of established osteoporosis. In this situation further bone loss is prevented and the skeletal status is stabilized (Table 1). In our study of postmenopausal osteoporotic women we evaluated the effects of estrogen (Premarin 0.625mg/day) prescribed with calcium supplementation to give a total intake of 1500mg/day compared with calcium given by itself. Women with an intact uterus were also given a progestogen (Provera 5mg/day for two weeks each calendar month. Bone mass was measured by dual photon absorptiometry at the lumbar spine and hip with corrections for source strength as we have described previously (33). The patients were randomly assigned to therapeutic groups, but turned out to be fairly well matched for age, height, weight, and years from menopause. The results are summarized in the table. Bone mass in the lumbar spine increased in the estrogen treated group compatible with relatively sudden inhibition of resorption while the osteoblast population continue to work and fill in the remodeling space. In contrast the calcium treated group lost bone. Similar but less marked effects were seen in the femoral neck.

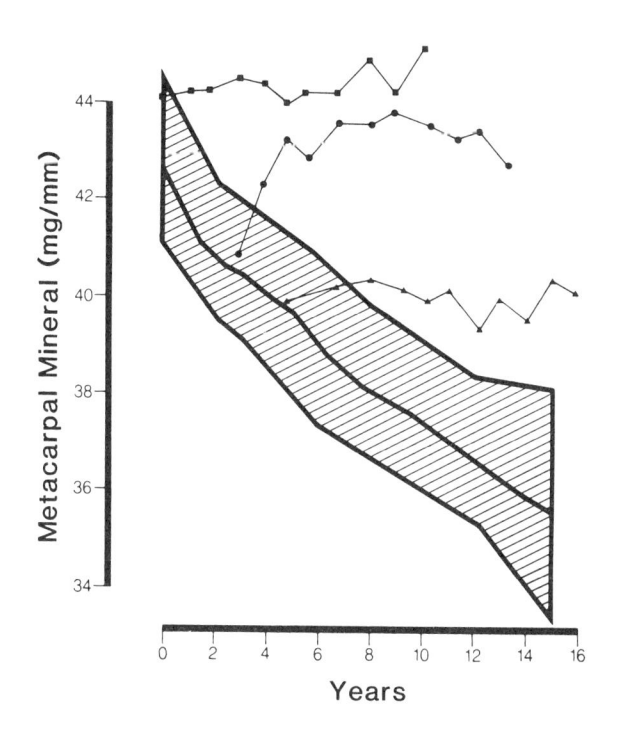

2. The effects of mestranol on bone mass in three groups of women in whom treatment was begun immediately, 3 years or 6 years after complete oophorectomy. The hatched area represents the pattern of bone loss in the placebo treated groups (mean + SD), while only the means of the three estrogen treated groups are shown.

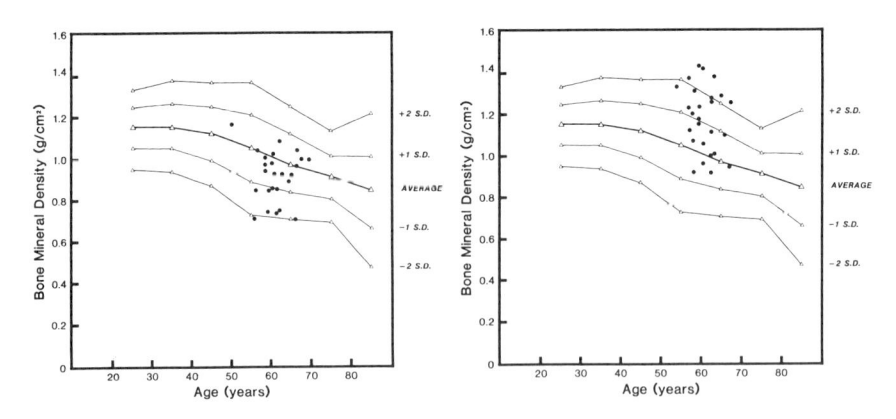

3. Lumbar bone mass in postmenopausal women treated with placebo for 10 years (left hand panel) and estrogen (right hand panel). Data from the patients are plotted in the normal distribution of bone mass with age from our institution.

TABLE 1

Bone Mass in Patients with Osteoporosis Treated with Estrogen (Group E) plus Calcium or Calcium alone (Group C).

	n	Lumbar Spine (gm/cm2)		Femoral Neck (gm/cm2)	
		Initial	Final	Initial	Final
Group E	22	0.85±0.03	0.92±0.05	0.61±0.03	0.64±0.04
Group C	20	0.86±0.04	0.79±0.04	0.65±0.05	0.61±0.03
		$p<0.01$		n.s.	

CONCLUSIONS

Estrogen therapy has a proven place in the prevention of postmenopausal bone loss. These effects have been demonstrated in multiple studies from many investigators. Since the skeletal effects of estrogen can be seen whenever estrogens are introduced to an estrogen deficient woman, these hormones also have a role to play in the treatment of the established disease. Studies have demonstrated that this is sufficient to reduce fracture recurrence.

At present, especially in the USA the use of an estrogen preparation in women with an intact uterus requires the addition of a progestogen to protect against the deleterious long-term effects of unopposed estrogen on the endometrium. The does not interfere in any way with the effects of estrogen on the skeleton, but does result in the return of menses, which reduces compliance among the older female population. In our group, estrogens are usually prescribed orally (0.625 mg Premarin or its equivalent) or by another route such as percutaneously or transdermally, provided circulating estradiol levels can be maintained in the midfollicular range. Estrogens are given continuously and for women with an intact uterus, a progestogen (Provera 5mg per day) is added for 12-14 days each month. We prefer to start the progestogen on the first day of each calendar month and continue for two weeks (36). If bleeding begins before the eleventh day of the month we increase the progestogen dose. All women should be followed by a gynecologist, and should follow guidelines for mammography appropriate to their age range (In USA we advise mammography before initiating treatment and annually there after if the patient is over 50 years).

In deciding who to treat, the judicious use of bone mass measurements is of value for asymptomatic patients. Reduced bone mass at the time of menopause probably indicates an individual who is at increased risk of osteoporosis. For those women who cannot or do not wish to take estrogen treatment, since estrogens are potent hormones that have multiple effects in the body, alternatives are becoming available. The best documented is calcitonin which has the advantage that it affects only the skeleton. Diphosphonates also fall into this category. For the first time the physician is faced with alternatives for the prevention and treatment of osteoporosis and can tailor treatment to the requirements of the patient.

Mechanism of Estrogen Action

Until recently estrogen receptors had not been detected in cells derived from bone, and it was assumed that estrogen action on the skeleton was mediated indirectly. The most popular hypothesis suggested that estrogen stimulated the production of endogenous calcitonin and that calcitonin was responsible for the inhibition of bone turnover that was seen after estrogen treatment. Indeed some data suggest do that calcitonin may well be an intermediary in the estrogen effect. Secretion of calcitonin from medullary carcinoma cells can be stimulated in vitro by low levels of estrogen. It has been shown that circulating calcitonin levels are lower in women than in men and tend to fall with age. However, in some laboratories calcitonin levels have been shown to be increased in patients with osteoporosis, the opposite of expectation if calcitonin is indeed a mediator of estrogen action, and clearly further data are required on this issue.

The recent demonstration that osteoblasts and osteoblast-like cells may express estrogen receptors has renewed the argument for a direct effect of estrogen on the skeleton (37,38). Osteoblasts in addition seem to respond physiologically to low levels of estrogen by increasing alkaline phosphatase, mRNA for procollagen and growth alterations. However, the effects of estrogen in vivo are compatible with reductions in bone remodeling, perhaps by reducing activation of new remodeling cycles, and also reduction in the activity of osteoclasts. As far as we know at present osteoclasts, the cells responsible for bone resorption do not appear to have estrogen receptors, although they have been insufficiently studied as yet. These cells appear only to be target cells for calcitonin, at least of the generally circulating hormones. If this is confirmed we must postulate a second messenger relaying information from the osteoblast to the osteoclast population. Possibilities include interleukin 1, transforming growth factor-beta, or prostaglandins, all of which can modulate osteoclast activity. Several indirect sources of evidence can be brought to support each of these factors.

REFERENCES

1. F. Albright, F. Bloomberg, and P.H. Smith, Trans. Assoc. Am. Phys. 55, 298-305 (1940).
2. F. Albright, Recent Prog. Horm. Res. 1, 293-353 (1947).
3. R. Lindsay in: Osteoporosis: Etiology, Diagnosis, and Management, B.L. Riggs and L.J. Melton III, eds. (Raven Press, New York 1988) pp. 333-358.
4. C.C. Johnson, S.L. Hui, R.M. Witt, R. Appledorn, R.S. Baker, and C. Longcope, J. Clin. Endocrinol. Metab. 61, 905-911 (1985).
5. J.M. Aitken, D.M. Hart, J.B. Anderson, R. Lindsay, and D.A. Smith, Brit. Med. J. i, 325-328 (1973).
6. L.S. Richelson, H.W. Wahner, L.J. Melton, and B.L. Riggs, N. Engl. J. Med. 311, 1273-1275 (1984).
7. C. Slemenda, S.L. Hui, C. Longcope, and C.C. Johnson, J. Clin. Invest. 80, 1261-1269 (1987).
8. S.L. Hui, W. Slemenda, and C.C. Johnston, J. Clin. Invest. 81, 1804-1809 (1988).
9. R.P. Heaney, R.R. Recker, and P.D. Saville, Am. J. Clin. Nutr. 30, 1603-1611 (1978).
10. R.P. Heaney, R.R. Recker, and P.D. Saville, J. Lab. Clin. Med. 92, 953-963 (1978).
11. R.P. Heaney, R.R. Recker, and P.D. Saville, J. Lab. Clin. Med. 92, 964-970 (1978).
12. I. Fogelman, J.W. Poser, M.L. Smith, D.M. Hart, and J.A. Bevan in: Osteoporosis, C. Christiansen, ed. (Aalborg, Denmark 1984) pp. 519-522.
13. C.E. Cann, M.C. Martin, and H.K. Genant, J. Am. Med. Assoc. 251, 626-629 (1984).
14. B.D. Drinkwater, K.L. Nilson, and C.H. Chesnut III, N. Eng. J. Med. 311, 277-281 (1984).
15. E.R. Gonzalez, J. Am. Med. Assoc. 248, 513-514 (1982).
16. A. Klibanski, R.M. Neer, I.Z. Beitins, C. Ridway, N.T. Zervas, and J. MacArthur, N. Engl. J. Med. 303, 1511-1514 (1980).
17. D.J. Barr, Arch. Dis. Child. 49, 821-822 (1974).
18. F.A. Conte, M.M. Grumbach, S.L. Kaplan, J. Clin. Endocrinol. Metab. 40, 670-674 (1975).
19. D.A.S. Smith and M.S. Walker, Calcif. Tissue Res. 22, 225-228 (1976).

20. R. Lindsay, J.R.T. Coutts, and D.M. Hart, Clin. Endocrinol. 6, 87-93 (1977).
21. R. Lindsay, G.M. Aitken, J.B. Anderson, D.M. Hart, E.B. MacDonald, and A.C. Clark, Lancet ii, 1038-1041 (1976).
22. R. Lindsay, D.M. Hart, P. Purdie, M.M. Ferguson, A.C. Clark, and A. Kraszewski, Clin. Sci. Mol. Med. 54, 193-195 (1978).
23. R. Lindsay, D.M. Hart, C. Forrest, and C. Baird, Lancet ii, 1151-1154 (1980).
24. R. Lindsay, D.M. Hart, and D.M. Clark, Obstet. Gynecol. 63, 759-763 (1984).
25. F. Al-Azzawi, D.M. Hart, and R. Lindsay, Br. Med. J. 1261-1262 (1987).
26. C. Christiansen, M.S. Christiansen, and P. McNcir, Europ. J. Clin. Invest. 10, 273-279 (1980).
27. C. Christiansen and P. Rodbro, Calcit. Tiss. Int. 35, 720-722 (1983).
28. R. Lindsay, D.M. Hart, A. McLean, A.C. Clark, A. Kraszewski, and J. Garwood, Lancet ii, 1325-1327 (1978).
29. B. Ettinger, H.K. Genant, and C.E. Cann, Ann. Intern. Med. 102, 319-324 (1985).
30. T.A. Hutchinson, J.M. Polansky, and A.R. Feinstein, Lancet ii, 705-709 (1979).
31. N. Kreiger, J.L. Kelsey, and T.R. Holford, Am. J. Epidemiol. 116, 141-148 (1982).
32. N.S. Weiss, C.L. Ure, and J.H. Ballard, N. Engl. J. Med. 303, 1195-1198 (1980).
33. R. Lindsay, A. Haboubi, and C. Fey, Calc. Tiss. Intl. 41, 293-294 (1987).

Prevention of Postmenopausal Bone Loss by Long-Term Parenteral Administration of 17β Estradiol: Comparison of Percutaneous and Transdermal Route

C. Ribot, F. Tremollieres, and J.M. Pouilles

Bone Mineral Unit, Endocrinology Department, CHU Purpan, Toulouse, France

ABSTRACT

This study aimed to evaluate the long term efficacy of parenterally administered 17ß estradiol (17ß E2) on postmenopausal bone loss. A two years prospective study was conducted in 94 early postmenopausal women, divided into 3 groups comparable for age, interval since menopause, height and weight: untreated group (U): n=31, Transdermal group (T): n=25, Percutaneous group (P): n=38. Treatment consisted of either 50 µg/d of transdermal 17ß E2, or 1.5 mg/d of percutaneous 17ß E2 (1 dose), 3 weeks monthly associated the last ten days of the estradiol cycle with an oral gestagen. Vertebral bone density (BMD - g/cm2) was measured by DPA (DP3 - Lunar Rad Corp) before, then every 6 months in treated women and every year in the untreated group. After 2 years, at the group level, BMD increased significantly in treated women (p<0.001, paired t test), without any differences between P (5.02%) and T (4.42%). In U a mean decrease of 4.4% (p<0.001) was observed during the same period. Mean concentrations of plasma E2 were in the same range in the treated groups (P: 62 to 69 pg/ml vs T: 44 to 55 pg/ml), with higher variations in the P group (SD: 45 to 65 pg/ml) than in the T group (SD: 22 to 30 pg/ml). The metabolic tolerance was the same in the two treated groups. The study of the individual rates of bone changes, using regression linear analysis versus time, showed that 13% of women in P (n=5), and 4% in T (n=1) had a significant bone loss after 2 years of treatment. These results indicate that the cutaneous way (percutaneous or transdermal) enables to prevent post menopausal bone loss, while maintaining a physiological level (early follicular phase) of plasma E2, and whithout the adverse metabolic effects related to the oral route. However a higher percentage of "non response" was observed using the percutaneous way, which in our experience could be related to the individual variations of the dose applied to the skin due to this mode of administration. On the other hand, some cutaneous reactions were observed in a few cases with the transdermal system.

INTRODUCTION

Postmenopausal administration of estrogens cannot be systematic. When it is necessary, in particular for osteoporosis prevention, this treatment must be continued for several years, be efficient and well-tolerated.
- The efficiency of prolonged administration of estrogens,

whatever the way of administration, on postmenopausal bone loss [1-4] and the subsequent risk of osteoporotic fractures (Colle's, hip fractures and vertebral crush fractures) is no longer the subject of debate.

Long-term tolerance is however a matter of controversy. Even in the absence of formal contraindications (such as the risk of breast cancer), postmenopausal use of estrogens remains limited for fear of the metabolic effects liable to increase the atherogenous risk in a population which is spontaneously exposed due to its age [5]. This is all the more so as the addition of certain progestogens (19-nor steroid derivatives), necessary to prevent the risk of endometrium cancer [6], is liable to add its own negative effects on lipid and carbohydrate metabolism [7].

Long-term tolerance to estrogen therapy must be considered with two essential parameters in mind: the chemical nature of the steroid used and the way of administration.

- Estrogens do not all have the same chemical structure, but act by the same mechanism at the cellular level: in the target cells, the hormone/cytoplasmic receptor complex is transferred to the nucleus where it binds with the chromatin. This binding is highly specific and the retention time in the nucleus, measured by means of dissociation constant, is a key factor in the cellular action mechanism of steroids. The comparison between three estrogens with different structures, at the level of the human endometrium receptors shows that, with respect to human estrogen, 17ß estradiol, 17ß dihydroequilinin, a conjugated estrogen of equine origin or ethynil estradiol have dissociation constants 5 to 10 times shorter, and therefore a more prolonged cellular action [8].

- The second point involves the means of administration: oral administration is by far the most common method. However, the low level of gastric absorption and the intestinal metabolism of steroids impose the use of doses or of estrogen molecules liable, due to their first-pass liver effect, to induce undesirable metabolic effects. Furthermore, this administration method results in a preferential metabolism of the estradiol into estrone. Parenteral administration, in particular cutaneous (transdermic or percutaneous) has the advantage of delivering a lower concentration of estradiol into the general circulation, of avoiding the first-pass liver and of maintaining an estradiol/estrone ratio corresponding to the premenopausal phase.

- Two types of cutaneous administration can be used at present, percutaneous or transdermal.

- Percutaneous administration has been used in France since 1975. The 17 ß estradiol is presented in the form of a gel (Oestrogel®, Besins-Iscovesco Laboratories). Each tube contains 80 g of gel, i.e. 48 mg of 17 ß estradiol. The use of a strip enables 2.5 or 5 g gel to be delivered, i.e. 1.5 or 3 mg of 17 ß estradiol. The gel is applied to the skin of the abdomen, the arms, shoulders or any other part of the body except the breasts. It must be applied fairly rapidly over a large surface. The application technique, which is very important for bio-availability, must be carefully explained to the patient who must be capable of accomplishing it correctly.

- Transdermal administration, a more recent development, is based on the use of a transdermal system or "patch" (TTS-E2 or Estraderm®, Ciba-Geigy Laboratories) which contains the estradiol in an alcohol gel solution in a reservoir. This reservoir consists of a transparent, impermeable external membrane and an internal membrane that controls estradiol release. Contact with the surface of the skin is established by a hypoallergenic adhesive substance.

3 different doses of TTS-E2 are available with different surface areas (5, 10 or 20 cm^2) and deliver doses of 0.025, 0.05 and 0.1 mg/day estradiol respectively. The system is applied to the skin of the lower abdomen or of the buttocks and has to be changed twice weekly. Following application of the system, estradiol level rises rapidly and stabilizes at mean values of 25, 50 or 75 pg/ml respectively for the 3 systems.

Advances in pharmacology mean that postmenopausal women can now be proposed a substitutive hormone therapy which is is as close as possible to the physiological conditions of ovarian production. This treatment is based on the use of the human hormone - 17 ß estradiol - administered parenterally, associated with natural progesterone or synthetic progestogens without androgenic effects but with a potent action on the endometrium. However, the efficiency of and tolerance to this type of administration are not as well documented as for oral administration.

In a prospective 2-year study the effect on vertebral post menopausal bone loss of these 2 types of administration was compared to that of untreated women monitored for the same period of time.

POPULATION AND METHODS

1 - Population :

The women who participated in this study were recruited from those sent to the menopause clinic for therapeutic proposal. All were early postmenopausal women, for 5 years at the most (mean 2.4 years). Their menopausal status was confirmed by an estradiol level lower than 20 pg/ml, and FSH level higher than 30 mU/ml and a progesterone test when necessary. They satisfied the same selection criteria (table 1).

Table 1: Criteria for selection

	Hormone Groups	Comparison group
Inclusion :		
ISM	Postmenopausal	Postmenopausal
Progesterone test	> 6 months	> 6 months
Plasma E2	no bleeding	no bleeding
FSH (mU/ml)	< 20 pg/l	< 20 pg/l
	> 30	> 30
Exclusion :	Counter indications to ERT	
	Obesity, osteoporosis	Obesity, osteoporosis
	Osteoarthrosis	Osteoarthrosis
	Chronic disease	Chronic disease
	No treatment with sex hormones or drug known to influence calcium and bone metabolism	No treatment with sex hormones or drug known to influence calcium and bone metabolism

- Following detailed questioning, clinical and biological examination, 110 women entered this study between January and December 1986. They were divided into 3 groups: (U): untreated (n = 36), (P): percutaneous treatment (n = 43), (T): Transdermic treatment (n = 31). The women were not randomly assigned, but allocated to the different groups according to contraindications to hormonal treatment and/or their personal choice.
31/36, 38/43 and 25/31 subjects in groups (U), (P) and (T) respectively were monitored for 2 years. Their clinical characteristics and initial bone mineral density values are given in table 2.

Table 2: Clinical characteristics and initial bone mass values.

	Untreated group (n = 31)	Percutaneous group (n=38)	Transdermal group (n = 25)
AGE (yr)	52.3±8.6	51.7±4.5	50.7±4.3
ISM (yr)	2.2±1.4	2.6±2.3	2.4±1.5
HEIGHT (cm)	159.8±5.8	159.2±5.3	162±6.3
WEIGHT (kg)	57.1±6.0	56.2±6.6	57.7±6.1
Bilateral Oophorectomy	3	6	11
BMD (g/cm2)	1.048±0.07	0.953±0.12*°	1.003±0.12*°

(m±SD) * $p < 0.001$ vs Untreated, ° NS within Treated women

. Percutaneous treatment was based on the application of one "dose" of gel per day (2.5 g, i.e. 1.5 mg estradiol), 3 weeks out of 4, after carefully explaining the prescription to the patient. As for transdermal treatment, a system delivering 0.05 mg/day was used, with twice-weekly change of the patch, 3 weeks out of 4. The last 10 days of the estradiol cycle were associated with administration of natural progesterone (200 mg/day) or dihydrogesterone (20 mg/day) or promegestone (250 mcg/day).
. The treated women were submitted to a clinical examination, blood and urine sampling before treatment and then every 6 months during two years.
Bone mass measurements were performed every 6 month in the treated women and every 12 months in the untreated women.

2 - Methods
- Biological measurements:
Serum estradiol was measured by radioimmunoassay using commercially available kits (3-H Estradiol Kit, Bio-Merieux France). The assay detection limit was 20 pg/ml with an intraassay and interassay variation of 8.3 ± 2.6 % and of 10 to 12 % respectively.

Serum osteocalcin was measured by a radioimmunoassay (OSTK-PR. Cis-France), the detection limit being 0.35 ng/ml. Plasma calcium, total cholesterol, triglycerides and urinary clacium and creatinin were measured by routine methods.

- Bone mass measurements:
Vertebral bone mass measurements were performed at the lumbar spine level (L2-L4) by Dual Photon Absorptiometry using a 1Ci 153 Gadolinium source (Lunar - model DP3). Results were expressed as Bone Mineral Density (BMD) in g/cm2. Long term reproducibility in our laboratory was 2.3 % [13]. The individual bone variation rates were calculated by linear regression of the bone mass values with respect to time using all the measurements for each subject. The confidence interval was calculated as a function of long term reproducibility and of the number of scans performed in each group, i.e. 5 for the treated women, 3 for the untreated women.

- Statistical analysis:
Paired or unpaired Student's t-tests were used as appropriate. A two-way analysis of variance was used for the percentage of BMD changes variable. The two studied factors were the bleeding pattern (regular or not), and the individual mean estradiol levels (higher or lower than 50 pg/ml). This analysis was completed by a Fisher's test and its validity controlled by homogeneity of variances and residual analysis.

RESULTS

1 - Trial compliance and side effects
5 women in the untreated group, 5 in the percutaneous group and 6 in the transdermal group dropped out of the study. In the untreated group, 4 for personal reasons, 1 for intercurrent hyperthyroidism. In the percutaneous group, 3 because they had difficulties in following the treatment correctly, and 2 due to mastodynia. In the transdermal group, 2 for personal reasons, 1 due to viral hepatitis, 1 due to somnolence and 2 due to cutaneous reactions. In this group 9 other women had slight and transient cutaneous reactions (redness, irritation) that did not compromise pursual of treatment after changing the application area (buttocks).

2 - Variations at group level (m±SEM)
In the untreated group, the BMD decreased on average by -0.016 g/cm^2 (±0.006), (-1.8%) after 1 year and by -0.051 g/cm^2 (±0.006) after two years (-4.4%).
But, in the treated groups, the BMD increased significantly ($p < 0.001$) after one year, by $+0.035$ g/cm^2 (±0.01) and by $+0.041$ g/cm^2 (±0.007) respectively for groups T and P. After two years this increase reached $+0.041$ g/cm^2 (±0.01) and $+0.046$ g/cm^2 (±0.008) without any significant differences between the two groups. After 12 and 24 months, the difference between the untreated and treated groups was highly significant ($p < 0.001$) (Fig. 1).

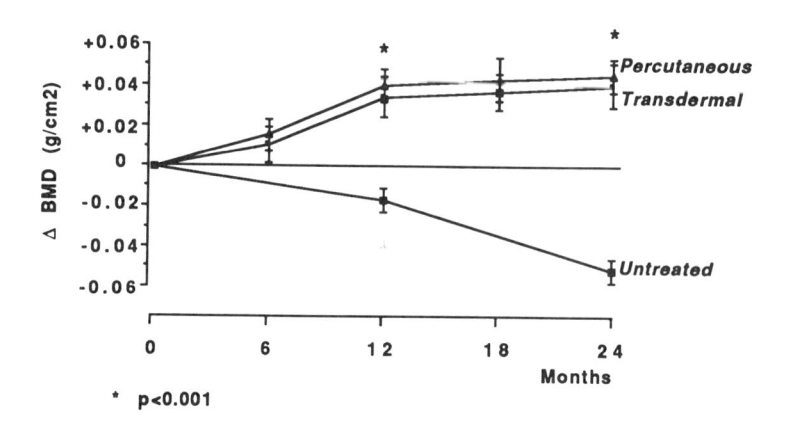

Fig.1: Evolution of BMD(g/cm2) in the groups

* p<0.001

- At the group level, the mean estradiol concentration remained stable throughout treatment, 62 to 69 pg/ml in group P, 44 to 55 pg/ml in group T, without any signicant difference between the two groups (Fig. 2).

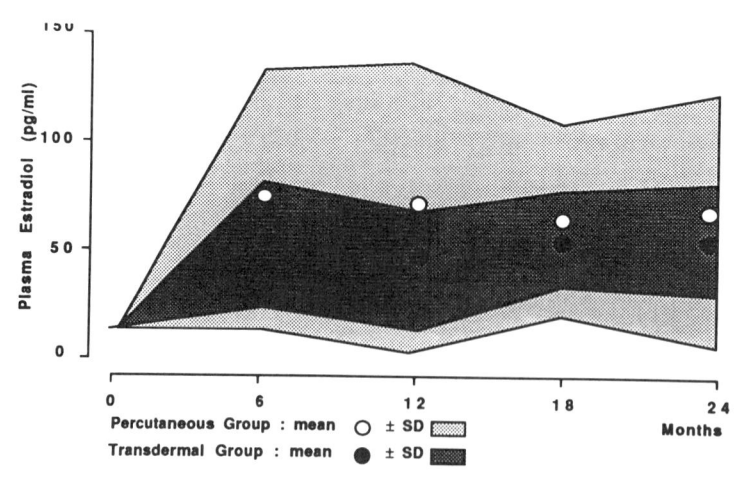

Fig 2: Variation of estradiol plasma levels during treatment.

3 - Individual variations

After two years, significant bone loss was observed in 23 untreated women (75%), but no significant bone loss was observed in 33 out of 38 women in group P (87%) nor in 23 out of 25 women in group T (96%) (Fig.3).

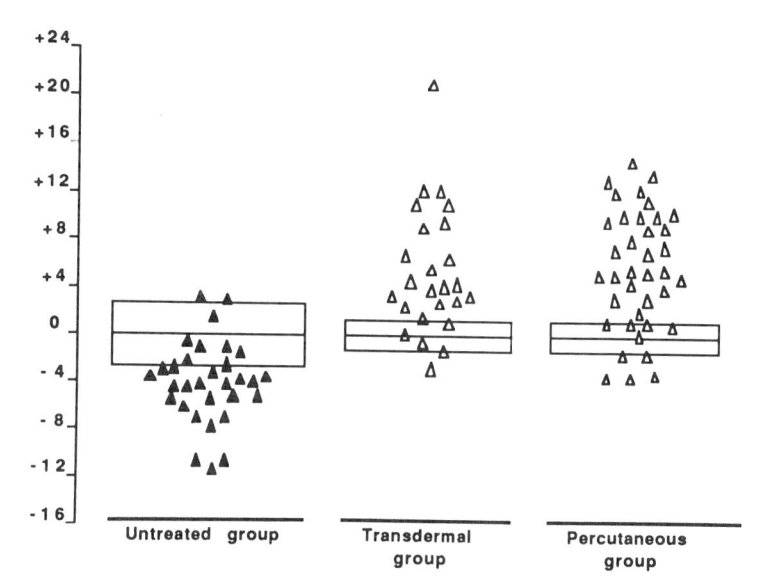

Fig.3: Individual rates of bone changes (%) after two years follow up.

- Although the mean estradiol concentrations did not differ significantly between the two treated groups, the inter-individual variations were twice as high in group P (SD = 45 to 65 pg/ml) as in group T (SD = 22 to 30 pg/ml) (Fig. 2).

4 - Predictive factors of bone response

None of the clinical characteristics nor the initial BMD or biological parameter values presented significant differences between subjects found to be "responsive" or "unresponsive" after two years.
The notion of regular withdrawal bleeding did not constitute an element for predicting bone response unlike a mean estradiol level higher than 50 pg/ml did ($p < 0.05$. ANOVA). For a sensitivity of 57%, a specificity of 70%, this parameter's positive predictive value was 93%. (Table 3).

Table 3: Predictive factors of bone response after two years of treatment.

	ANOVA	Sensitivity	Specificity	PPV	NPV
Regular Bleeding (A)*	NS				
Estradiol level >50 pg/ml (B)**	p<0.05	0.57	0.70	0.93	0.18
Interaction (AxB)	NS				

* Regular withdrawal bleeding following the estrogen cycle during the two years of treatment
** Mean individual estradiol levels during the two years of treatment

PPV: Positive Predictive Value
NPV: Negative Predictive Value

5 - Lipid metabolism

No significant variations in the plasma levels of total cholesterol and of triglycerides were observed during treatment.

CONCLUSION

The results of this study show that transdermal administration of 17 ß estradiol using a system delivering 0.05 mg/day or the percutaneous application of 1.5 mg estradiol, associated with orally administered progestogen present the same comparable efficiency in preventing post menopausal vertebral bone loss. Furthermore, we observed a transient bone gain which was at its highest after one year, as has been observed in other studies of the same type [15, 16, 17]. With these doses, which enable estradiol levels to be obtained that are equivalent to an early follicular phase, 90% of the treated women did not present any significant bone loss. According to our study, a serum estradiol level of at least 50 pg/ml appears sufficient for providing a protective effect on bone in virtually all cases. The clinical and metabolic tolerances to these therapeutic plans appeared highly satisfactory, which probably explains the good compliance to treatment. Some cutaneous reactions were observed in patch-treated women, but only in a few cases the treatment had to be stopped. The only noteworthy difference between the two ways of administration was the inter-individual estradiol levels, which were higher with percutaneous treatment than with the transdermal system. These variations would seem to be linked not with the bio-availability of the product, but rather with dose variations inherent to the this mode of administration in daily use. These variations could explain the higher percentage of non-response in the percutaneously treated group than in the transdermally treated group.

REFERENCES

1. S. Meema, M.L. Bunker, H.E. Meema. Preventive effect of estrogen on postmenopausal bone loss. Arch.Intern. Med. 135, 1436-1440 (1975).
2. L.E. Nachtigall, R.H. Nachtigall, R.D. Nachtigall, E.M. Beckman. Estrogen replacement therapy I : a 10 year prospective study in the relationship to osteoporosis. Obstet. Gynecol. 53, 277-291 (1979).
3. G.F. Jensen, C. Christiansen, I.B. Transbol. Fracture frequency and bone preservation in postmenopausal women treated with estrogen. Obstet. Gynecol.60, 493 496 (1982).
4. D.P. Kiel, D.T. Felson, J.J. Anderson, P.W.F. Wilson, M.A. Mosrowitz. Hip fracture and the use of estrogens in postmenopausal women. The Framingham Study. N. Engl. J. Med.317, 1170-1174 (1987).
5. C.B. Hammond, F.R. Jelovsek, K.L. Lee et al. Effects of long term estrogen replacement therapy I. Metabolic effects. Am. J. Obstet. Gynecol. 133, 528-527 (1979).
6. R.D. Gambrell, F.M. Massey, T.H. Castaneda et al. Use of the progestogen challenge test to reduce the risk of endometrial cancer. Obstet. Gynecol. 55, 732-738 (1980).
7. W.N.Spellacy, W.C. Buhi, S.A. Burk. Effects of norethindrone on carbohydrate and lipid metabolism. Obstet. Gynecol. 46, 560-563 (1975).
8. B.R. Bhavnani. The saga of the ring B unsaturated equine estrogens. Endocrine Reviews. 9, 396-416 (1988).
9. R. Lindsay, M. Hart, M. Clark. The minimum dose of estrogen for prevention of postmenopausal bone loss. Obstet. Gynecol. 63, 759-763 (1984).
10. B. De Lignières, A. Basdevant, G. Thomas et al. Biological effects of estradiol 17 ß in postmenopausal women. Oral versus percutaneous administration. J. Clin. Endocr. Metab. 62, 536-541 (1986).
11. J.A. Simon, J.A. Leal, J.D. Hodgen. Skin and serum pharmacokinetics of percutaneous estradiol absorption in postmenopausal women and non human primates. in : Osteoporosis 1987, C. Christiansen eds. pp.1101-1112.
12. M.S. Powers, L. Schenkel, P.E. Darley et al. Pharmacokinetics and pharmacodynamics of transdermal dosage forms of 17 ß estradiol : comparison with conventional oral estrogens used for hormone replacement. Amer. J. Obstet. Gynecol. 152, 1099-1106 (1985).
13. L.R. Laufer, J.L. De Fazio, J.K.H. Lu et al. Estrogen replacement therapy by transdermal administration. Am. J. Obstet. Gynecol. 21, 26-28 (1983).
14. J.M. Pouillès, F. Tremollières, J.P. Louvet, B. Fournie, G. Morlock and C. Ribot. Sensitivity of dual photon absorptiometry in spinal osteoporosis. Calcif. Tissue. Int. 43, 329-334 (1988).
15. B.J. Riis, D. Thomsen, V. Strom, C. Christiansen. The effect of percutaneous estradiol and natural progesterone on postmenopausal bone loss. Am. J. Obstet. Gynecol. 156, 61-65 (1987).
16. B. Ettinger, H.K. Genant, C.E. Cann. Postmenopausal bone loss in prevented by treatment with low-dosage estrogen with calcium. Ann. Int. Med. 106, 40-45 (1987).

Prophylaxis of Bone Loss: Long-Term Effects of Continuous and Sequential Estrogen/Progestin Administration and Identification of Women at Risk

S. Pors Nielsen, N. Munk-Jensen, E.B. Obel, and O. Barenholdt

Department of Clinical Physiology & Nuclear Medicine, Hillerød Central Hospital, Hillerød, Denmark

ABSTRACT

Oral estrogen/progestin administration, continuous or sequential, given during 12 months, can reverse the "physiological" postmenopausal bone loss to a gain in bone mass. Bone histomorphometry studies have suggested that this effect might be temporary. We have performed a study over 30 months (including a six months run-in period) to investigate this problem. It was an additional aim of the study to investigate whether "fast losers" exist, and to develop methods for identification of women at risk of developing fractures later in life. The following observations were made:

1. Hormone treatment over two years reversed bone loss from both the forearm and the lumbar spine, the changes being most pronounced in the spine, where the difference in BMD (g/cm^2) between the hormone groups and the placebo group approached 10%.
2. Continuous and sequential treatment produced identical results.
3. The mean rise in BMD was higher during the first than during the second year, where it approximated zero for both the lumbar spine and the forearm.
4. There was no subpopulation of "fast losers" when active treatment was not given, the distribution of changes in BMD being Gaussian, both for the forearm and the lumbar spine.

Women losing bone at a high rate at the beginning do not appear to continue to do so. We suggest that identification of women needing prophylactic treatment with hormones should not be based on sequential measurements, but rather on one BMD measurement, carried out if one or more of the classical risk factors are present.
Since vertebral compression fractures do not depend on lumbar BMD alone, but also on the body height and weight load per square unit, we suggest the introduction of a vertebral fracture risk index (FRI) including BMD, body surface and vertebral diameter. In a population of 96

normal women, aged 42-62 years, referred to BMD measurement due to classical risk factors, the use of FRI rather than a lumbar BMD limit (BMD < 0.900 g/cm^2) put 8 women into the risk zone, and removed 5 women from it. By both methods around one fourth of the women were at risk.

INTRODUCTION

Population studies have shown that the risk of vertebral crush fractures augments with the reduction in vertebral bone density (1). We have previously shown that oral continuous or sequential estrogen/progestin administration in normal early postmenopausal women during 12 months significantly reversed the "physiological" early postmenopausal bone loss from the lumbar spine and the forearm to an absolute gain in bone mass over 12 months (2). This investigation, comprising 151 normal postmenopausal women with a mean menopausal age of 93 weeks (randomization after a six months run-in period), studied in a placebo controlled double-blind trial during one year after which the code was broken, is being extended to a total of five years of hormone administration. The reason for the extension is the simple fact that it is unknowm whether the rise in lumbar spine and forearm bone density (L-BMD and F-BMD, respectively), levels off, perhaps approaching values of non-treated women. We here present data on BMD during two years of active treatment compared with placebo values.

It has been suggested that normal postmenopausal women at risk of fractures later in life could be identified by serial measurements of BMD, determining the rate of bone loss, or by measurements of chemical markers of bone turnover in the blood or urine (3). Selection of women for prophylactic treatment with estrogen/progestin on the basis of measurement of the rate of bone loss rather than on one absolute measurement seems doubtful. The measurement of the rate of bone loss, directly or indirectly, presupposes the existence of a subgroup of "fast losers", or the existence of some postmenopausal women maintaining a high rate of bone loss over years. Perhaps rapid bone loss does not continue, but takes place in all women for a period immediately after the onset of the menopause (4). Furthermore, the precision of the measurement of the rate of bone loss might not suffice for measurement in one individual (5).

It is obvious that selection criteria for prophylactic treatment with hormones are of paramount importance. We therefore decided to investigate, with high-precision bone absorptiometry, 1) whether a subpopulation of "fast losers" exist; 2) whether those losing bone at a relatively fast rate initially continue to do so, and 3) whether fracture risk can be estimated more meaningfully by one measurement of L-BMD and subsequent corrections for body weight, height, and vertebral width, the rationale being that a high load on the vertebral bodies and a low horizontal vertebral surface would increase the risk of development of crush fractures. The importance of vertebral size has been stressed by the recent observation that vertebral body diameter remains unchanged in women after the menopause, while in men, having larger vertebrae than women, it increases with age (Lis Mosekilde, personal communication). We have previously shown that it is characteristic of women with crush fractures that they have a low vertebral body diameter (6).

METHODS

Part I. Effects of hormones.

As described earlier (2) 151 normal postmenopausal women were allocated to three groups by block randomization after a six months run-in period. All were given tablets of identical colour and size (28 days cycles), and no extra calcium was supplied. Group A took estrogen/progestin continuously (one tablet daily containing 2 mg oestradiol and 1 mg norethisterone acetate); group B took estrogen/progestin sequentially - (first 12 days one tablet daily containing 2 mg oestradiol; next 10 days one tablet daily containing 2 mg oestradiol and 1 mg norethisterone acetate; last six days one tablet daily containing 1 mg oestradiol); group C took placebo tablets.

The following variables were measured every six months from time 0 to 30 months: renal excretion of calcium and hydroxyproline, serum concentrations of calcium, inorganic phosphate, alkaline phosphatase, follicle stimulating hormone (FSH), blood pressure, and body weight. Bone mineral content was assessed by dual photon absorptiometry (lumbar spine) and single photon absorptiometry (forearm).

Part II. Identification of women at risk.

Ninety-six consequtive women aged 42-62 years (mean menopausal age 52 years), referred for measurement of L-BMD due to known risk factors (family story of osteoporosis, sedentary work, slimness etc.) were included. L-BMD was measured with a BMC-LAB 23 (NOVO, SCAN DETECTRONIC). With this apparatus mean lumbar vertebral body diameter (side-to-side) was measured (D). Also relative body surface (RBS) was estimated as

$$RBS = H^{0.725} \times W^{0.425} \times 0.007184/1.73,$$

where H is body height (cm) and W is body weight (kg) (Courvoisier's equation).

D and RBS were used to calculate a vertebral fracture risk index (FRI):

FRI = BMD x D/ RBS, which has the dimension of g/cm.

It can be seen that the lower the FRI the higher the risk of crush fracture, like for L-BMD. Also, according to the FRI equation small vertebrae and high RBS predispose to crush fracture. Interestingly, in Courvoisier's equation for calculation of body surface, body height is weighted stronger than body weight e.g. tallness 10% over normal would predispose more to crush fracture than a 10% overweight. The physical laws determing whether a crush fracture occurs are not very different from those valid for concrete columns or tall buildings: The moment of inertia (I) is crucial:

$$I = M \times H^2$$

where M denotes mass (or weight) and H^2 denotes the square of the distance from the axis about which rotation takes place.

RESULTS

Part I. Effects of hormones.
The mean values of L-BMD are shown in *Fig. 1*.

It can be seen that 1) there was an absolute gain in bone mass; 2) the net gain in L-BMD approached 10% after two years of hormone administration; 3) continuous and sequential treatment acted alike; and 4) the fall in the placebo group was linear. The changes in L-BMD are shown in more detail in *Fig. 2*, which demonstrates that the absolute gain in bone mass was higher immediately after the beginning of treatment than later.

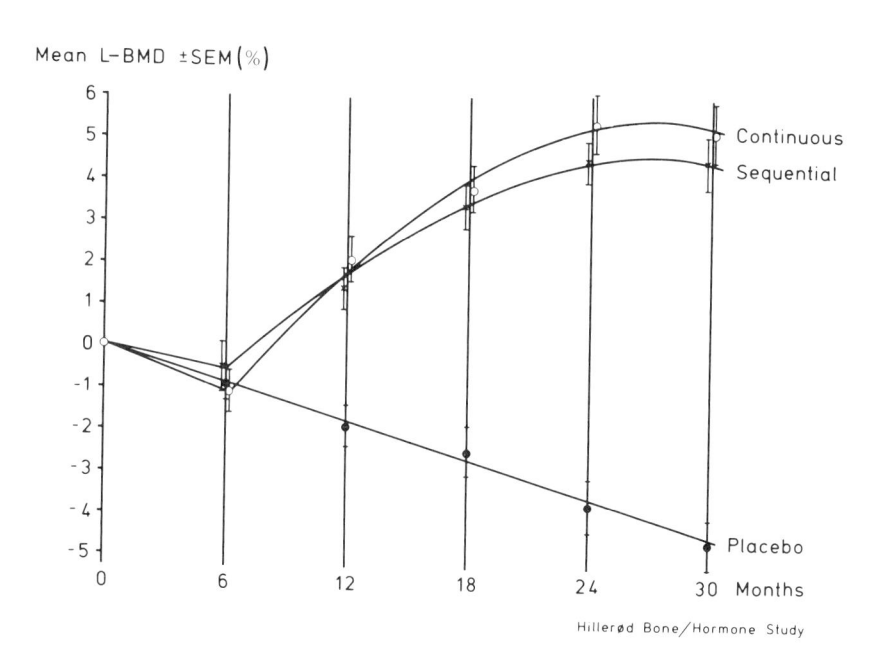

Fig. 1. Mean lumbar bone density during continuous and sequential estrogen/progestin administration.

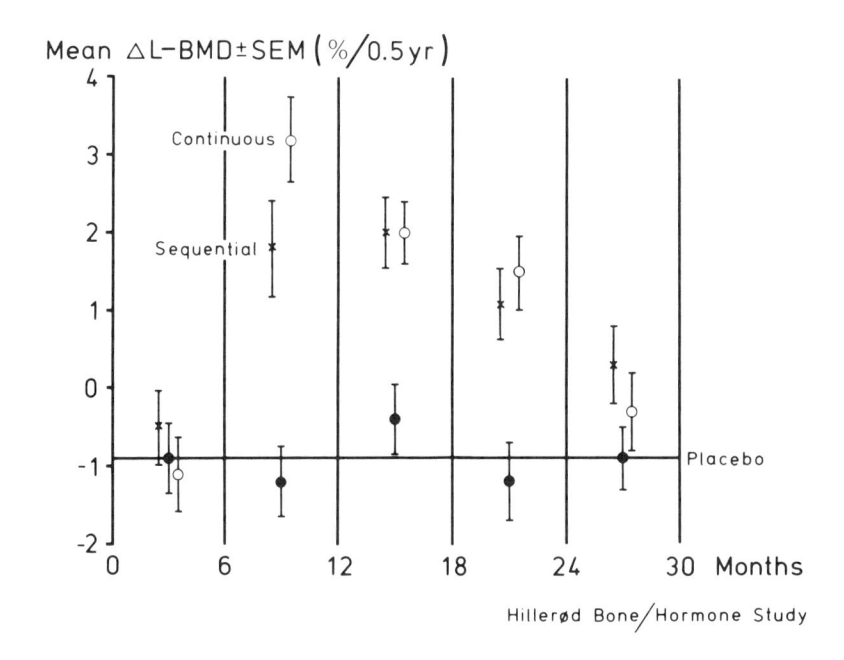

Fig. 2. Mean rate of change in lumbar bone density during continuous and sequential estrogen/progestin administration.

The absolute values of F-BMD and the changes of F-BMD are depicted in *Fig. 3* and *Fig. 4*, respectively.

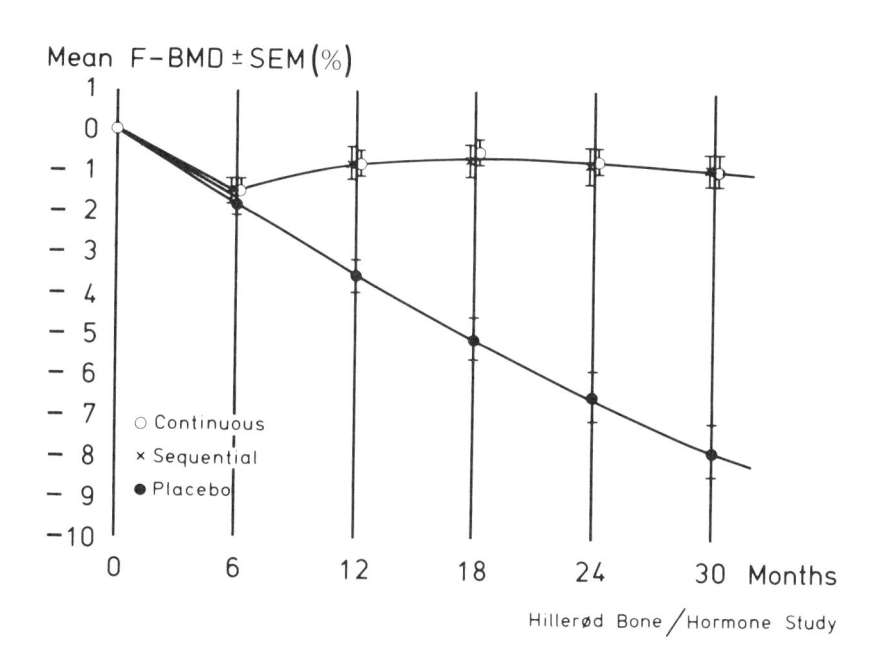

Fig. 3. Mean forearm bone density during continuous and sequential estrogen/progestin administration.

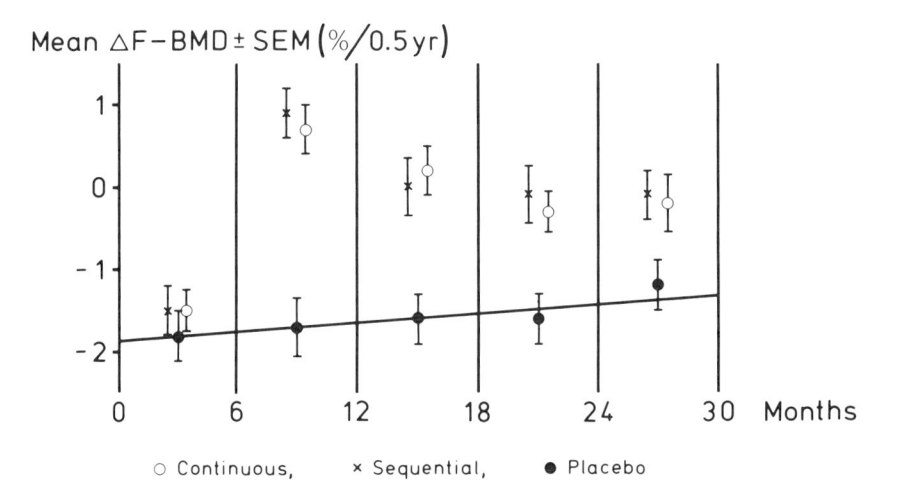

Fig. 4. Mean rate of change in forearm bone density during continuous and sequential estrogen/progestin administration.

It can be seen that 1) the percentage net gain for the forearm is smaller than for the lumbar spine; 2) the effect seems to last longer; 3) the two types of hormone treatment acted alike; and 4) the fall in the placebo group was higher, particularly during the first year (non-linear decline).

Treatment comparison was done by parametric analysis of variance. The groups A and B were each compared to group C (placebo) (6-30 months). Highly significant differences ($p<0.001$) were observed for: L-BMD and F-BMD (increase), and for renal excretion of calcium (Ca/creatinine ratio), renal excretion of hydroxyproline (hydro-

xyproline/creatinine ratio), serum calcium, serum alkaline phosphatase, serum inorganic phosphate, and serum FSH (reduction). There was no statistically significant difference for any of those variables between groups A and B. Blood pressure and body weight were not influenced by the administration of hormones.
Analysis of baseline comparability (Kruskal-Wallis or Pearson's Chi-squared test) revealed no evidence to suggest that the three treatment groups were not comparable at baseline (all the variables mentioned above).

Part II. Identification of women at risk.
Analysis of the distribution of the changes in F-BMD and L-BMD did not confirm the existence of a subpopulation of "fast losers". (Fig. 5 and Fig. 6).

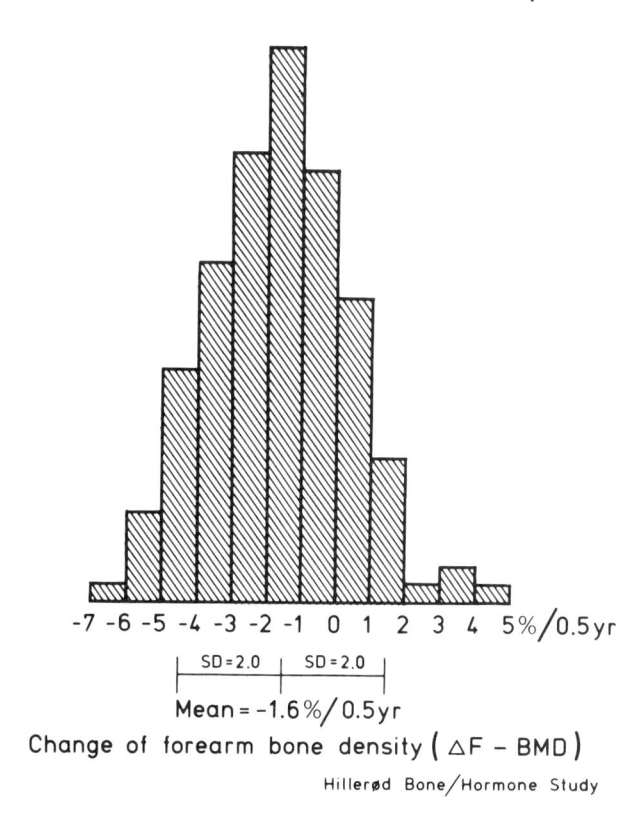

Fig. 5. Distribution of spontaneous changes in forearm bone density during the run-in period. Note: Gaussian distribution.

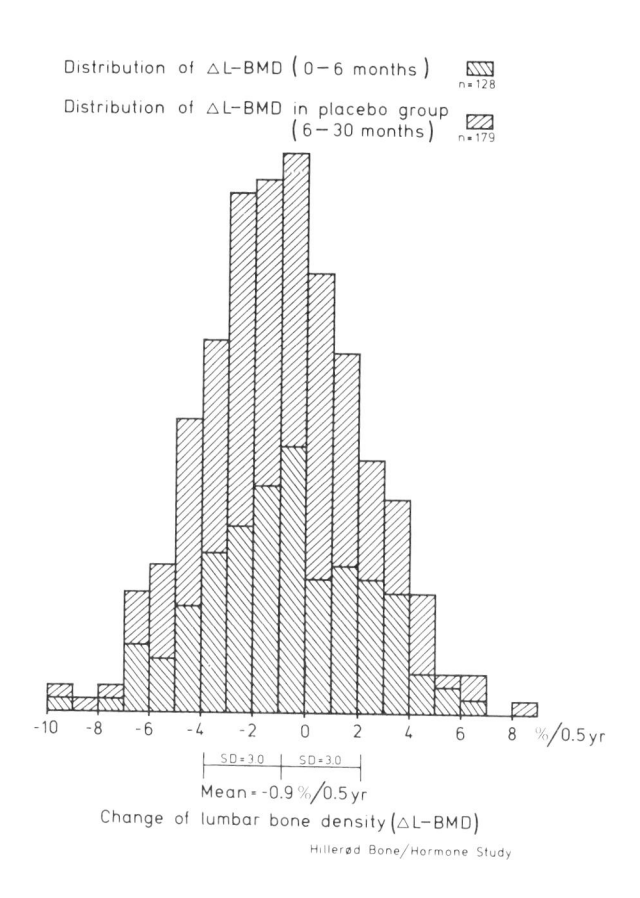

Fig. 6. Distribution of spontaneous changes in lumbar bone density (no hormone administration). Note: Gaussian distribution.

This would not encourage selection of candidates for hormone replacement on the basis of sequential measurements of L-BMD. Furthermore, there was no obvious sign that those losing bone at a fast rate at the beginning continue to do so.

In a populaiton of 96 normal women aged 42-62 years, referred to the hospital for L-BMD measurement on the basis of classical risk factors one fourth had values below 0.900 g/cm². Calculation of FRI, and a hereof derived FRI risk limit of 3.75 g/cm put 8 women with L-BMD values above 0.900 g/cm² into the fracture risk zone, and removed 5 women with L-BMD values below 0.900 g/cm² from it. This might suggest that in case of extreme values of vertebral diameter and body surface the use of FRI might be an appropriate supplement to a L-BMD fracture risk limit (*Fig. 7*).

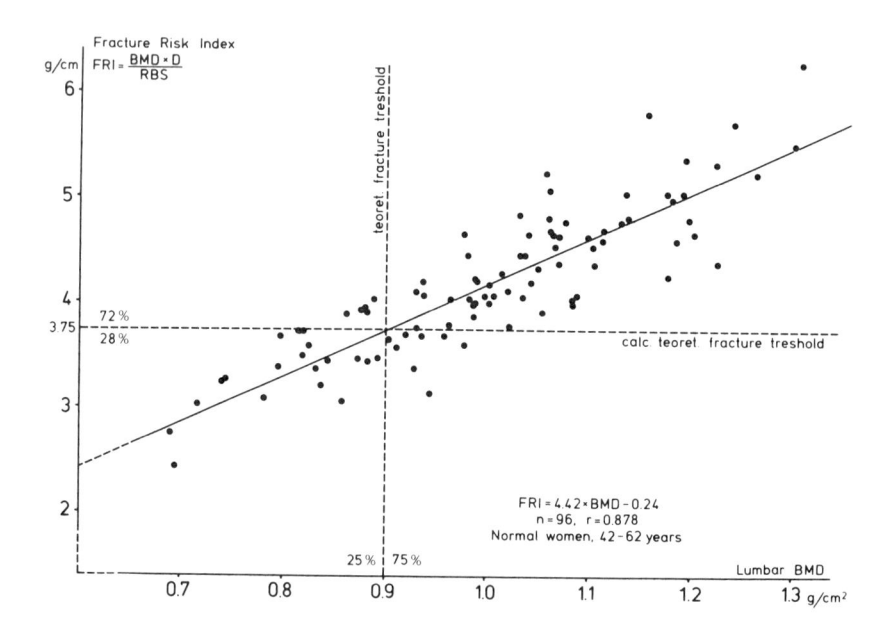

Fig. 7. Lumbar bone density versus calculated fracture risk index (FRI) in 96 normal women aged 42-62 years.

It should be mentioned that, as expected, FRI is correlated to L-BMD (r=0.878), since L-BMD is part of the expression of FRI, but neither vertebral diameter (D) nor relative body surface (RBS) are correlated to L-BMD.

COMMENTS

The results suggest that the effects of estrogen/progestin administration on bone density, though pronounced over two years, might level off, but it is so far unknown whether forearm and lumbar spine bone density approach placebo values after another few years. It seems safe to assume that the time of occurence of fractures might be postponed by a number of years. Side-effects of long-term hormone replacement therapy were few (2), but there seems to be a moderately increased risk of breast cancer during long-term hormone administration (7). Continuous and sequential hormone administration produced the same results regarding bone density and biochemical markers of bone resorption. Continuous hormone therapy has the advantage of producing an atrophic endometrium, and reduce the risk of endometrial cancer.

Although our method for measurement of L-BMD is as precise as current methods for measurement of F-BMD (8), it does not seem safe to trust longitudinal measurements of bone density in one individual (5). Furthermore, since we could find no evidence of the existence of a subpopulation of "fast losers", as claimed by others (3), and we do not believe that those losing bone at a rapid rate immediately after the menopause, continue to do so (4), we recommand that candidates for hormone replacement therapy be chosen among those having low L-BMD, after referral to bone density measurement according to classical risk factors. Also, we suggest corrections for body surface and vertebral diameter, when fracture risk estimation is the problem.

REFERENCES

1. H. W. Wahner: Bone mineral measurements. Nucl. Med. Ann. *1986*, 195-226.

2. N. Munk-Jensen, S. Pors Nielsen, E. B. Obel & P. Bonne Eriksen: Reversal of postmenopausal vertebral bone loss by oestrogen and progestogen: A double blind placebo controlled trial. Brit. Med. J. *296*, 1150-1152, 1988.

3. C. Christiansen, B. J. Riis & P. Rødbro: Prediction of rapid bone loss in postmenopausal women. Lancet *1987 (1)*, 1105-1110.

4. S. Pors Nielsen & B. Krølner: Photonbeam absorptiometry. In : Osteoporosis. A multidisciplinary problem. Roy. Soc. Med. Int. Congr. Symp. Ser. *No. 55*, 105-108, 1983. Academic Press.

5. J. A. Kanis, F. Caulin & R. G. G. Russell: Problems in the design of clinical trials. In : Osteoporosis. A multidisciplinary problem. Roy. Soc. Med. Int. Congr. Symp. Ser. *No. 55*, 205-221, 1983. Academic Press.

6. B. Krølner: Osteoporosis and normality: how to express the bone mineral content of lumbar vertebrae. Clin. Physiol. *2*, 139-146, 1982.

7. M. Ewertz: Influence of non-contraceptive exogenous and endogenous sex hormones on breast cancer risk in Denmark. Int. J. Cancer *42*, 832-838, 1988.

8. S. Pors Nielsen & O. Barenholdt: A novel high-precision dual-photon absorptiometer. Proc. symp. osteoporosis & bone mineral measurements. Bath, England, 18-19 April, 1988 (in press).

A Current Perception of HRT Risks and Benefits

T.M. Mack and R.K. Ross

University of Southern California, Los Angeles, California

ABSTRACT

The goal of a contemporary decision about hormone replacement is to minimize <u>net</u> predictable lifetime risks. Estrogens ameliorate menopausal symptoms, maintain bone integrity, and produce endometrial cancer; the quantitative aspect of each of these is familiar. Other links are becoming clear: estrogens consistently increase biliary disease, but prevent heart disease, and stroke. Well designed studies suggest that breast cancer is increased by estrogen use; the increase is modest as a risk factor but substantial in absolute terms. The impact of an added progestin cannot yet be empirically assessed; there is concern about breast cancer, heart disease, stroke, and the magnitude of the expected reduction in endometrial cancer. We have used a simple model to insert estimates of the regimen-specific relative risk for each outcome, and have translated all outcomes into common denominators of morbidity and mortality. We conclude that largely because of protection against heart disease, the net impact of estrogen in modest dose will be highly beneficial to women to age 75 or longer; hormone replacement which includes systemic progestin supplemention may be really harmful, depending on how it modifies the estrogen effects on the breast and heart. While conventional wisdom dictates that estrogens be supplemented with progestin, important considerations mitigate against it.

INTRODUCTION

Although the emphasis in discussion has shifted gradually from the merits of endometrial cancer epidemiology to the need for adding a progestin to estrogen replacement, opinions about hormone replacement are still diverse, but still strongly held

[1-2], and "consensus" conference statements [3-5] still hedge and thereby betray a lack of unanimity. Such whistling in the dark is adequate justification for a periodic update of the evidence.

There is now less need to act on faith alone. Estrogen use has been shown to prevent stroke and post-menopausal rheumatoid arthritis, and additional information about the putative links between estrogens and gall bladder disease, ischemic heart disease, and breast cancer has appeared. More accurate estimates of survival after osteoporotic fracture have been published. While there is still no empiric assessment of the long term impact of added progestin, predictions should periodically be updated.

Moreover, an adequate method of synthesis is still needed. The single published cost-effectiveness analysis [6] is outdated, and cost information is not very generalizable. An attempt to reduce all outcomes to common units of "quality-adjusted" life expectancy [7] did not consider breast cancer, and in any case has not proved useful to clinicians, possibly because they are unused to basing decisions on longevity, and are unwilling to take the results on faith, especially if it means giving the same weight to the same event in women of very different age. Decisions continue to be made on a basis which emphasizes a single positive or negative outcome, usually that paramount in the decision-maker's specialty, without accounting for the relative probability of occurence of the various diseases [8]. While endocrinologists and especially gynecologists uniformly recommend replacement treatment [9], a minority of eligible women are taking it at any given time [10], and consumers exhibit real confusion about the pertinent issues [11]. We propose here not just to provide a packaged recommendation, but to describe a framework into which updated information about risks and benefits can be translated into net losses and gains, and used to alter policies.

METHODS

At present, the frequency of eight common conditions is known to be influenced by estrogen usage. In addition to the climacteric itself, these include osteoporosis and osteoporotic fractures, acute (and therefore presumably chronic) ischemic heart disease, stroke, rheumatoid arthritis, gallbladder disease, endometrial cancer and breast cancer. In our judgement, the evidence suggesting links between hormone replacement and liver disease, other neoplasms, and serious psychiatric outcomes, including suicide, is not sufficiently suggestive to warrant adding any of these conditions to the list.

The Model and the Outcomes

It is difficult to select a single outcome to serve as a common indicator of therapeutic success or failure. While survival of the patient must be considered the most important outcome, it does not serve as an adequate measure of either the quality of life or the economic cost of illness. Without very expensive and time-consuming special studies, these latter can only be assessed through the use of surrogate outcomes; here we have chosen respectively the estimated cumulative number of days of disability and the number of hospitalizations to be anticipated.

To estimate the net effect of estrogen replacement, we consider a cohort of 100,000 women entering menopause at age 50 and followed to age 75, treated continuously with estrogens in moderate dose (.625 mgm daily), and cumulate the outcomes that would result. We apply the available outcome-specific estimates of age-specific relative risk for each condition to the baseline frequency, sum the net changes across conditions, and express them in absolute terms and as a percentage of the summed baseline frequency.

We then introduce a number of alternative adjustments. We reduce the size of the aging population over the period on the basis of competing causes of mortality. Because a diagnosis anticipated tomorrow creates more concern than one expected after many years, we discount all outcomes at an annual level of 5%. We extend the computation to age 85. We produce an alternative estimate ignoring long term links with less severe and less easily counted chronic conditions, namely rheumatoid arthritis and gallbladder disease. We also make estimates under various alternative therapeutic assumptions; that treatment be continued for only 5 years, that women all recieve hysterectomy prior to beginning therapy, that only the 10% at highest (three-fold) prior risk of preventable outcomes (fracture and myocardial infarction) be treated, that the 10% at highest baseline risk (again, three-fold) of breast cancer be denied treatment, and that both of these latter policies be observed simultaneously.

In the absence of empiric evidence to the contrary, we assume that protection from estrogen therapy appears rapidly, is maintained at a constant level despite the duration of past use, is relatively insensitive to increases in dose, and gradually wanes in the years following cessation. In contrast, we assume that the carcinogenic hazard posed by estrogens is a function of both dose and duration of use, is slow to appear (especially in the case of breast cancer), and does not regress. The state of the available information is such that, except for variations in potency, we found no reason to distiguish between synthetic and natural estrogens, or between various preparations.

Mortality rates were taken from US age-specific, cause-specific mortality for 1986 [12], incidence from cited well-designed population-based surveillance studies or by applying adjusted consensus case-fatality ratios to mortality rates. Rates of hospitalization derive from clinical estimates or from the published results of the National Health Survey [13]. Days of disability were obtained from the latter source, with the exception of those attributable to cancer, which were calculated by adding standard estimates of post-operative morbidity days to those of cancer in recurrence. The origin of the estimates of incidence and mortality are discussed disease by disease.

Menopausal Symptoms

Climacteric symptoms are assumed to afflict 80% of the population, largely before age 55, and on the basis of randomized trials [14] are assumed to be relieved in 30% of those treated.

Osteoporotic Fracture

Osteoporotic fractures are assumed to occur from an annual baseline rate of 150/100,000 at age 50, to 10 times that rate at age 80 [15-16]. Most of those with fractures of the femoral neck are hospitalized; it is assumed that 10% (younger) to 15% (older) would die as a result [17], and that a substantial period of disability, increasing in duration with age at fracture, would prevail. The several consistent studies [18-19] that have quantified the strength of the protective effect are in general agreement; we assume that estrogen therapy would prevent 60% of the fractures to be otherwise expected.

Heart Disease

Ischemic heart disease is the most common single lethal condition of post-menopausal American women, newly affecting 350 (younger) to 1500 (older) of every 100,000 women [20] and killing from 25% (younger) to 67% (older) of them. All victims are candidates for hospitalization and considerable disability occurs among survivors.

Observations that women of premenopausal age are relatively endangered by atheromata and ischemic heart disease after castration [21] led to the hypothesis that estrogen replacement might also protect. Estrogen use has been shown to be clinically related to angiographic abnormalities [22].

TABLE 1. COMMUNITY STUDIES OF ERT AND HEART DISEASE

1st Author	RR-CU*	1st Author	RR-CU*	1st Author	RR-CU*
Wilson	1.9	Pfeffer	0.7	Ross	0.4
Bain	0.7	Stampfer	0.3	Bush	0.4
Criqui	0.7	Pettiti	0.5	Henderson	0.6

*CU = Current Use, when available.

Excluding those in which the subjects were compared to hospital patients with unrepresentative access to medical care, studies to-date which bear on the strength and direction of this link are in general agreement [23-31] (Table 1). With one exception [27], a protective effect of moderate size has been found; the exceptional results are from a cohort study which employed cross-sectional information about estrogen use gathered only as an afterthought, and a method of analysis that has been vigourously criticized [32]. Perhaps the most convincing results have come from a cohort of nurses [28], who can be presumed to have accurately recorded their exposure and to have sought competent medical care; in these women protection was apparent at all ages after 40.

On the basis of the combined experience, we have assumed that estrogen therapy prevents 50% of subsequent ischemic heart disease episodes. It must be noted in passing that heart disease is acknowledged to be particularly complex in its etiology [20], and interpretations of the evidence to date must be tentative. Behavioral factors are among the determinants and must be assumed to also determine access to and acceptance of estrogen therapy.

Stroke

A large cohort study of individually identified hormone users and non-users in a retirement community has offered an opportunity to evaluate the impact of estrogen use on mortality from non-hemorrhagic stroke [33], taking into consideration not only the details of hormone use but the other predictors of individual risk. Protection against fatal stroke prevailed at all ages more than 10 years after menopause, and was unaffected by adjustment for hypertension, smoking, alcohol, body mass and habits of exercise. The magnitude of the reduction prior to age 70 was estimated at greater than 20% (accordingly we have assumed the protective factor to be .80), and was presumed to operate against non-fatal as well as fatal stroke. Observation of one other prospectively followed cohort [34] has produced a similar result. Like that of ischemic heart disease, the baseline annual incidence of stroke has declined [35]; population-based studies have projected it to now range from 50/100,000 in the immediate postmenopausal age group to about 1400/100,000 in octogenarians. Case-fatality has been estimated at 30% (younger) to 60% (older) [36], and disability following non-fatal stroke is substantial.

Rheumatoid Arthritis

In few populations can an unbiased estimate of rheumatoid arthritis incidence be produced; in one such, the Minnesota county containing the Mayo clinic, a secular decrease has been observed and tentatively attributed to the use of contraceptives or replacement hormones [37]. One well-designed analytic study of replacement hormone use and newly incident rheumatoid arthritis has been conducted using the patients attending arthritis clinics in the city of Rotterdam [38]; estrogen use was estimated to diminish the incidence rate by a factor of .34, and we have conservatively used a figure of 0.4. The first appearance of rheumatoid arthritis in the postmenopausal period is not common; it has been estimated to occur at an annual rate of 12 (younger) to 20 (older) per 100,000 women. Mortality can be attributed directly or indirectly to the disease in a small proportion of patients; we estimate this to be 7% [39]. Disability among survivors is moderate.

Gallbladder Disease

Endogenous and exogenous estrogens increase the cholesterol content of bile and increase the residual volume of the gallbladder [40], both leading to the expectation that the prevalence of cholesterol gallstones and the incidence of symptomatic gallbladder disease would be increased among users. Empirically the latter [41], but not the former [42], has been consistently observed, with roughly a 2-3 fold increase in the rates of symptomatic episode, hospitalization, and cholecystectomy. The annual frequency of gallbladder disease has been estimated in many settings [43-44], and varies greatly, certainly on the basis of ethnicity and probably on that of socio-economic class; the figures used here are estimates for non-Latino white US residents. While mortality from gallbladder disease is essentially restricted to that from operative anesthesia, and disability is negligible, the surgical treatment and the required days of hospitalization make gallbladder disease an important category of medical expense.

Endometrial Cancer

Concerns about the dangers of estrogen replacement were initially sparked by the appearance of endometrial cancer in women with premorbid conditions associated with high levels of endogenous estrogens [45], and by the appearance of hyperplasia in long-term users [46]. Literally dozens of case-control and cohort studies have now documented a high relative risk of endometrial cancer following replacement hormone usage [47]. Several have demonstrated that high risk follows usage of even moderate dosages taken for long periods [48-49], and that risk remains elevated many years after cessation [50-51].
While the overall mortality among afflicted users is much lower than among non-users who get endometrial cancer [52], the incidence of aggressive disease is also increased by estrogen usage [53], and the apparently favorable survival experience of user cases is likely in part to patients with estrogen-induced benign hyperplasia mislabeled as cases, and in part to an earlier diagnosis among patients closely followed after treatment with a drug known to induce vaginal bleeding. The annual incidence of endometrial cancer normally reaches a level after menopause of 150-200/100,000 [54], and the 5-year mortality is about 20% [55]. Disability is substantial on a population basis, but is mostly attributable to post-operative convalescence. For purposes of these calculations, we have assumed the relative risk after 5 years of usage to be 7, and the 5-year mortality among estrogen-associated excess cases to be 15%.

Breast Cancer

Breast cancer occurs at an annual rate of 220 (younger) to 800 (older) cases/100,000 women [54], and kills roughly a third of affected women within 5 years [55]. It has long been presumed to have a hormonal etiology, because risk was recognized early on to vary with type of menopause and age at menopause, menarche and first full-term pregnancy [56], and because the pattern of occurence in families [57] and populations [58] correlates with patterns of serum estrogen level and menarcheal age. Several anecdotal studies of the rare cancers of the male breast suggest links with estrogens taken for either cosmetic [59] or therapeutic [60] reasons.
Although the role of endogenous estrogen provides a solid basis for suspecting exogenous estrogens, it has proved very difficult to evaluate this link, because the usage of hormonal replacement is linked to these same breast cancer risk factors, and because the relatively high social class of breast cancer patients (due in large part to the same risk factors) affords preferential access to sources of replacement therapy. An estimate of the strength of the expected link with moderate

levels of usage, based on the risks from cumulative endogenous estrogen exposure, has predicted a modest increase in risk, well under twofold [56]. Such an increase would still produce an important impact, given the high incidence and gravity of this cancer, but it does offer a difficult target for epidemiologists, who must distinguish it from the inevitable minor effects of chance, errors of classification, and bias.

TABLE 2. COMMUNITY STUDIES OF ERT AND BREAST CANCER

1st Author	RR-LTU*	1st Author	RR-LTU*	1st Author	RR-LTU*
Craig	1.0	Brinton	1.5	Hiatt	1.8
Mack	1.6	Rohan	0.9	Hulka	1.7
Hoover	2.0	Nomura	1.9, 1.3	Buring	1.5
Ross	1.9	Hunt	1.6	Bergkvist	1.7
Evertz	1.6	Wingo	1.7	McDonald	1.2
				LaVeccia	2.1

*LTU = Long Term Use, when available.

By now, quite a substantial number of studies have employed comparisons explicitly designed to minimize differences in access to replacement therapy [47,61-75], usually by means of choosing controls from the same community that gave rise to the cases. These studies are quite variable with respect to other aspects of design, including the method of ascertaining the details of estrogen treatment. The results are summarized in Table 2. Most are weakly positive, at a level of risk quite compatible with that predicted.

None of these studies is perfect; some results are compatible with the null hypothesis, and there is substantial inconsistency between and even within them with respect to the designation of subgroups especially subject to estrogen effects.

On the other hand, there is fair consistency between the net results of the better designed studies (again with emphasis on the comparability of control subjects), and there is a disturbing tendency for reports from those same studies to suggest that higher risk follows longer usage (insufficient time has elapsed to properly evaluate risk after lengthy use and a truly long latent period). While we are unable to accurately specify the precise magnitude of the factor, or to designate those women who are at higher risk from estrogen usage, or even to state with absolute certainty that breast cancer is produced by estrogens, it does seem prudent to assume that it sometimes is, at least at the modest level of increase predicted. We have here assumed that a 20% increase in risk first appears after 5 years of treatment and that a peak increase of 40% prevails after 10 more years.

We have assumed that survival experience is unaffected by estrogen use, although it has already been observed [76] that estrogen-treated cases might survive longer than breast cancer cases in general.

RESULTS

TABLE 3 : NET CHANGES AFTER ERT: OUTCOMES FROM 50-74 IN THOUSANDS /100,000 WOMEN TREATED

	Hosp Adm	Deaths	Days of Restriction
Baseline frequency, 8 affected conditions	52	9.5	961
Net change	+73.7%	-14.3%	+17.2%
Baseline frequency, all conditions	420	17.7	2280
Net change	+9.1%	-7.7%	-0.3%

Overview

When combined, these 8 conditions account for slightly more than half of the deaths to be expected in women between 50 and 75, a bit less than half of all the days of disability, and about one in every 8 hospitalizations. Thus any given proportion of deaths from estrogen-related diseases represents about twice that proportion of all deaths.

The net effects of estrogen replacement are summarized in Table 3. We estimate that hospitalizations are made more frequent by an increment of about 75%, and that the days of disability are also more frequent among the treated, but by a smaller factor of about 17%. More than balancing this net impact on morbidity is a reduction of about 14% in the number of deaths to be expected in members of the cohort, confirming the net benefit of treatment with estrogen replacement. This result is quite compatible with that found earlier by means of a more sophisticated model [7].

The increase in hospitalization is largely attributable to an increase in the demand for cholecystectomy and hysterectomy; the extra disability is attributable to post-operative recovery from these operations plus the added breast cancer morbidity.

Over half of the anticipated reduction in mortality derives from the prevention of heart disease; stroke accounts for about a fourth of it and the consequences of osteoporosis account for another eighth.

Results under Alternative Assumptions

Exclusion of gallbladder disease and rheumatoid arthritis from the calculation produces a substantial reduction in the expected hospitalizations (Table 4), but otherwise has little effect, as does excluding women from the cohort as they die from other causes. Discounting the importance of outcomes in proportion to the time that will pass before occurance, however, cuts the impact of both the net benefits and the net risks in half. If the women are followed to age 85 rather than only to 75, the magnitude of the increase in both hospitalizations and days of disability is halved, largely as a result of the number of events to be expected from other medical problems. This longer follow-up, however, has virtually no effect on the proportional reduction in mortality.

TABLE 4. EFFECTS OF ADJUSTMENT ON NET CHANGE FROM ERT

Adjustment:	Hosp Adm	Deaths	Days of Restriction
None	+73.7%	-14.3%	+17.2%
-RA, GB Effects	+13.2%	-14.6%	+10.9%
+Competing Mortality	+73.4%	-14.3%	+16.5%
+ Discount Adjustment	+37.4%	- 6.9 %	+4.8%
+Follow to 84 years	+24.4%	-14.7%	+ 3.1%

Alternative estrogen replacement policies also have been considered. It appears that stopping treatment at the end of 5 years, usually after symptoms have abated, would produce a moderate reduction in the expected hospitalizations, whereas it would virtually eliminate the savings in long term mortality (Table 5). Women with no uterus would enjoy a slightly greater reduction in mortality and a substantial reduction in hospital admissions and convalescence; the impact of the hysterectomy itself on morbidity and mortality has not been considered.

Finally, the table demonstrates the absence of a strong rationale for allowing treatment to be determined by screening for characteristics marking high risk of osteoporotic fracture or ischemic heart disease on the one hand, or low risk of breast cancer on the other. With our limited ability to predict risk, treating a small proportion of the potential beneficiaries is to deny substantial benefits to the majority. With respect to breast cancer, even those with strong risk factors, such as a family history of breast cancer or a history of benign breast disease, are likely to receive more protection against death from heart disease than they are to be endangered by estrogens, which in the absence of coherent information now must be presumed to act independently of other known determinants.

TABLE 5. EFFECT OF CLINICAL ERT POLICIES: OUTCOMES 50-74

Policy:	Hosp Adm	Deaths	Days of Restriction
Rx for All	+73.7%	-14.3%	+17.2%
Rx 5 yrs	+53.3%	-2.1%	+21.3%
Hysterectomy	+51.0%	-18.9%	-0.5%
Screen Hi Rsk	+12.8%	-6.2%	+1.5%
Screen Lo Rsk	+66.8%	-12.2%	+16.7%
Screen Both Hi/Lo	+11.6%	-5.4%	+1.6%

As a check on the credibility of the results of these calculations, it is of interest to examine the one population of estrogen users in which most outcomes on our list have been simultaneously followed. Rèsidents of a large retirement community in Southern California were surveyed for hormone use in 1984 [77], and have been comprehensively monitored since then for all hospitalizations, cancers, and deaths [78]. The current approximate relative risk estimates for the various outcomes are: fractures 0.9, myocardial infarction 0.6, stroke 0.8, gallbladder disease 3.0, endometrial cancer over 10.0, and breast cancer 1.2. With the surprising exception of the protective effect against osteoporotic fractures, all estimates are consistent with those used in the model. The measured protection against fractures is much weaker than the estimates quoted above and thus far cannot be explained; it is not, for example, entirely due to a longer average interval since cessation of usage [79]. Nonetheless, the net observed reduction in mortality of 20% is quite consistent with that predicted by the model, and other estimates of the reduction in mortality following long term estrogen replacement [19-21] are consistent in both direction and magnitude.

DISCUSSION

The benefits of estrogen therapy appear to far outweigh the risks when measured in terms of mortality, if not in terms of either hospitalization or subsequent days of disability. These benefits are mostly attributable to protection against heart disease, stroke, and, to a considerably smaller extent, death after osteoporotic fracture. The substantial increase in endometrial cancer results in a minor offset to the savings in mortality, although it does produce a substantial increment in hospitalizations. Using the best available estimates, the contribution to mortality from estrogen-related breast cancer is unlikely to offset the protection against deaths from heart disease.

Most replacement therapy is prescribed by or on the recommendation of gynecologists, and gynecologists are especially aware of the effects of long term estrogens on the endometrium. In a desire to oppose these effects, many recommend that replacement therapy include a progestin, usually medroxyprogesterone, to be given in sequence with estrogens. While this regimen is now common, it has only recently become so in the chronology of these long term investigations, and reliable empirical estimates of the effects of combined therapy are unavailable. Nonetheless it is very important to predict the impact of this policy upon the net effect of hormone replacement.

Progestins do not interfere with the therapeutic efficacy of estrogens [80], and may even enhance protection against osteoporotic fracture [81]; there is no basis for predicting any substantial impact upon rheumatoid arthritis. However, it is not clear why sequentially administered progestin should be expected to eliminate estrogen-induced endometrial cancer, and there is a basis for concern about adverse effects on the risk of vascular disease, breast cancer, and gallbladder disease, and about long-term compliance with replacement therapy.

Progestins and Endometrial Cancer

The cellular mechanism of progestin antagonism in the uterus is essentially protective in nature; its actions block estrogenic activity by inducing conjugation and excretion, and by reducing the density of estrogen receptors [82]. It must also be presumed that the cells acted upon by estrogens are, or at least include, undifferentiated stem cells near the basement membrane, cells which are not shed periodically. Empirically, the intracellular effects of estrogen are not completely reversable by sequential therapy [83]. Moreover, the rapid increase in endometrial cancer risk precedes the cessation of ovulatory cycles [54], and sequential oral contraception causes premenopausal endometrial cancer [84], while combination pills prevent it [85]. The increased risk produced by unopposed postmenopausal estrogens continues long after cessation of estrogen use [50,51]. Taken together, these observations suggest that estrogenic causation of endometrial cancer will only be prevented when progestin is given concomitantly with estrogens; since sequential administration leaves the tissue unprotected during two-thirds of the period of estrogen administration, only one-third of the excess cases are likely to be prevented.

Progestins and Breast Cancer

In contrast with the compelling evidence of antagonism between estrogens and progestins in the endometrium, the information available does not indicate pharmacological antagonism in breast ductal tissue. Like estrogens, progestins induce ductal growth in the embryo [86]. Mitotic activity peaks in the luteal, not the follicular phase [87], suggesting either that there is stimulation by progesterone as well as estrogens, the simplest explanation, or that a complex and site-specific scenario prevails, in which the effect of estrogens is cumulative or follows a period of latency. As with endometrial cancer, age-specific breast cancer risk increases at a slower rate after regular cycles have stopped. Unlike endometrial cancer, breast cancer is not prevented by combined oral contraceptives. On the contrary, the latest careful estimate of risk in young women who long used combined oral contraceptive formulations [88] shows an increase in breast cancer risk. Moreover, long term oral contraceptive users followed through ages up to that of menopause also tend to show high risk [89-90], although the number of subjects in any single study is small. These age-disparate risk increases are most easily explained if cancer were produced by the combination of estrogen and progestin, since the pill is the same at all ages, and it is at these extremes of age that non-ovulatory cycles with little endogenous progesterone characterize the women not on contraceptives. In addition, the follow-up of cohorts receiving depot medroxyprogesterone as contraception [91-93] has not revealed the decrease in risk that was to have been expected on the basis of prolonged anovulation. While the highly publicized early studies of the empirical effects of combined replacement showed protection against breast cancer [94], they were poorly designed [95]. The first well controlled sizable follow-up of women receiving combined replacement therapy [61] has shown a strongly suggestive increase in risk.

Progestins and Vascular Disease

Nor is it safe to assume that estrogenic benefits to the heart will go unaffected by the addition of a progestin. Combined oral contraceptives produce longstanding increases in cardiovascular risk [96] which are related to progestin potency as well as to estrogen dose [97]. 19-nor progestins strongly alter lipoprotien profiles (both HDL and LDL) in an adverse direction, and while this seems to be much less true of medroxyprogesterone [98] (and not true at all of micronized progesterone [99]), the beneficial alterations in the profile produced by estrogens may well be diminished by any progestin.

Moreover, it is not clear that the potential cardiovascular liability of progestins is mediated by, or solely by, lipoprotiens. Even though production of angiotensinogen is stimulated to varying degrees by estrogens [100], increases in blood pressure seem to appear rarely and unpredictably in estrogen users [101], and the majority of women respond with a reduction in pressure [102], the degree of reduction depending on the kind of estrogen [103]. In contrast, some progestins produce hypertension of clinical significance [104]. The increase in blood flow produced in some vessels by estrogens is opposed by progesterone [105]. Blood flow and vascular volume are modulated by the prostaglandin system [106], and hormones may initiate such changes in part by differentially inducing the production of either vasoconstrictory thromboxane or vasodilatory prostacyclin [107]. Thromboxane and prostacyclin also are in dynamic opposition with respect to platelet aggregation. By means of this or other mechanisms, steroid hormones also act upon platelet aggregation [108] as well as on other clotting factors [109], although the specific conditions under which such effects occur are not well defined. Finally, estrogens and especially progestins have long-lasting effects upon glucose metabolism that vary with compound and potency as well as hormonal class [110]. It would be imprudent to assume that the net direction or magnitude of the estrogen-modified incidence of vascular disease will go unaffected by a progestin.

Miscellaneous Concerns

Progestin preparations are unlikely to mitigate the increase in gallbladder disease, since they also promote bile lithogenicity and stasis [111-112]. Finally. a substantial number of women are discomforted by progestin-induced systemic symptoms [113], or by withdrawal bleeding [114]. Sequential replacement is associated with a notably low compliance [115], and it is quite possible that the benefits of estrogen, or the follow-up of women on estrogen, will be lost in some by virtue of an unwillingness to continue the combined regimen.

TABLE 6. SUMMARY OF CONCERNS: SENSITIVITY TO RR's

Net Change Deaths		Breast Cancer Relative Risk			
		1.0	1.4	1.6	1.8
Heart Disease Relative Risk	0.6	-25.7%	-18.9%	-10.9%	- 6.0%
	0.8	-18.2%	-11.4%	- 3.4% (+ 1.3%)*	+ 1.5%
	1.0	-10.7%	- 3.9 %	+ 4.1%	+ 9.0%
	1.2	- 3.2%	+ 3.6%	+11.5%	+16.5%
	1.4	+ 4.2 %	+11.0%	+19.0%	+24.0%

* If sequential progestin usage were to prevent only 25% of endometrial cancer

Conclusions

Table 6 demonstrates the interaction of these various concerns. If the estimated impact on breast cancer and heart disease is accurate, 14.3% of the lives otherwise lost to these conditions will be spared by estrogen therapy, and if no additional endometrial cancer at all were to be produced by a regimen, the savings would increase to 18.9%. If the assumption about a 40% excess risk of breast cancer after 10 years of therapy is unduly conservative, and breast cancer risk is unaffected by the regimen, but the heart disease estimate is accurate, fully 25.7% of the deaths before 75 would be saved, and any hormonal impact upon the heart short of a 40% increase in risk would still produce a net saving of lives.

If, alternatively, the assumption about breast cancer is correct, then at the very least, the regimen must be neutral with respect to heart disease if lives are to be saved. If a regimen produces not a 40%, but an additional boost in breast cancer risk. to 80% or larger (i.e. to a relative risk of 1.8 from 1.4), the net saving in lives also would be reversed. If there were an adverse heart disease risk as great as 40%, with or without a further increase in breast cancer risk, the proportion of women in the cohort lost solely because of treatment easily could be as high as 25%. Note that all of the figures used as examples to describe these concerns lie within the range of the findings to date from individual studies of estrogen alone shown in Tables 1-2..

Are there any treatment strategies which will provide the valuable benefits while playing it safe? Probably not. From the tables provided one can see that neither screening out high risk women, preferentially treating only those most likely to benefit, treating only those with no uterus, nor treating women only for the short term will provide major benefit without a major risk.

It would seem prudent to provide estrogen replacement and to avoid the use of progestin for the time being. To do so in a woman with a uterus is clearly to risk iatrogenic, and patently iatrogenic, endometrial cancer. Repeated uterine biopsy after each episode of bleeding [116] will be expensive, and will result in large numbers of patients recieving unnecessary follow-up curettage, some under general anesthesia. More importantly, repeat procedures will doubtless induce non-compliance and even non-follow up, and the policy will probably not produce any substantial impact on survival from early estrogen-induced endometrial cancer, which is a largely curable disease even when symptomatic.

An alternative that might protect the endometrium with progestagen without risk of systemic effect should be considered; it is the employment of a progestagen-dispensing intra-uterine device [117]. Once in place it would provide protection to the endometrium, and at virtually no risk of infection in the postmenopausal woman.

Perhaps a prudent course in any event is to assume the role of medical fiduciary rather than that of decision-maker, to insist that the patient fully participate in the choice of therapy, and to make sure that whatever the choice, she explicity acknowledge the measure of uncertainty. In any case, both doctor and patient must place high priority on surveillance for unexplained bleeding and breast lumps, emphasizing follow-up for the former and follow-through for the latter.

BIBLIOGRAPHY

1. P.M. Sarrel, Obstet.Gynecol. 72, 2S-5S (1988).
2. P.C. MacDonald, N.Engl.J.Med. 315, 959-961 (1986).
3. Natl.Inst.Health Consensus Development Conference Summary, 2 #8 (1979).
4. Conference Report, Brit.Med.J. 295, 914-915 (1987).
5. M. Whitehead and R. Lobo, Lancet ii, 1243-1244 (1988).
6. M.C. Weinstein, and I. Schiff, Obstet.Gynecol.Surv. 38, 445-455 (1983).
7. B.E. Hillner, J.P. Hollenberg, and S.G. Pauker, Am.J.Med. 80, 1115-1127 (1986).
8. A.S. Elstein, G.B. Holzman, M.M. Ravitch, W.A. Metheny, M.M. Holmes, R.B. Hoppe, M.L. Rothert, and D.R. Rovner, Am.J.Med. 80, 246-258 (1986).

9. R.K. Ross, A. Paganini-Hill, S. Roy, A. Chao, and B.E. Henderson, Am.J.Public Health 78, 516-519 (1988).
10. E. Hemminki, D.L. Kennedy, C. Baum, and S.M. McKinlay,Am.J.Publ.Health 78, 1479-1481 (1988).
11. K.J. Ferguson, C.Hoegh, and S. Johnson, Arch.Intern.Med. 149, 133-136 (1989).
12. U.S. Natl.Cent.Health.Stat., 1986 Vital Statistics of the U.S, Volume II, Mortality, Part A, (U.S.D.H.H.S, Hyattsville, 1988)
13. U.S. Natl. Cent. Health Stat., Vital and Health Statistics Series 10, Nos. 154, 155, 158 (U.S.Public Health Service, Washington, 1986).
14. S. Campbell and M. Whitehead, Clin Obstet Gynaecol. 4, 31-47 (1977).
15. B.L. Riggs, and L.J. Melton III, N.Engl.J.Med. 314, 1676-1686 (1986).
16. J.G. Rodriguez, R.W. Satten, and R.J. Waxweiler, Am.J.Prev.Med. 5, 175-181 (1989).
17. J. Magaziner, E.M. Simonsick, T.M. Kashner, J.R. Hebel, and J.E. Kenzora, Am.J.Public Health 79, 274-278 (1988).
18. N.S. Weiss, C.L. Ure, J.H. Ballard, A.R. Williams, and J.R. Daling, N.Engl.J.Med. 303, 1195-1198 (1980).
19. A.Paganini-Hill, R.K. Ross, V.R. Gerkins, B.E. Henderson, M. Arthur, and T.M. Mack, Ann.Intern.Med. 95, 28-31 (1981).
20. S Johansson, A. Veden, and C. Wilhelmsson, Epidemiol.Rev. 5, 67-95 (1983).
21. J.C.M.Witteman, D.E.Grobbee, F.J.Kok, A.Hofman, and H.A. Valkenburg, Brit.Med.J. 298, 642-644 (1989).
22. J.M. Sullivan,R. VanderZwaag, G.F. Lemp, J.P. Hughes, V. Maddock, F.W. Kroetz, K.B. Ramanathan, and D.M. Mirvis, Ann.Int.Med. 108, 358-363 (1988).
23. R.I. Pfeffer, G.H. Whipple, T.T. Kurosaki, and J.B. Chapman, Am.J.Epidemiol. 107, 479-487 (1978).
24. C. Bain, W. Willett, C.H. Hennekens, B. Rosner, C. Belanger, and F.E. Speizer, Circulation 64, 42-46 (1981).
25. R.K. Ross, T.M. Mack, A. Paganini-Hill, M. Arthur, and B.E. Henderson, Lancet i, 858-860 (1981).
26. T.L. Bush, L.D. Cowan, E. Barrett-Connor, M.H. Criqui, J.H. Karon, R.B. Wallace, A. Tyroler, and B.M. Rifkind, J.A.M.A. 249, 903-906 (1983).
27. P.W.F. Wilson, R.J. Garrison, and W.P. Castelli, N.Eng.J.Med. 313, 1038-104, (1985).
28. M.J. Stampfer, W.C. Willett, G.A. Colditz, B. Rosner, F.E. Speizer, and C.H. Hennekens, N.Engl.J.Med. 313, 1044-1049 (1985).
29. D.B. Pettiti, J.A. Perlman, and S. Sidney, Obstet.Gynecol. 70, 289-293 (1987).
30. M.H. Criqui, L. Suarez, E. Barrett-Connor, J. McPhillips, D.L. Wingard, and C. Garland, Am.J.Epidemiol. 128, 606-614 (1988).
31. B.E. Henderson, A. Paganini-Hill, and R.K. Ross, Am.J.Obstet.Gynecol. 159, 312-317 (1988).
32. Correspondence, N.Engl.J.Med. 315, 131-136 (1986)
33. A. Paganini-Hill, R.K. Ross, and B.E. Henderson, Brit Med. J. 297, 519-522 (1988).
34. T.L. Bush, E. Barrett-Connor, L.D. Cowan, M.H. Criqui, R.B. Wallace, C.M. Suchindran, H.A. Tyroler, and B.M. Rifkind, Circulation 75, 1102-1109 (1987).
35. J.P. Broderick, S.J. Phillips, J.P. Whisnant, W.M. O'Fallon, and E.J. Bergstrahl, Stroke 20, 577-582 (1989).

36. R. Bonita, R. Beaglehole, and J.D.K. North, Am.J.Epidemiol. 120, 236-243 (1984).
37. A. Linos, J.W. Worthington, W.M. O'Fallon, and L.T. Kurland, Am.J.Epidemiol. 111, 87-98 (1980).
38. J.P. Vandenbroucke, J.C.M. Witteman, H.A. Valkenburg, J.W. Boersma, A. Cats, J.J.M. Festem. A. Hartman. P. Huber-Bruning, J.J.Rasker, and J. Weber, J.A.M.A. 255, 1299-1303 (1986).
39. P. Allebeck, A. Ahlbom, and E. Allander, Scand.J.Rheumatology 10, 301-306 (1981).
40. L.J. Bennion, R.L. Ginsberg, M.B. Garnick, and P.H. Bennett, N.Engl.J.Med. 294, 189-192 (1976).
41. D.B. Pettiti, S. Sidney, and J.A. Perlman, Gastroenterology 94, 91-95 (1988).
42. R.B. Everson, D.P. Byar, and A.J. Bischoff, Gastroenterology 82, 4-8 (1982).
43. G.D.Friedman, W.B. Kannel, and T.R Dawber, J. Chronic Dis. 19, 273-292 (1966).
44. A.K. Diehl, M.P. Stern, V.S. Ostrower, and P.C. Friedman, South.Med.J. 73, 438-441 (1980).
45. S.B. Gusberg, Am.J.Obstet.Gynecol. 54, 905-927 (1947).
46. I. Schiff, H.K. Sela, D. Cramer, D. Tulchinsky, and K.J.Ryan, Fertil.Steril. 37, 79-82 (1982).
47. WHO Technical Report #670, (WHO, Geneva, 1981)
48. C.M.F. Antunes, P.D. Stolley, N.B. Roseshein, J.L. Davies, J.A. Tonascia, C. Brown, L. Burnett, A. Rutledge, M. Pokempner, and R. Garcia, N.Engl.J.Med. 300, 9-13 (1979).
49. N.S. Weiss, D.R. Szekely, D.R. English, and A. Schweid, J.A.M.A. 242, 261-264 (1979).
50. S. Shapiro, J.P. Kelly, L. Rosenberg, D.W. Kaufman, S.P. Helmrich, N.B. Rosenshein, J.L. Lewis Jr., R.C. Knapp, P.D. Stolley, and D. Schottenfeld, N.Engl.J.Med. 313, 969-972 (1985).
51. A. Paganini-Hill, R.K. Ross, and B.E. Henderson, Br.J.Cancer 59, 445-447 (1989).
52. N.S. Weiss, V.T. Farewell, D.R. Szekely, D.R. English, and N. Keviat, Maturitas 2, 185-190 (1980).
53. T.M. Mack, M.C. Pike, M.E. Henderson, R.I. Pfeffer. V.R. Gerkins, M. Arthur, and S.E. Brown, N.Engl.J.Med. 294, 1262-1267 (1976).
54. S.S. Devesa, D.T. Silverman, J.L. Young, Jr, E.S. Pollack, C.C. Brown, J.W. Horm, C.L.Percy, M.H. Myers, F.W. McKay, and J.F. Fraumeni,Jr, J.N.C.I. 79, 701-770 (1987).
55. L.G.Ries, E.S.Pollack, and J.L. Young, Jr, J.N.C.I. 70, 693-707 (1983).
56. M.C. Pike, M.D. Krailo, B.E. Henderson, J.T. Casagrande, and D.G. Hoel, Nature 303, 767-770 (1983).
57. M.C. Pike, J.T. Casagrande, J.B. Brown, V. Gerkins, and B.E. Henderson, J.Natl.Cancer Inst. 59, 1351-1355 (1977).
58. D. Trichopoulos, S. Yen, J. Brown, P. Cole, and B. MacMahon, Cancer 53, 187-192 (1984).
59. W.St.C. Symmers, Brit.Med.J. ii, 83-85 (1968).
60. O.K. Schlappack, O. Braun, and U. Maier, Cancer Detect.Prevent. 9, 319-322 (1986).
61. L. Bergkvist, H-O Adami, I. Persson, R. Hoover, and C. Schairer, N.Eng.J.Med. 321, 293-297 (1989).
62. L.A. Brinton, R. Hoover, and J.F. Fraumeni,Jr, Br.J.Cancer 54, 825-832 (1986).
63. J.E. Buring, C.H. Hennekens, R.J. Lipnick, W. Willett, M.J. Stampfer, B. Rosner, R. Peto, and F.E. Speizer, Am.J.Epidemiol. 125. 939-947 (1987).

64. T.J. Craig, G.W. Comstock, and P.B. Geiser, J.Natl.Cancer Inst. 53, 1577-1581 (1974).
65. M. Ewertz, Int.J.Cancer 42, 832-838 (1988).
66. R.A. Hiatt, R. Bawol, G.D. Friedman, and R. Hoover, Cancer 54, 139-144 (1984).
67. R. Hoover, A. Glass, W.D. Finkle, D. Azevedo, and K. Milne, J.N.C.I. 67, 815-820 (1981).
68. B.S. Hulka, L.E. Chambless, D.C. Deubner, and W.E. Wilkinson, Am.J.Obstet.Gynecol. 143, 638-644 (1982).
69. K. Hunt, M. Vessey, K. McPherson, and M. Coleman, Br.J.Obstet.Gynecol. 94, 620-635 (1987).
70. C. LaVecchia, A. Decarli, F. Parazzini, A. Gentile, C. Liberati, and S. Franceschi, Int.J.Cancer 38, 853-858 (1986).
71. J.A. McDonald, N.S. Weiss, J.R. Daling, A.M. Francis, and L. Polissar, Breast Cancer Research and Treatment 7, 193-199 (1986).
72. A.M.Y. Nomura, L.N. Kolonel, T. Hirohata, and J. Lee, Int.J.Cancer 37, 49-53 (1986).
73. T.E. Rohan, and A.J. McMichael, Med.J.Austral. 148, 217-221 (1988).
74. R.K. Ross, A. Paganini-Hill, V.R. Gerkins, T.M. Mack, R. Pfeffer, M. Arthur, and B.E. Henderson, J.A.M.A. 243, 1635-1639 (1980).
75. P.A. Wingo, P.M. Layde, N.C. Lee, G. Rubin, and H.W. Ory, J.A.M.A. 257, 209-215 (1987).
76. L. Bergkvist, H-O. Adami, I. Persson, R. Bergstrom and U.B. Krusemo, Am.J.Epidemiol. 130, 221-228 (1989).
77. A. Paganini-Hill, and R.K. Ross, Am.J.Epidemiol. 116, 1635-1639 (1982).
78. B.E. Henderson, R.K. Ross, A. Paganini-Hill, and T.M. Mack, Am.J.Obstet.Gynecol. 154, 1181-1186 (1986).
79. A. Paganini-Hill, R.K. Ross, B.E. Henderson, Personal communication, (1989).
80. I. Schiff, D. Tulchinsky, D. Cramer, and K.J. Ryan, J.A.M.A. 244, 1443-1445 (1980).
81. C. Christiansen, Eur.J.Clin.Invest. 10, 273-279 (1980).
82. B.E. Henderson, R.K. Ross, R.A. Lobo, M.C. Pike, T.M. Mack, Fertil.Steril. 49, 9S-15S (1988).
83. Z. Rosenwaks, A.C. Wentz, G.S. Jones, M.D. Urban, P.A. Lee, C.J. Migeon, T.H. Parmley, and J.D. Woodruff, Obstet.Gynecol. 53, 403-410 (1979).
84. S.G. Silverberg, E.L. Makowski, and W.D. Roche, Cancer 39, 592-598 (1977).
85. C.D.C. Cancer and Steroid Hormone Study Group, J.A.M.A. 257, 796-800 (1987)
86. S. Nandi, J.Nat.Cancer Inst. 21, 1039-1063 (1958).
87. T.J.A. Key, M.C. Pike, Eur.J.Cancer Clin. Oncol., 24, 29-43, (1988).
88. UK National Case-Control Study Group, Lancet i, 973-982, (1989).
89. M. Vessey, J. Baron, R. Doll, K. McPherson, and D. Yeates, Br.J.Cancer, 47 455-462 (1983).
90. C.R. Kay and P.C. Hannaford, Br.J.Cancer 58, 675-680 (1988).
91. A.P. Liang, A.G. Levenson, P.M. Layde, J.D. Shelton, R.A. Hatcher, M. Potts, M.J. Mechelson, J.A.M.A. 249, 2909-2912 (1983).
92. WHO Collab.Study of Neoplasia and Steroid Contraceptives, Bull.W.H.O. 63, 513-519 (1985).

93. N.C. Lee, L Rosero-Bixby, M.W. Oberle, A.S. Whatley, and E.Z. Rovira, J.N.C.I. 79, 1247-1254 (1987).
94. R.D. Gambrell, Maturitas 8, 169-176 (1986).
95. V.L. Ernster, and S.R. Cummings, Obstet.Gynecol. 68, 715-717 (1986).
96. D. Slone, S. Shapiro, D.W. Kaufman, L. Rosenberg, O.S. Miettinen, and P.D. Stolley, N.Engl.J.Med. 305, 420-424 (1981).
97. T.W. Meade, G. Greenberg, and S.G. Thompson, Br.Med.J. 1, 1157-1161 (1980).
98. E. Hirvonen, A. Lipasti, M. Malkonen, J. Karkkainen, J. Nuntila, H. Timonen, and V. Manninen, Maturitas 9, 69-79 (1987).
99. U.B. Ottosson, B.G. Johansson, and B. von Schoultz, J.Obstet. Gynecol. 151, 746-750 (1985).
100. C.A. Mashchak, R.A. Lobo, R. Dozono-Takano, P. Eggena, R.M. Nakamura, P.F. Brenner, and D.R. Mischell, Am.J.Obstet.Gynecol. 144, 511-518 (1982).
101. M.G. Crane, J.J. Harris, and W. Winsor 3rd, Ann.Intern.Med. 74, 13-21 (1971).
102. H. Luotola, Ann.Clin.Res. Suppl 38, 9-121 (1983).
103. B.G. Wren and A.D. Routledge, Maturitas 5, 135-142 (1983).
104. C.R. Kay, Am.J.Obstet.Gynecol. 142, 762-765 (1982).
105. R.Risnik, G.W.Brink, and M.H.Plumer, Am.J.Obstet.Gynecol. 128, 251-254 (1977).
106. B. Pitt, M.J. Shea, J.L. Romson, and B.R. Lucchesi, Ann.Intern.Med. 99, 83-93 (1983).
107. O. Ylikokala, A. Puolakka, and L. Viinikka, Maturitas 5, 201-205 (1984).
108. G.N. Mileikowsky, J.L. Nadler, J. Huey, R. Francis, and S. Roy, Am.J.Obstet.Gynecol. 159, 1547-1552 (1988).
109. E.F. Mammen, Am.J.Obstet.Gynecol. 142, 781-790 (1982).
110. L.D. Cowan, R.B. Wallace, E. Barrett-Connor, D. Hunninghake, P. Pomrehn, P. Wahl, and G. Heiss, J.Reproduct.Med. 27, 275-282 (1982).
111. R.H.L. Down, M.J. Whiting, J. McK. Watts, and W. Jones, Gut 24, 253-259 (1983).
112. P.F. Keane, A.S. Clanachan, and G.W. Scott, Surgical Forum 35, 467-468 (1984).
113. L. Dennerstein and G. Burrows, Maturitas 8, 101-106 (1986).
114. R.G.Hahn, R.D. Nachtigall, and T.C.Davies, J.Family Practice 18, 411-414 (1984).
115. V.A. Ravnikar, Am.J.Obstet.Gynecol. 156, 1332-1334 (1987).
116. M.H. Thom, P.J. White, R.M. Williams, D.W. Sturdee, M.E.L. Paterson, T. Wade-Evans, and J.W.W. Studd, Lancet ii, 455-457 (1979).
117. T.K. Hagenfeld, B.M. Landgren, K. Edstrom, and E. Johansson, Contraception 16, 183-197 (1977).

FLUORIDE

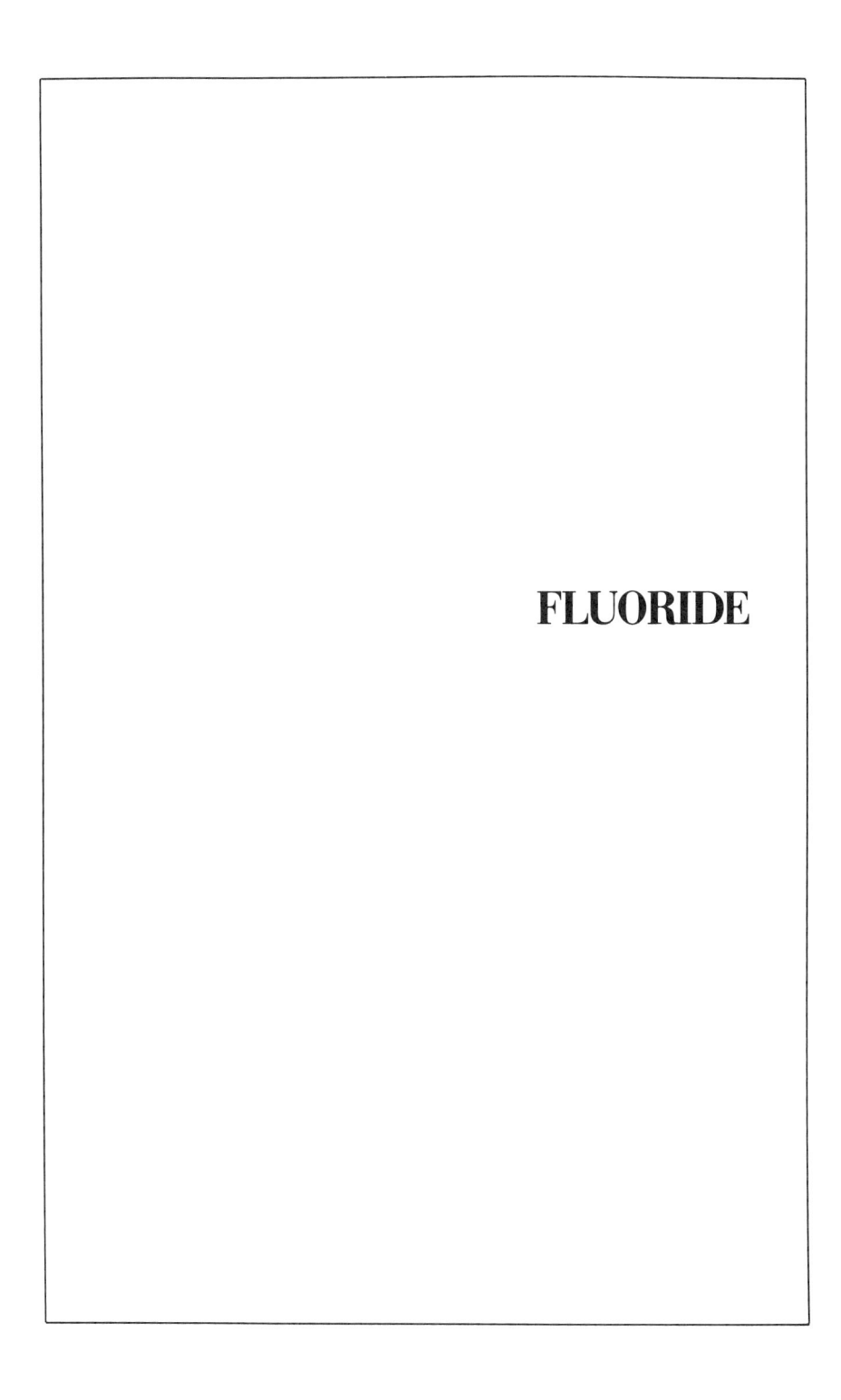

Benefit-Risk Ratio of Fluoride Therapy in Vertebral Osteoporosis: Comparison of Sodium Fluoride to Monofluorophosphate

P.J. Meunier,[*] N. Mamelle,[†] P.D. Delmas,[*] R. Dusan,[†] and J. Dupuis[*]

[*]INSERM, Hôpital Ed. Herriot, Lyon, France
[†]INSERM, Lyon, France and GETOP

ABSTRACT

In the past 28 years several open and uncontrolled studies have shown that fluoride (F) has an anabolic effect on trabecular bone mass in the axial skeleton, but doubts persisted about the effectiveness of this treatment in decreasing the vertebral fracture rate. We elected to examine prospectively in 446 patients with at least one vertebral fracture, the benefit-risk ratio of combined fluoride-calcium therapy in primary vertebral osteoporosis. 257 patients were randomized to receive sodium fluoride (NaF) 25 mg twice daily plus elemental calcium 1 g daily and a vitamin D_2 supplement, and 209 received one of the alternative therapies usually prescribed in France. After a follow-up of 24 months the fluoride group showed a significantly lower rate of new vertebral fractures between 12 and 24 months (18.8 per cent in F group vs 31.6 per cent in non F group) and between 0 and 24 months (39.2 per cent vs 50.8 per cent). The main adverse effect of the regimen was a higher incidence of osteoarticular pain in the ankle and foot (15 per cent in F group vs 5 per cent in non F group). The risk of non vertebral fractures was not increased and digestive disorders arose with equal frequency in the two groups. NaF 50 mg daily seems to represent a reasonable compromise in terms of antifracture effectiveness and side-effects. Further studies comparing the benefit-risk of 200 mg daily of monofluorophosphate (MFP) (26 mg F-ion) to 50 mg of NaF (22 mg F-ion) showed a greater increase in lumbar bone mineral density measured by DPA with MFP than with NaF, but associated with a higher incidence of osteoarticular pain syndrome. Bioavailability of F is better with MFP than with NaF and, beside the dose, this factor should be taken into account in the evaluation of benefit-risk of fluoride treatment in osteoporosis where the therapeutic window is rather narrow.

INTRODUCTION

Sodium fluoride (NaF) was introduced 28 years ago for the curative treatment of vertebral osteoporosis (1), and since 1961 several prospective open studies have shown that NaF is effective in increasing trabecular bone mass in the spine because of its ability to stimulate osteoblastic bone formation. This was shown first by radiological techniques (2,3), then by histomorphometric analysis of iliac bone biopsies (4,5), by measurements of the mineral bone density of the axial skeleton with dual photon absorptiometry (6-10), quantitative computed tomography (11), neutron activation analysis (12), and most recently by serum osteocalcin measurement (10). There is general agreement that NaF, combined with adequate calcium supplementation, has an anabolic effect on vertebral bone mass, but uncertainties persist, however, about the quality of the newly synthesized bone, the effectiveness of this treatment in decreasing the vertebral fracture rate, the effects on non vertebral fractures and on cortical bone mass (13,6). Furthermore side-effects are common and have limited the clinical usefulness of fluoride treatment, especially of high doses which induce a higher incidence of gastrointestinal disorders and of lower extremity pain syndromes (4,14). In order to evaluate the benefit-ratio of combined fluoride-calcium therapy in vertebral osteoporosis, we examined prospectively the rate of new vertebral fractures and of side effects in patients with at least one non traumatic vertebral crush fracture, and treated either with sodium fluoride and calcium or with other alternative therapies usually prescribed in France (15). In addition, in order to analyze the influence of the dose and of the bioavailability of fluoride salts, we compared the efficacy and the occurence of side-effects in two other groups of patients with vertebral osteoporosis and treated with fluoride administered either as monofluorophosphate or as sodium fluoride (16). Monofluorophosphate (MFP or $Na_2 PO_3 F$) is a highly soluble fluoride salt which forms with calcium carbonate a soluble salt which is readily absorbed in the duodenum and the small intestine. In contrast, NaF forms with calcium salts poorly soluble salts (CaF_2) which account for a mild reduction of fluoride intestinal absorption (17). Despite the potential advantages of MFP there are still few documented reports on the effects of this compound in vertebral osteoporosis (18,19).

PROSPECTIVE STUDY ON THE BENEFIT-RISK OF SODIUM FLUORIDE TREATMENT

Materials and Methods (16)

The target population consisted of 466 adult patients aged between 50 and 92 years consulting one of 94 physicians who had agreed to participate in the study. All had a diagnosis of primary osteoporosis with at least one non traumatic vertebral crush fracture, and expressed their willingness to accept the medication for 2 years. 257 patients (229 women and 28 men were treated with NaF and took 25 mg NaF twice a day, just before lunch and dinner (ie 50 mg NaF/day). They also received 1 gram elemental calcium per day, to be taken between meals, and a vitamin D_2 supplement of 800 IU per day. NaF was given in the form of enteric-coated tablets, each containing 25 mg, ie 11.3 mg fluoride-ion. 209 patients (192 women and 17 men) received one of the other regimens prescribed by French physicians after diagnosis of osteoporosis : calcium 1 g/day and vitamin D_2 800 IU/day (93 patients), calcitonin 50 U/day for 5 days every 3 weeks and phosphorus 1-1.5 g/day (85 patients) ; calcium plus phosphorus (17 patients) ; calcitonin plus calcium (12 patients) ; phosphorus and sodium etidronate (2 patients). Follow-up visits were at 3,6,12,18 and 24 months and included radiographs of thoracic and lumbar spine from T3 to L5.

Results

Of the 466 patients enrolled in the study, 316 (68 %) were followed for a full 24 months. The reasons for discontinuation of treatment did not differ between the two groups. Among the patients with 24 months follow-up, the crush fracture rate per year was found significantly lower in the NaF group and the mean number of new crush fractures per year was also lower in the group treated with fluoride, the difference being statistically significant between 12 and 24 months (Table I). A new vertebral crush fracture was characterized by the deformation of a normal vertebra to a biconcave one, a fractured plate, an evident wedging or a collapse of the vertebral body.

Table I. Antifracture efficacy of NaF in the subgroup followed for 24 months.

	NaF treatment (n : 180)	Non NaF treatment (n : 136)	p
Proportion with ≥ a new crush fracture/year			
0-24 months	39.2 %	50.8 %	<0.05
0-12 months	30.1 %	37.2 %	ns
12-24 months	18.8 %	31.6 %	<0.05

On the total randomized group (466 patients), a descriptive analysis of all patients followed for at least 6 months indicated the percentage of patients who had at least one new crush fracture during each period. As calculated by the product limit method, the probability of absence of crush fracture between 0 and 24 months was 0.60 in patients treated with NaF compared with 0.47 in patients who were not treated with NaF (p < 0.01). Use of the Cox model to compare the two treatments confirms the result obtained by the product limit method with a risk of a new crush fracture 1.39 times higher in patients without NaF treatment than in patients treated with fluoride (p = 0.03). After adjustment for the pronostic variables (age and number of vertebral fracture on entry) , the relation between crush fractures and treatment persists and the relative risk increases to 1.44 (p = 0.02).

Among side-effects, episodes of osteoarticular pain were frequent in both groups of patients followed for 2 years : 37 % of NaF treated patients versus 30 % of non-NaF subjects (not a significant difference). But pain in the lower limbs located in the ankle and foot were more often noted among NaF-treated patients than in the non-NaF group (39/180 versus 10/136). 27 patients (15 %) in the NaF group, compared with 7 (5 %) in the non-NaF group, had at least one episode of pain in the ankle and foot (p < 0.01). In the total sample the relative risk of pain located in the ankle and foot between non-NaF and NaF was of 0.34, significantly different from 1 (p = 0.01).

Non-vertebral fractures, both traumatic and spontaneous, occurred with equal frequency (13 %) in the two group followed for 2 years. The fracture sites were also similar. 24 fractures were noted in the NaF group and 22 in the non-NaF group, including 6 femoral neck fractures in the NaF group and 4 in the non-NaF group. These figures represent an annual incidence of 1.7 and 1.5 % in patients treated with NaF and in those not treated with NaF respectively. In the total sample, 28 fractures were reported in each group, including 7 femoral neck fractures in the NaF group and 8 in the non-NaF group.

Digestive disorders were frequent in both groups and were responsible for a drop-out rate in the NaF and non-NaF groups, respectively, of 24 % and 38 %. In the total sample, use of the Cox model set the relative risk of gastrointestinal disorders (non-NaF/NaF) at 1.08 (non significant), after adjustment for history of digestive disorders.

COMPARISON OF BENEFIT-RISK OF SODIUM FLUORIDE TREATMENT TO BENEFIT-RISK OF DISODIUM MONOFLUOROPHOSPHATE TREATMENT.

Materials and Methods (17)

We studied 81 consecutive women (65 ± 8 year old), with vertebral osteoporosis and at least one non traumatic vertebral crush fracture. 71 had postmenopausal osteoporosis and 10 a corticosteroid induced osteoporosis. All the patients had a normal serum creatinine level. Monofluorophosphate was given as effervescent tablets containing 100 mg of NaPO3F - i.e. 13.2 mg fluoride ion - and 1250 mg of CaCO3 - i.e. 500 mg elemental calcium - twice a day (Fluocalcic® from Beytout). Sodium fluoride was given as enteric-coated tablets containing 25 mg of NaF - i.e. 11.3 mg fluoride ion -, twice a day (Osteofluor® from Merck-Clevenot). Patients treated with NaF were supplemented with 1 g of elemental calcium per day taken apart from NaF. All patients received a vitamin D2 supplementation of 800 to 8000 IU per day.

Clinical assessment made every 6 months included any traumatic or spontaneous vertebral or non vertebral fractures, gastro-intestinal disorders, osteo-articular pain and any other associated disorders. In case of lower extremity pain syndrome, the suspicion of stress micro-fractures was always substantiated with X-rays of the painful area and by radionuclide bone scan. Bone mineral density (BMD) was measured from L2 to L4 with a Novo Lab 22a device and the data were expressed as g/cm2 or as Z score. The precision in vivo measured on volunteers was 2.1 % (18).

Results

Fluoride treatment resulted in a progressive increase of BMD with time which was significant earlier with MFP than with NaF (Table II). This BMD increase was significantly higher in the MPF group than in the NaF group after 6, 12 and 18 months of treatment.

Urinary fluoride was significantly higher in the MFP group than in the NaF group during the treatment with a mean value being 50 % higher throughout the entire study. As an example urinary fluoride, measured after 12 months of treatment was 6.8 ± 3.4 mg/24 hrs in NaF group and 9.6 ± 3.5 mg/24 hrs in MFP group (p : 0.003).

Table II. Increase in lumbar BMD in women with vertebral osteoporosis treated either with sodium fluoride or with monofluorophosphate. The increase is expressed in percent pre-treatment BMD.

Months of Treatment	Relative increase of BMD NaF (n)	MFP (n)	p <
6	+ 1.5 ± 7.8 * (36)	+ 6.6 ± 7.2 (28)	0.01
12	+ 4.2 ± 10.7 (36)	+ 10.5 ± 6.9 (23)	0.02
18	+ 6.1 ± 12.3 (27)	+ 20.5 ± 10.3 (12)	0.002
24	+ 11.5 ± 14.5 (21)	+ 18.4 ± 7.4 (6)	ns

* mean ± 1 SD

Among the 81 treated women, 3 out of 52 on NaF had new crushed vertebrae during treatment (one in 2 patients and 2 in the third one). In the MFP group 7/29 patients had new vertebral fracture (one vertebra in each one), a proportion not significantly different from the NaF group. The analysis of the side effects has shown that after correction for the duration of treatment, the incidence of lower extremity pain syndrome related to stress microfractures were significantly more frequent with MFP than with NaF (Table III). The treatment was sometimes interrupted for 3 to 4 weeks during the painful episode but definitive withdrawal of the treatment was never necessary because of this lower extremity pain syndrome.

Table III. Incidence of lower extremity pain syndrome related to stress microfractures (SMF) in 81 osteoporotic females treated with fluoride.

	NaF Group	MFP Group	p <
No of patients	52	29	
No of patients with SMF	8/52 (15.4 %)	10/29 (34.5 %)	0.05
No of episodes/patient-years of treatment	9/72 (12.5 %)	14/38 (36.8 %)	0.01
No of episodes/patient First 6-12 mths of treat.	2/44 (4.5 %)	10/25 (40 %)	0.001

Patients who developed SMF had a higher increase of BMD than those without SMF. The difference was significant when all women on NaF and MFP were analyzed together but also when women on NaF were analyzed separately (17). Two patients -one on NaF, one on MFP- developed osteomalacia during treatment revealed by severe long bones pain and in one case by bilateral impacted femoral neck fracture. The diagnosis of osteomalacia was confirmed in both cases by histomorphometric analysis of a transiliac bone biopsy and treatment was interrupted. A patient in the NaF group had a femoral neck fracture during treatment, without osteomalacia. Gastro-intestinal side-effects were rare -1/37 patients on NaF and 3/29 patients on MFP- consisting of transient gastric pain, nausea or constipation, but did not require interruption of the treatment.

DISCUSSION

The above results confirm that treatments with sodium fluoride or disodium monofluorophosphate increase bone mass in the axial skeleton. But vertebral fracture rate is a more relevant end-point than bone mass, and our large randomized controlled trial has shown that the proportion of patients with new vertebral fractures was significantly reduced at 24 months, from 51 per cent in patients receiving other therapies to 39 per cent in patients treated with 50 mg/day enteric coated sodium fluoride (15). When other risk factors were taken into account, the risk of new vertebral fractures was 39 per cent greater in the non-fluoride-treated patients. These results are consistent with a large body of evidence from uncontrolled previous studies. Fracture results from two other larged randomized and controlled trials, just completed at Mayo Clinic and Henry Ford Hospital where a daily dose of 75 mg of sodium fluoride has been given for 4 years are not yet available. This regimen represents a cumulative dose delivered to bone much greater than the total dose given to our patients treated with 50 mg/day of sodium fluoride given for two years.

We also found that despite an almost similar fluoride content, MFP induces a greater increase of lumbar bone mineral density and a higher incidence of osteoarticular pain syndrome of lower limbs than enteric-coated NaF (16). This difference is probably related to a higher intestinal absorption and to a better bioavailability of MFP than NaF.

In conclusion, the overall risk/benefit ratio of low dose fluoride treatment of vertebral osteoporosis is favourable, but there is a clear correlation between the efficacy and the incidence of osteo-articular side effects according to the dose. The therapeutic window is rather narrow, and the bioavailability of the fluoride salt used, in conditions of routine prescription, should be taken into account when establishing the optimum therapeutic dose.

REFERENCES

1. C. Rich and J. Ensinck, Nature 191, 184-185 (1961).
2. K. Chlud, Z. Rheumatol 36, 126-139 (1977).
3. M.A. Dambacher, T. Lauffenburger, B. Lämmle and H.G. Haas in : Fluoride and Bone, B. Courvoisier, A. Donath and C.A. Baud eds (Hans Huber, Bern, 1978) pp. 238-241.
4. D. Briancon and P.J. Meunier, Orthop Clin N Am 12, 629-648 (1981)
5. E.F. Eriksen, L. Mosekilde and F. Melsen, Bone 6, 381-389 (1985).
6. B.L. Riggs, S.F Hodgson, J. Muhs and H.W. Wahner in : Osteoporosis 1987, C. Christiansen, J.S. Johansen and B.J. Riis eds (Osteopress, Copenhagen 1987) pp. 817-823.
7. C. Nagant de Deuxchaisnes, J.P. Devogelaer, P. Resimont and J.P. Huaux, Louvain Med 106, 407-432 (1987).
8. J.A. Raymakers, C.F. van Dijke, A. Hoekstra and S.A. Duursma, Bone, 8, 143-148 (1987).
9. T. Hansson and H.T. Roos, Calcif Tissue Int, 40, 315-317 (1987).
10. C.Y.C. Pak, K. Sakhaee, J.E. Zerwekh, C. Parcel, R. Peterson and K. Johnson, J Clin Endocrinol Metab, 68, 150-159 (1989).
11. F.R. Singer, C.F. Sharp, R.K. Rude in Calcium Regulation and Bone Metabolism, D. Cohn, T.J. Martin and P.J. Meunier eds (Elsevier Science Publishers, Amsterdam 1987) p. 861.
12. J.E. Harrison, K.G. Mc Neill, W.C. Sturtridge, T.A. Bayley, T.M. Murray, C. Williams, C. Tam and V. Fornastier, J Clin Endocrinol Metab, 52, 751-758 (1981).
13. M.A. Dambacher, J. Ittner and P. Ruegsegger, Bone, 7, 199-205 (1986).
14. C.M. Schnitzler and L. Solomon, Skeletal Radiol 14, 276-279 (1985).
15. N. Mamelle, P.J. Meunier, R. Dusan, M. Guillaume, J.L. Martin, A. Gaucher, A. Prost, G. Ziegler, P. Netter, Lancet, 361-365 (1988).
16. P.D. Delmas, J. Dupuis, F. Duboeuf, M.C. Chapuy and P.J. Meunier, J Bone Min Res (in press).
17. E.F. Eriksen, S.F. Hodgson, B.L. Riggs in : Osteoporosis, etiology, diagnosis and management, B.L. Riggs and L.J. Melton III eds (Raven Press, New York 1988) pp. 415-432.
18. D. Dressler, Therapiewoche 34, 1843-1852 (1984).
19. V.I.D. Ringe, Fortschr Med 105, 379-382 (1987).

Fluoride and Calcium Therapy for Osteoporosis Increases Trabecular Vertebral Bone Density Above the Fracture Threshold

S.M.G. Farley[*], V. Perkel[*], L.A. Tudtud-Hans[*], M.R. Mariano-Menez[*], C.R. Libanati[*], E.E. Schulz[‡], and D.J. Baylink[*]

[*]*Departments of Medicine and Research, Loma Linda University and Jerry L. Pettis Memorial Veteran's Hospital, Loma Linda, California*
[‡]*Department of Radiology, Loma Linda University, Loma Linda, California*

ABSTRACT

41 postmenopausal osteoporotic females were treated with fluoride 32 +/- 6 mg/day (equivalent to 71 +/- 12 mg NaF daily) plus calcium 1500 mg/day for 32 +/- 10 months. Serial measurements of trabecular vertebral bone density were made at 10 +/- 4 month intervals by quantitative computed tomography. Compared to pretreatment values, vertebral bone density was significantly increased by 25% ($p<.001$) after six months of therapy and continued to increase at a linear rate throughout the study ($r = 0.40$, $p<.001$). The average rate of increase was 1.25 +/- 0.91 mg/cc/month. The rate of increase in vertebral bone density was related to the dose of fluoride ($r=.34$, $p<.03$); patients on the higher doses of fluoride increased at a rate of 1.73 mg/cc/month compared to the rate of .92 +/- .74 mg/cc/month observed in patients on lower doses of fluoride. Vertebral bone density was increased above the fracture threshold of 100 mg/cc in 44% of patients. Compared to these patients, the remaining 56% of the patients had a lower pretreatment spinal bone density and a slower rate of increase in vertebral bone density, suggesting that longer treatment might be required to correct the greater bone deficit. We conclude that fluoride plus calcium is an effective therapy for increasing vertebral bone density above the risk for fracture but that a long period of treatment (i.e. > three years) and/or large doses of fluoride (i.e. > 72 mg/NaF/day) may be required to effect this outcome in the majority of osteoporotic patients.

INTRODUCTION

Current therapies for osteoporosis (e.g., calcium, estrogen, and calcitonin) are useful for reducing bone loss in perimenopausal women but may be of less value in treating older osteoporotic women whose bone loss has slowed and whose remaining bone is of inadequate quantity to prevent fractures [1]. Optimum treatment for these millions of elderly women who have already suffered significant bone loss and spontaneous fractures requires a therapy which can promote a large increases in bone density sufficient to reduce the risk for fracture.

Fluoride, a bone cell mitogen [2], is one of the few agents known with the potential to substantially increase spinal bone density. Fluoride therapy for osteoporosis has consistently been shown to increase both trabecular bone formation and bone volume in the iliac crest [3-4]. With the recent introduction of dual photon absorptiometry [5] and quantitative computed tomography (QCT) [6] the efficacy of therapies for osteoporosis can now be measured directly in the spine. Only a few studies thus far have reported results of fluoride therapy with either of these methods; but findings indicate that fluoride therapy does indeed promote a significant increase in bone density of the osteoporotic spine [8-11]. Depending largely on the densitometric method used and perhaps to some extent on other variables in these studies (e.g., sex of the patients, pretreatment spinal bone density, dose of fluoride, treatment duration, and treatment combinations) the spinal bone response to fluoride has ranged from a 3% to 42% increase after one year of therapy.

In the current study, serial measurements of spinal bone density were made by QCT over a 1 to 4 year period of treatment with fluoride and calcium to determine if the rate and magnitude of the spinal bone response was sufficient to increase vertebral bone density above the risk for fracture. The findings indicate that fluoride and calcium therapy increases trabecular vertebral bone density above the fracture threshold value of 100 mg/cc [12] in 44 % of patients treated for 32 +/- 10 months, and suggest that longer therapy may benefit the remaining patients who tended to have a greater deficit in spinal bone density and/or a slower response to therapy.

METHODS

Patient Selection

41 females, aged 70 +/- 9 years (range: 48 - 88 years) were selected from an ongoing clinical study of fluoride therapy. These subjects included all patients who had been on treatment sufficient time to have had at least two post-treatment measurements of spinal bone density and who satisfied the following inclusion/exclusion criteria. All subjects were ambulatory, post-menopausal (either surgical or natural menopause) females with primary osteoporosis. Osteoporosis was evident by the presence of one or more non-traumatic vertebral fractures (i.e., a minimum collapse in anterior or central vertebral body height of 15%) and low spinal bone density (i.e., less than 100 mg/cm3 by QCT). Osteoporosis associated with glucocorticoid therapy, ethanol abuse, anticonvulsant therapy, or malabsorption syndrome was reason for exclusion. Concurrent metabolic bone disease, treatment with other therapies for osteoporosis (e.g., vitamin D or estrogen), or impaired renal function were also reasons for exclusion.

Treatment

All patients received treatment with fluoride, as either sodium fluoride or monofluorophosphate 10 mg elemental fluoride per capsule, 3 to 4 capsules daily in divided doses as tolerated. In addition, dietary calcium intake was supplemented with calcium carbonate tablets for a total calcium intake of 1500 mg/day. Patients were treated for 32 +/- 10 months (range: 12 to 48 months).

Variation in the dosage of fluoride occurred as management of G.I. and/or peri-articular pain required decreasing the dose of fluoride and/or interrupting fluoride therapy briefly (i.e., 1 - 4 weeks) in 68% of the patients and the dose of fluoride was inadvertently increased above the recommended for a short time by one patient. This resulted in an average intake of fluoride, calculated as the total amount of fluoride ingested divided by the time on the study, ranging from 15 to 43 mg/day; the mean dose for the group was 32 +/- 6 mg/day (equivalent to 71 +/- 12 mg NaF daily).

Assessment

Trabecular bone density in the spine was measured by single energy QCT of five vertebrae, T-12 to L-4 inclusive, using a mineral reference for calibration [7]. Compressed vertebrae were not included in the analysis. Results are give for the mean of the unfractured vertebrae and expressed in mineral equivalents of K2PO4 in mg/cc. The coefficient of variation for duplicate measurements ranged from 3% in 9 normal volunteers to 5% in 5 osteoporotic subjects.

Spinal bone density measurements were obtained prior to therapy and at 10 +/- 4 month (range: 6 to 24 month) intervals thereafter. The number of measurements made (including the pretreatment measurement) averaged 4 +/- 1 (range: 3 - 6) per patient. Results in each patient were plotted as a function of time on treatment to calculate the rate of change in spinal bone density by linear regression analysis. Results are given for the slope of this analysis, expressed as mg/cc/month.

Aggregate data are expressed as mean +/- S.D. Quantitative data were compared by Student's two-tailed t-test, paired or unpaired as appropriate and regression analysis were performed using Microstat, a commercial statistical computer program (Echosoft, Indianapolis, IN). For all results, a p value less than .05 was required for statistical significance.

RESULTS

Prior to treatment, spinal bone density averaged 51 +/- 20 mg/cc (range: 12 - 88 mg/cc) in this group of 41 female osteoporotics. During treatment with fluoride and calcium, trabecular bone density of the spine was significantly increased throughout four years of observation compared to pretreatment values (Figure 1). The increase in spinal bone density occurred at a linear rate (r = 0.40; p < .001).

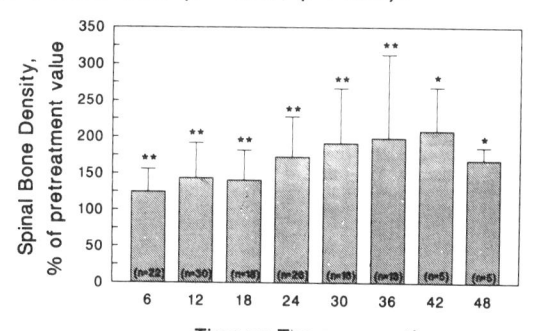

FIG. 1. Change in spinal bone density measured by QCT during treatment with fluoride and calcium. Values represent the mean +/- S.D. Numbers in parenthesis indicate the number of patients from the study group of 41 osteoporotic females with a measurement at that time point.
 * Significantly different from baseline, p<.01
 ** Significantly different from baseline, p<.001

The rate of increase in spinal bone density, determined from regression analysis of results from serial measurements in each patient, averaged 1.25 +/- .91 mg/cc/month for the group, but varied widely between patients (range: .006 - 3.65 mg/cc/month). This interpatient variation in the skeletal response to fluoride could be explained in small part by variation in the dose of fluoride (r = .34, p<.03) (Figure 2), but was not related to the patients' age (r = .07) or pretreatment spinal bone density (r = .30, p<.058). Further examination of the dose response to fluoride revealed that patients treated with a high dose of fluoride (i.e., 33 - 43 mg/F/day, comparable to 73 - 95 mg/NaF/day) increased spinal bone density at a rate nearly twice that of patients treated with smaller doses of fluoride (i.e., 15 - 32 mg/F/day, comparable to 33 - 70 mg/NaF/day) (1.73 +/- 94 mg/cc/month, n= 17 compared to .92 +/- .74, n = 24, respectively; p < .01).

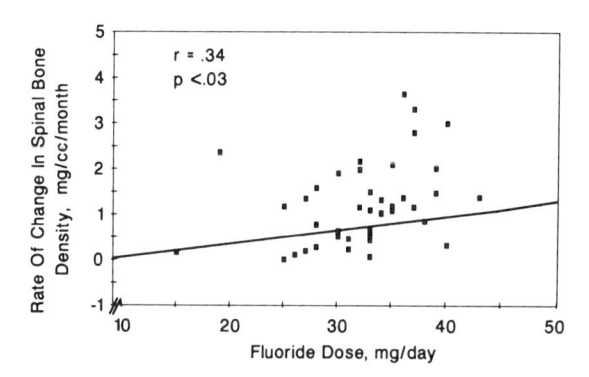

FIG. 2. Relationship between the rate of change in spinal bone density and the dose of fluoride. Each point represents the slope from the plot of serial measurements of spinal bone density as a function of time on therapy and the average daily intake of fluoride for each patient in the study.

After treatment with fluoride and calcium, spinal bone density was equal to or greater than 100 mg/cc in 44% (18/41) of the patients (Figure 3). Maximum spinal bone density observed in these patients during 32 +/- 11 months of observation was 126 +/- 22 mg/cc (range: 100 - 169 mg/cc). Spinal bone density in the remaining patients (23/41 or 56%) was significantly increased during fluoride therapy compared to pretreatment values (e.g., change in spinal bone density at 12 months was 14 +/- 13 mg/cc, p <.001) but the maximum spinal bone density attained during the study was 66 +/- 21 mg/cc (range: 19 - 96 mg/cc). This difference in the therapeutic outcome was not due to differences in the duration of treatment or the dose of fluoride, but was associated with a lower pretreatment spinal bone density and a slower rate of increase in spinal bone density in the group with the lower post-treatment spinal bone density (Table 1).

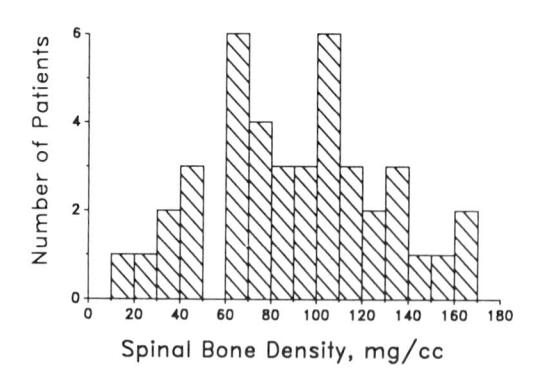

FIG. 3. Distribution of the maximum spinal bone density observed after treatment with fluoride and calcium in 41 female osteoporotics. Table 1: Clinical parameters as a function of post-treatment spinal bone density in 41 female osteoporotics treated with fluoride and calcium.*

	Post-treatment Spinal Bone Density, mg/cc		
	< 100	=> 100	p
Number	23 (56%)	18 (44%)	
Age, years	71 +/- 8	68 +/- 10	n.s.
F dose, mg	32 +/- 6	35 +/- 7	n.s.
Treatment Time, months	31 +/- 10	32 +/- 11	n.s.
Pretreatment Spinal Bone Density, mg/cc	42 +/- 17	62 +/- 20	<.001
Rate of Change in Spinal Bone Density, mg/cc/month	.76 +/- .51	1.88 +/- .94	<.001

* Values shown are the mean +/- S.D.

DISCUSSION

Previous studies have shown that vertebral fracture risk is related to trabecular vertebral bone density [13-14] and that a threshold value can be observed above which fractures are rare and below which fractures occur with increasing frequency [12,15]. This threshold value serves as a useful therapeutic goal for treating patients with osteoporosis. Since we found that the fracture threshold using QCT was 100 mg/cc for females, we proposed that treatment for post-menopausal osteoporosis must raise trabecular vertebral bone density to at least this level to eliminate risk for fracture [12].

In the current study, trabecular vertebral bone density was progressively increased during treatment with fluoride and calcium. We have previously demonstrated that this response to therapy is fluoride-dependent, as spinal bone density was unchanged in osteoporotics treated with calcium only [11]. These recent data extend our earlier findings, demonstrating the effectiveness of fluoride therapy to increase spinal bone density to 100 mg/cc or greater in 44% of treated patients within 32 +/- 11 months of therapy. Furthermore, since the increase in spinal bone density was related to the time on therapy, the data indicate that further treatment may benefit those patients who failed to achieve this level of spinal bone density. Spinal bone density was significantly increased in this subgroup of patients and the rate of change was positive in all patients but pretreatment spinal bone density was lower, suggesting that the greater bone deficit may require a longer time on therapy to correct.

The success of fluoride therapy to increase spinal bone density above the fracture threshold was also dependent upon the speed at which bone density was increased in response to treatment. This varied widely within the group of fluoride treated patients, ranging from .006 - 3.647 mg/cc/month. In the subgroup of patients whose post-treatment spinal bone density remained below 100 mg/cc, the rate of increase in spinal bone density was less than half that of patients who increased spinal bone density above the fracture threshold (i.e., .76 mg/cc/month compared to 1.88 mg/cc/month, respectively).

It is not clear why the osteogenic effect of fluoride differs so greatly between patients. Previous studies have linked at least part of this variation to variations in the absorption and retention of fluoride [16-19]. Those data suggest that increased skeletal exposure to fluoride may improve the skeletal response. Consistent with that conclusion, we found a weak but significant positive correlation between the rate of increase in spinal bone density and the dose of fluoride (r = 0.34; p<.03).

In summary, this study of post-menopausal osteoporotic females treated with fluoride and calcium found that patients on larger doses of fluoride had the fastest improvement in spinal bone density, and that those with a fast rate of improvement and/or a smaller deficit in pretreatment spinal bone density were most likely to increase trabecular vertebral bone density above a fracture threshold value of 100 mg/cc. Based on these findings, we recommend fluoride as an effective therapy for increasing vertebral trabecular bone density above the fracture threshold of 100 mg/cc, but suggest a dose of 40 mg/day for those with severe osteoporosis (e.g., spinal QCT values less than 50 mg/cc) and a dose of 20 - 30 mg/day for those with less severe bone loss.

ACKNOWLEDGMENTS

This work was supported by the Department of Medicine, Loma Linda University and the Veterans' Administration.
We wish to express our thanks to the staff of the Dept. of Endocrinology in the Faculty Medical Offices for coordination of the patient studies, to George Javier and Ellen Imperio for their assistance in data analysis, and to Linda Carrillo and the Medical Media Staff of the Jerry L. Pettis Memorial Veterans' Hospital for their assistance in the preparation of the manuscript.

REFERENCES

1. N.M. Resnick and S.L. Greenspan, JAMA 261, 1025-1029 (1989).
2. J.R. Farley, J.E. Wergedal and D.J. Baylink, Science 227, 320-332 (1983).
3. D.J. Baylink and D.J. Bernstein, Clin Orthop 55, 51-85 (1967).
4. M.A. Dambacher, T. Lauffenburger, B. Lammle and H.G. Haas, in: Fluoride and Bone B. Courvoisier, A. Donath and C.A. Boud, eds. (Hans Huber, Bern 1978) pp. 238-241.
5. D. Briancon and P.J. Meunier, Orthop Clin of North America 12, 629-648 (1981).
6. W.L. Dunn, H.W. Wahner and B.L. Riggs, Radiology 136, 485-487 (1980).
7. C.E. Cann and H.K. Genant, J Comput Assist Tomogr 4, 493-500 (1980).
8. J.A. Raymakers, C.F. van Dijke, A. Hoekstra and S.A. Duursma, Bone 8, 143-148 (1987).
9. T. Hansson and B. Roos, Calcif Tissue Int 40, 315-317 (1987).
10. C.Y. Pak, K. Sakhaee, J.E. Zerwekh, C. Parcel, R. Peterson and K. Johnson, J. Clin. Endocrin. & Metab. 68, 150-159 (1989).
11. S.M.G. Farley, C.R. Libanati, M.R. Mariano-Menez, L.A. Tudtud-Hans, E.E. Schulz and D.J. Baylink, J. Bone & Min. Res. (In Press).
12. C.V. Odvina, J.E. Wergedal, C.R. Libanati, E.E. Schulz and D.J. Baylink, Metabolism 37, 221-228 (1988).
13. G.H. Bell, O. Dunbar, J.S. Beck, et. al., Calcif. Tissue Res. 1, 75-88 (1967).
14. V.M. Nokso-Koivsto, E.M. Alhava and H. Olkkonen, Ann. Clin. Res. 8, 399-402 (1976).
15. C.E. Cann, H.K. Genant, F.O. Kolb and B Ettinger, Bone 6, 1-7 (1985).
16. R.G. van Kesteren, S.A. Duursma, W.J. Visser, J. van der Sluysveer and O. Backerdirks, Metab. Bone Dis. & Rel. Res. 4, 31-37 (1982).
17. S.A. Duursma, J.H. Glerum, A. van Dijk, R. Bosch, H. Kerkhoff, J. van Putten and J.A. Raymakers, Bone 8, 131-136 (1987).
18. F.H. Budden, T.A. Bayley, J.E. Harrison, R.G. Josse, T.M. Murray, W.C. Sturtridge, R. Kandel, R. Vieth, A.L. Strauss and S. Goodwin, J. Bone & Min. Res. 3, 127-132 (1988).
19. M.E. Kraenzlin, C. Kraenzlin, S.M.G. Farley, R.J. Fitzsimmons and D.J. Baylink, J Bone & Min Res (In Press).

VITAMIN D

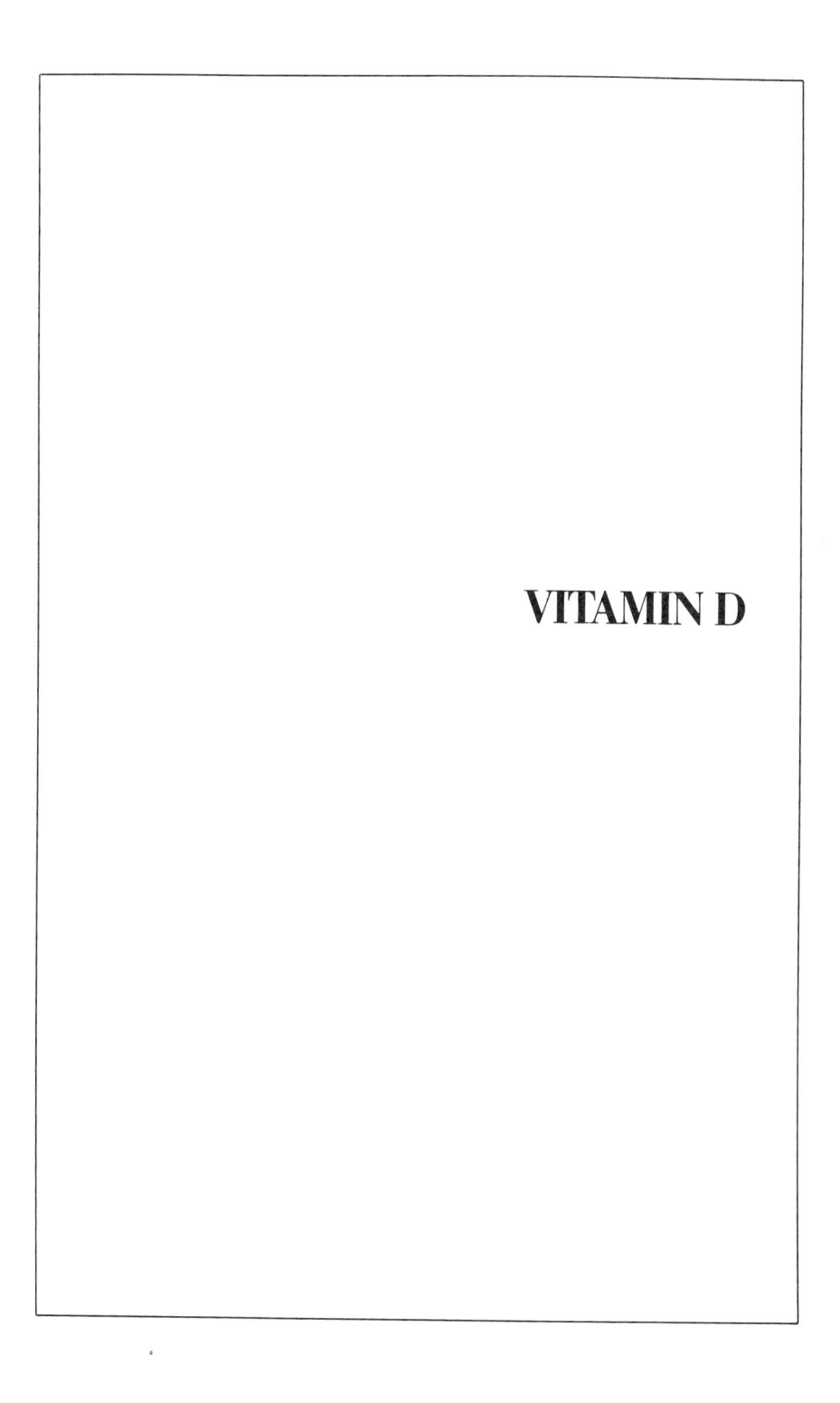

The Basis for 1,25 Dihydroxyvitamin D Therapy in the Treatment of Osteoporosis

J.C. Gallagher

Creighton University School of Medicine, Omaha, Nebraska

ABSTRACT

Vitamin D analogues prevent bone loss in osteoporotics and can increase bone density in some patients. There appears to be a dose related effect on bone. However, with increasing dose there is increased potential for toxicity (hypercalcuria and hypercalcemia). When using these compounds, the chances of toxicity can be reduced by limiting the daily calcium intake to less than 500mg. No long term adverse effects on creatinine clearance have been noted in long term studies.

INTRODUCTION

It is well accepted now that most patients with osteoporosis, particularly with postmenopausal or Type 1 osteoporosis, suffer from an impairment of calcium absorption [1-3]. In a substantial proportion of these patients calcium balance studies have shown that fecal calcium exceeds the calcium intake, thus implying a severe absorptive problem [2]. There is some evidence that the most severe calcium absorption defect occurs in the patients with the most severe osteoporosis, that is, those with the largest number of fractures [4]. Because 1,25 dihydroxyvitamin D is the major vitamin D metabolite that controls calcium absorption, one would expect to find reduced levels of serum 1,25(OH)$_2$D in patients with malabsorption of calcium. In general, reduced levels of 1,25(OH)$_2$D have been found in patients with osteoporosis [2, 5-9], although there are occasional reports of normal 1,25(OH)$_2$D levels in some osteoporotics. These discrepant findings could be explained by differences in the types of osteoporotic patients seen in different centers, or to variations in calcium intake. Although there is a significant correlation between serum 1,25(OH)$_2$D and calcium absorption in normal subjects, the correlation between these two parameters is not significant in the osteoporotics [2]. The lack of correlation between calcium absorption and serum 1,25(OH)$_2$D in osteoporotics could be explained by the fact that most of the values lie at the low end of the normal range, or there may be a subgroup of patients who have an intrinsic abnormality of calcium absorption within the intestinal cell but in whom serum 1,25(OH)$_2$D levels are normal [2, 10]. Further investigation of

postmenopausal osteoporotics by Tsai et al. [11] have shown
that the serum 1,25(OH)$_2$D level increases after injections of
parathyroid hormone whereas in older patients with senile
osteoporosis or hip fracture there is a failure of serum
1,25(OH)$_2$D to increase after parathyroid hormone injection.
These findings suggest that the abnormality in the parathyroid
hormone - 1,25(OH)$_2$D axis in postmenopausal osteoporotics
occurs because of a breakdown in the homeostatic control
mechanisms. A number of studies have now shown that serum
parathyroid hormone levels are lower in postmenopausal
osteoporotic patients [12, 13]. As a result of these hormonal
findings, two strategies may be employed in the correction of
these problems. First, one could increase serum parathyroid
hormone levels and thereby increase serum 1,25(OH)$_2$D levels.
However, studies along these lines have shown that injections
of parathyroid hormone down regulate 1,25(OH)$_2$D production
[14]. An alternative strategy is to treat patients with
synthetic analogues of 1,25(OH)$_2$D. On theoretical grounds this
mode of treatment should increase calcium absorption, reduce
negative calcium balance and prevent further loss of bone.
Some of the studies which used this approach will be discussed
in the next section.

THE USE OF VITAMIN D ANALOGUES IN THE TREATMENT OF OSTEOPOROSIS

The first use of vitamin D analogues in the treatment of
osteoporosis involved 1α OHD$_3$, and early studies showed that
this analogue must first be hydroxylated to 1,25(OH)$_2$D in the
liver. 1α OHD$_3$ was shown to be effective in increasing calcium
absorption and improving calcium balance [15]. Because calcium
absorption did not always increase on 1µg of 1α OHD$_3$, the dose
that was recommended for use was 2µg daily. Further increase
of the dose to 5µg/day caused hypercalcuria and increased the
degree of negative calcium balance. A number of studies have
shown an increase in bone mineral density of the radius on this
metabolite [16, 17]. Studies in Japanese patients have shown a
reduction in the vertebral fracture rate [18, 19].
Furthermore, discontinuing the treatment led to an increase in
the vertebral fracture rate.

Parallel studies using synthetic 1,25(OH)$_2$D$_3$ (Rocaltrol)
showed that this therapy increased calcium absorption and
improved calcium balance [20]. A comparison of these studies
suggests that 0.5µg of 1,25(OH)$_2$D$_3$ is bioequivalent to 1-2µg of
1α OHD$_3$. One possible explanation for the greater potency of
1,25(OH)$_2$D$_3$ on calcium absorption may be that 1,25(OH)$_2$D has a
first pass effect on calcium absorption in the intestinal cell
before being absorbed into the enterohepatic circulation. It
is possible that the bioequivalence is different for the gut
than for other target organs in the body. Various studies have
been carried out using Rocaltrol in the management of
osteoporosis with variable results. In a two center study
lasting one year a significant reduction in the vertebral
fracture rate was reported [21]. The long term effect of
Rocaltrol on bone density in osteoporotic patients has shown
variable results. In one study using an average dose of 0.4µg
daily of Rocaltrol no significant difference in bone density
was seen between the patients treated with Rocaltrol or placebo
(the placebo group had the calcium intake fixed at
1000mg/day)[22], however, the major finding of this study was

that there was no bone loss in the placebo group. In a study from another center where the average daily dose of Rocaltrol was 0.8µg , significant increases in total body calcium and spine density were reported [23]. In a similar study by our own group where the average daily dose of Rocaltrol was 0.68µg, we found a significant increase in total body calcium in Rocaltrol treated patients and significant decrease in the placebo group [24]. There has been only one study reported with the daily use of 1µg of Rocaltrol in osteoporotic patients. In this study a significant increase in total body calcium was seen in the osteoporotic patients [25]. Closer examination of all results suggested that the response of osteoporotic patients to Rocaltrol was dose related. Using total body calcium measurements there was no significant change in total body calcium on 0.4µg daily, on 0.68µg-0.80µg daily the increase was about 2% and on 1µg/day it was 4%. Bone histomorphometric examination of patients treated with 0.68µg daily or 0.8µg daily has not shown a significant increase in bone formation parameters or tetracycline labeling, however, in a study of osteoporotic patients treated with 2µg daily there were significant increases in bone formation parameters and tetracycline labeling [26]. Again, these results support the concept that there may be a dose related effect of Rocaltrol on bone.

From a therapeutic viewpoint, it is difficult to treat patients with a dose greater than 0.5µg daily without developing signs of toxicity. Hypercalcuria and hypercalcemia are not usually seen on the 0.5µg dose whereas they occur in about one third of patients treated with 0.75µg daily. The only way that larger doses of Rocaltrol can be administered to patients with osteoporosis without causing toxicity is by maintaining a calcium intake of less than 500mg/day. In countries where the calcium intake is traditionally low, such as in Italy or Japan, the use of high doses of vitamin D metabolites has led to few problems, but in countries such as the USA where the calcium intake is higher, toxicity with vitamin D compounds has been observed.

CONCLUSIONS

The available evidence suggests that vitamin D analogues have efficacy in the management of osteoporotic patients. There appears to be a dose related effect on bone, however, the incidence of toxicity increases with increasing doses of vitamin D analogues. Provided that the calcium intake can be maintained at levels of 500mg/day or less, the use of larger doses of vitamin D analogues can be administered safely. A major clinical problem in the USA is in maintaining the compliance of patients on a low calcium intake when there is frequent publicity in the media about the need for increasing the amount of calcium in the diet. For those patients who are intolerant of dairy products the use of vitamin D analogues presents less of a management problem. Available data suggest that maintaining a high serum level of 1,25(OH)$_2$D would have a beneficial effect on bone, and the development of a vitamin D analogue that has less effect on intestinal absorption while maintaining high serum levels of 1,25(OH)$_2$D could represent an improvement in therapeutic management with this group of compounds.

REFERENCES

1. Caniggia, A., Gennari, C., Bianchi, V., and Guideri, R. (1963): Intestinal absorption of Ca in senile osteoporosis. Acta. Med. Scand., 173:613.
2. Gallagher, J.C., Aaron, J., Horsman, A., Marshall, D.H., Wilkinson, R., and Nordin, B.E.C. (1973): The crush fracture syndrome in postmenopausal women.. Clin. Endocrinol. Metab., 2:293-315.
3. Gallagher, J.C., Riggs, B.L., and DeLuca, H.F. (1980): Effect of estrogen on calcium absorption and serum vitamin D metabolites in postmenopausal osteoporosis. J. Clin. Endocrinol. Metab., 51:1359-1364.
4. Nordin, B.E.C., Peacock, M., Aaron, J., Crilly, R.G., Heyburn, P.J., Horsman, A., and Marshall, D. (1980): Osteoporosis and osteomalacia. Clin. Endocrinol. Metab., 9:1.
5. Aloia, J.F., Cohn, S.H., Vaswani, A., Yeh, J.K., Yuen, K., and Ellis, K. (1985): Risk factors for postmenopausal osteoporosis. Am. J. Med., 78:95-100.
6. Caniggia, A., Nuti, R., Lorie, F., and Vattimo, A. (1984): The hormonal form of vitamin D in the pathophysiology and therapy of postmenopausal osteoporosis. J. Endocrinol. Invest., 7:373-378.
7. Bishop, J.E., Norman, A.W., Coburn, J.W., Roberts, P.A., and Henry, H.L. (1980): Studies in the metabolism of calcified 16. Determination of the concentration of 25 hydroxyvitamin D 24-25 dihydroxyvitamin and 1,25 dihydroxyvitamin D in a single 2 milliliter plasma sample. Miner Electrolyte Metab., 3:181-189.
8. Lawoyin, S., Zerwekh, J.E., Glass, K., and Pak, C.Y.C. (1980): Ability of 25-hydroxyvitamin D3 therapy to augment serum 1,25- and 24, 25-dihydroxyvitamin D in postmenopausal osteoporosis. J. Clin. Endocrinol. Metab., 50:593-596.
9. Lund, B., Sorensen, O.H., Lund, B., and Agner, E. (1982): Serum 1,25-dihydroxyvitamin D in normal subjects and in patients with postmenopausal osteopenia. Influence of age, renal function and oestrogen therapy. Horm. Metab. Res., 14:271-274.
10. Francis, R.M., Peacock, M., Taylor, G.A., Storer, J.H., and Nordin, B.E.C. (1984): Calcium malabsorption in elderly women with vertebral fractures: Evidence for resistance to the action of vitamin D metabolites on the bowel. Clin. Sci., 66:103-107.
11. Tsai, K.S., Heath, H. 3d, Kumar, R., Riggs, B.L. (1984): Impaired vitamin D metabolism with aging in women. J. Clin. Invest., 73:1668-72.
12. Gallagher, J.C., Riggs, B.L., Jerpbak, C., and Arnaud, C.D., (1980): The effect of age on serum immunoreactive parathyroid hormone in normal and osteoporotic women. The Journal of Laboratory and Clinical Medicine, 95:373-385.
13. Kotowicz, M.A., Klee, G.G., Kao, P.C., Gonchoroff, D.G. and Riggs, B.L. (1989): Serum Intact PTH in Type 1 (Postmenopausal) Osteoporosis Assessed by Sensitive Immunometric Assays. Endocrine Soc. Abstr. #450.
14. Slovik, D.M., Adams, J.S., Neer, R.M., Hollick, M.F., Potts, J.T. Jr. (1981): Deficient production of 1,25-dihydroxyvitamin D in elderly osteoporotic patients. N. Engl. J. Med., 305:372-4.

15. Marshall, D.H., Gallagher, J.C., Guha, P., Hanes, F., Oldfield, W., and Nordin, B.E.C. (1977): The effect of 1 alpha-hydroxycholecalciferol and hormone therapy on the calcium balance of post-menopausal osteoporosis. Calcif. Tissue. Res., 225:78-84.
16. Lund, B., Sorensen, O.H., Andeersen, R.B., Lund, B., Mosekilde, L., Egsmose, C., Storm, T.L., and Nielsen, S.P. (1985): Long-term treatment of senile osteopenia with 1 di-hydroxycholecalciferol. In: Vitamin D. a Chemical, Biochemical and Clinical Update, edited by A.W. Norman, K. Schaefer, H. -.G. Grigoleit, and D.V. Herrath, pp. 1039-1040. Walter de Gruyter & Co., Berlin-New York.
17. Lindholm, T.S., Nilsson, O.S. Kyhle, B.R., Elmstedt, E., Lindholm, T.C., and Eriksson, S.A. (1981): Failures and complications in treatment of osteoporotic patients treated with 1 di-hydroxyvitamin D3 supplemented by calcium. In: Osteoporosis, edited by C. Christiansen, C.D. Arnaud, B.E.C. Nordin, A.M. Parfitt, W.A. Peck, and B.L. Riggs, pp. 351-357. Aalborg Stiftsbogtrykkeri, Glostrup, Denmark.
18. Spencer, H., Jacob, M., Lewin, I., and Samachson, J. (1964): Absorption of calcium in osteoporosis. Am. J. Med., 37:223-234.
19. Orimo, H., Shiraki, M., Hayashi, R., Nakamura, T. (1987): Reduced occurrence of vertebral crush fractures in senile osteoporosis treated with 1α(OH)-vitamin D3. Bone and Mineral, 3:47-52.
20. Gallagher, J.C., Jerpbak, C.M., Jee, W.S.S., Johnson, K.A., DeLuca, H.F., and Riggs, B.L. (1982): 1,25-Dihydroxyvitamin D3: Short- and long-term effects on bone and calcium metabolism in patients with postmenopausal osteoporosis. Proc. Natl. Acad. Sci., 79:3325-3329.
21. Gallagher, J.C., Riggs, B.L., Recker, R.R., and Goldgar, D. (1989 in press) The Effect of Calcitriol on Patients with Postmenopausal Osteoporosis with Special Reference to Fracture Frequency. Soc. Experim. Med. and Biology.
22. Ott, S.M., Chestnut, C.H. (1989): Calcitriol Treatment Is Not Effective in Postmenopausal Osteoporosis. Annals of Internal Medicine, 110:267-274.
23. Aloia, J.F., Vaswani, A., Yeh J.K., Ellis, K., Yasumura, S., Cohn, S.H. (1988): Calcitriol in the treatment of postmenopausal osteoporosis. Am. J. Med., 84:401-8.
24. Gallagher, J.C., Goldgar, D., O'Neil, J. (1988): Prevention of Postmenopausal Bone Loss by 1,25 Dihydroxyvitamin D3 Therapy in Osteoporosis. VIIth Vitamin D Meeting. Chemical, Biochemical, and Clinical Update. Ed. A.W. Normal, et al.
25. Caniggia, A., Nuti, R., Lore, F., Martini, G., Righi, G., and Turchetti, V. (1989 in press): Long-term Calcitriol Treatment in Post-menopausal Osteoporosis: Follow-up of Two Hundred Patients.
26. Gallagher, J.C., and Recker, R.R. (1985): A comparison of the effects of calcitriol or calcium supplements. In: Vitamin D, A Chemical, Biochemical and Clinical Update, edited by A.W. Norman, K. Schaefer, H.-.G. Grigoleit, and D.V. Herrath, pp. 971-975. Walter de Gruyter & Co., Berlin-New York.

Pathophysiological Study in Women with Postmenopausal Osteoporosis on Long-Term Treatment with Calcitriol

A. Caniggia, R. Nuti, F. Loré, G. Martini, V. Turchetti, and G. Righi

Institute of Clinical Medicine, University of Siena, Siena, Italy

ABSTRACT

Calcitriol was administered at the dose of 1 µg/day for 1-8 years to 270 women with symptomatic, histologically proven postmenopausal osteoporosis, without calcium supplementation. The treatment resulted in remarkable relief from pain, with improvement of ambulancy. Intestinal calcium absorption increased significantly and remained higher than the basal value as long as calcitriol was administered. Urinary calcium excretion also increased, but hypercalcemia occurred, exceptionally and transiently, only in a few patients. Urinary hydroxyproline excretion did not increase, so indicating that hypercalciuria was not of resorptive origin. Total body density, determined by dual-photon total body absorptiometry in 56 patients, showed an increase after 18-24 months in the majority of them. The occurrence of non-traumatic, clinically relevant fractures decreased noticeably as compared with the period preceding calcitriol treatment. No change occurred in renal function and no renal stone developed. Calcitriol was shown to represent an effective and safe treatment of postmenopausal osteoporosis.

INTRODUCTION

Several experimental results have implicated a decrease in the circulating levels of the active vitamin D metabolite, 1,25-dihydroxyvitamin D (1,25(OH)2D) as the main cause of the impaired calcium absorption which characterizes postmenopausal osteoporosis (1). In fact, low serum levels of 1,25(OH)2D3 have been described in this condition (2-11) and this finding has been accounted for by an impaired endogenous production of the vitamin D metabolite.

Estrogens represent one of the physiologic endocrine stimulators of 1,25(OH)2D synthesis, as it has been demostrated in experimental animals (12) and in humans (2,13). Therefore, the decrease in 1,25(OH)2D production is likely to be due to postmenopausal estrogen deficiency: the administration of estrogen to postmenopausal osteoporotic women restores normal calcium absorption (14). The possibility of abnormalities in responsiveness of the 1-alpha-hydroxylase enzyme to parathyroid hormone has also been suggested (15,16).

Based on the above findings several clinical trials have been carried out concerning the treatment of osteoporosis with synthetic 1,25(OH)2D3 (calcitriol).

Caniggia and Vattimo (17) administered a daily dose of 1 µg of calcitriol to 11 postmenopausal osteoporotic patients for 10 days and reported a significant improvement of intestinal radiocalcium absorption.

This finding was confirmed by Gallagher et al. (3), who treated 10 patients with 0.5 µg per day of calcitriol for 6 months and obtained a significant increase in calcium absorption.

In a subsequent paper Gallagher (18) et al. presented 12 postmenopausal osteoporotic patients given calcitriol (0.5 µg/day) for 2 years; they reported increases in calcium absorption and trabecular bone volume.

Caniggia et al. (19) studied 28 women with postmenopausal osteoporosis in a double-blind placebo-controlled trial aimed to compare the effect of a one-year treatment with calcitriol (0.5 µg per day) and estrogen given alone or in combination. Calcitriol proved to be sufficiently effective in terms of intestinal calcium absorption and increase in mean trabecular diameter at the histomorphometric examination of bone biopsies from the iliac crest. Nevertheless, 9 patients, who, after completion of the trial with 0.5 µg/day, were given calcitriol 1 µg per day for 1 year, showed a greater increase in calcium absorption.

Riggs and Nelson (20) gave 0.5-0.75 µg/day of calcitriol to 48 patients for 6-12 months and to 29 patients for 24 months. They reported a significant increase in fractional calcium absorption and a decrease in urinary hydroxyproline (HOP) excretion and serum parathyroid hormone. No significant clinical complications were reported.

Twelve postmenopausal osteoporotic patients have recently been studied by Aloia et al. (21): these patients were given calcitriol at a mean dose of 0.8 µg/day for 24 months, without calcium supplementation, starting from a dose of 1 to 2 µg per day. Total body calcium, as measured by neutron activation analysis, bone mineral content of the radius and bone density of the spine increased.

Ten years ago we began a long-term study on the effects of 1,25(OH)2D3 (calcitriol) treatment at physiological doses and without calcium supplementation in postmenopausal osteoporosis. The treatment was based on the encouraging results obtained in short term studies (17) and on the following pathophysiological hypothesis: negative calcium balance of postmenopausal osteoporotic women is due to the impairment of intestinal calcium transport as a consequence of a reduced 1,25(OH)2D synthesis, resulting from the impaired activity of renal 25OHD-1alpha-hydroxylase no longer stimulated by estrogens. The positive results obtained (8, 22) led us to proceed with this kind of therapy.

At the present time, we have by far the biggest experience with calcitriol therapy available in the world, in terms of both the number of patients treated and the duration of treatment. The results obtained are here reported.

PATIENTS AND METHODS

Two hundred and seventy women with symptomatic post-menopausal osteoporosis, aged 49-78 years (mean age 63 years) entered the study. A rigid selection of the cases was performed.

Criteria for admission to the study were: back pain and difficulty in walking; a radiographic finding of vertebral translucency with one or more non-traumatic vertebral fractures; decreased bone mineral density in comparison with age-matched non osteoporotic women; a typical histologic pattern of osteoporosis as determined by microscopic inspection of undecalcified bone biopsies from the iliac crest; impaired intestinal radiocalcium transport; normal renal function; normal values of serum calcium; phosphate, alkaline phosphatase and 24 h urinary calcium, phosphate and hydroxyproline excretion.

Criteria for exclusion were represented by renal diseases; heart failure and major respiratory insufficiency; endocrine disease; diseases of the alimentary tract, liver and biliary ducts; osteomalacia and mixed forms of osteoporosis and osteomalacia (ruled out by iliac crest biopsy); primary and secondary neoplastic bone disease; spondyloarthritis; long-term treatments with glucoactive corticosteroids, anticonvulsants or heparin.

The patients were given calcitriol at the oral dose of 0.5 μg twice a day without calcium supplementation. The treatment was never discontinued. No other drug was given (including analgesics!). The patients were allowed their usual diet. The estimated daily intake of calcium and vitamin D was 580 ± 120 mg and 0.5 ± 0.2 μg, respectively.

All the patients of the present study (270) were treated for at least one year, 181 were treated for at least two years, 117 for three years, 70 for four years, 42 for five years, 24 for six years, 13 for seven years, and 4 for eight years.

Blood samples and 24 h urine were collected for the determination of the following parameters: plasma and urinary calcium (atomic absorption spectrophotometry, Perkin-Elmer model 2280); serum and urinary phosphate, serum alkaline phosphatase, urinary hydroxyproline (HOP) (standard methods). To assess renal function, urine analysis, blood urea nitrogen, serum creatinine and 24 h urinary creatine clearance were assessed by standard methods.

Fractional radiocalcium absorption was measured as follows: 10 μC_i of radiocalcium was given orally in 80 mg of $CaCl_2$ as non radioactive carrier; plasma radioactivity was assessed for 4 h and the circulating fraction of the dose (fx) calculated according to Marshall and Nordin (23). Normal range in our laboratory: 0.170-0.270.

Urine cAMP/Cr ratio was determined as a parathyroid function index (The Radiochemical Centre, Amersham, U.K.).

The aforementioned parameters were usually determined before, every other other month during the first year of treatment and every 4-6 months thereafter.

Serum osteocalcin (BGP) was evaluated in 72 patients before and after one year of calcitriol treatment, using an assay kit (ImmunoNuclear, Stillwater, Minn, USA).

Single-photon absorptiometry (241Am source) was used at the beginning of the study to evaluate the bone mineral content at the distal forearm: the results obtained with this technique have been published elsewhere and are not reported in this paper (24).

In the last two years bone mineral density (BMD) of the entire skeleton was measured by dual-photon absorptiometry (Lunar DP4, Madison, USA). The presence of two separate photon energies from 153Gd (peaks at 44 and 100 KeV) avoids the need for a uniform soft tissue thickness surrounding the bone. This technique, completely devoid from repositioning problems, enabled us to measure bone density and bone mineral content of the whole skeleton: the variation coefficient for total body density (TBD) estimated in our department in 25 patients was found to be as low as 0.66 % (25).

TBD was measured after 12 months of calcitriol treatment in 31 patients, after 18 month in 17 patients and after 24 months in 8. TBD was also assessed before and after a one year period in a control group of 7 untreated post-menopausal osteoporotic women (aged 55-68 years).

X-ray films of the spine and abdomen were obtained yearly for detection of new fractures and renal stones.

The rate of fracture occurrence during calcitriol treatment was compared with that of the period between menopause and the initiation of therapy, and expressed as number of fractures/100 patients x year. Only vertebral collapses easily distinguishable on X ray films and generally accompanied by sudden acute pain, were considered.

Statistical analyses were based on the determination of the probability density functions (26). The significance of differences was evaluated by analysis of variance and paired Student's t test.

RESULTS

Prior to the beginning of treatment in the women of the present study, intestinal radiocalcium absorption, expressed as fx values, was significantly lower than the normal range (fx: 0.128 $\pm$ 0.02). Within two months calcitriol treatment promoted a significant increase in fractional calcium absorption (fx), as indicated by the changes in mean values and the probability density functions (Fig. 1). The normalization of intestinal calcium transport persisted throughout the treatment, for 1 to 7 years or more, as long as calcitriol was administered (Fig. 2).

Fasting plasma calcium did not differ from normal controls in basal conditions. During the study the mean values averaged slightly higher (Fig. 2); differences were statistically significant only during the first years of treatment. Hypercalcemia was observed exceptionally (14 cases) and transiently: however, in no patient the treatment needed to be discontinued.

The 24 h urinary calcium excretion showed baseline levels lower in osteoporotic women (152 mg/24 h $\pm$ 68) than in controls (187 mg 24 h $\pm$ 90). Within two months calcitriol promoted a significant increase in urinary calcium (Fig. 1): hypercalciuria was constantly appreciated throughout the treatment (Fig. 2).

In basal conditions no significant correlation was found between fractional calcium absorption and urinary calcium excretion (r = 0.05; n.s.); calcitriol treatment promoted a statistically significant correlation between these two parameters, as long as the study was continued (e.g. after two years r = 0.308; p<0.001) (Fig. 3).

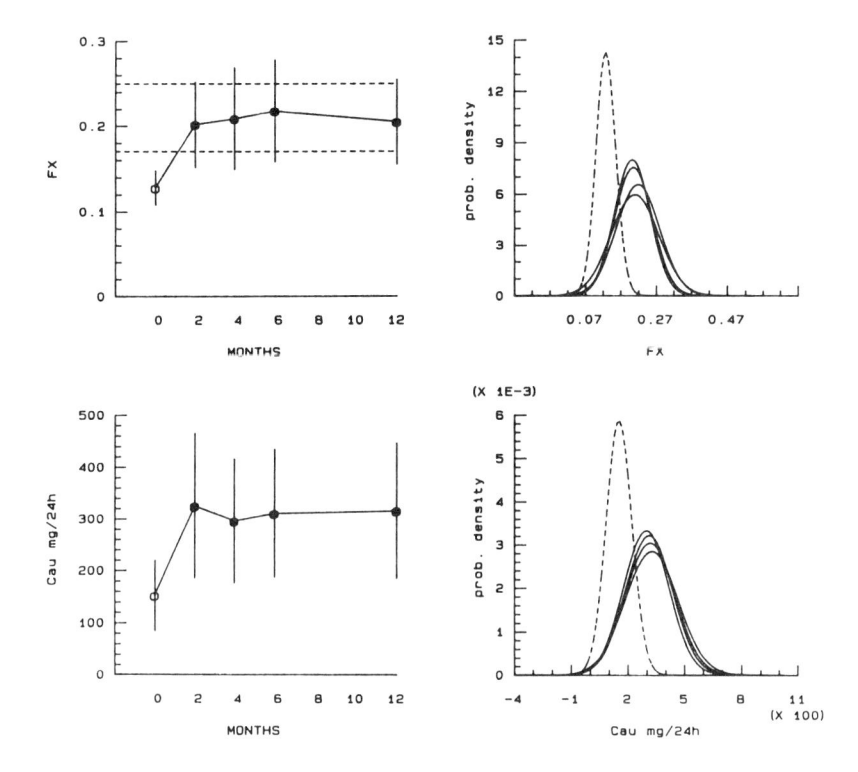

FIG. 1. Changes in radiocalcium absorption (fx) (p<0.001) and urinary calcium excretion (CaU) (p<0.001) during the first year of calcitriol treatment, expressed as mean ± SD (left) and probability density functions (right) (---- basal values, —— 2-12 months).

A similar correlation, although of lower statistical significance, was observed between fasting plasma calcium and urinary calcium.

The 24 h urinary HOP excretion did not differ in basal condition from that of controls and did not change significantly during long-term calcitriol treatment, whereas the ratio calcium/HOP in urine increased remarkably (Fig. 2). A statistically significant correlation was found between 24 h urinary calcium and 24 h urinary HOP in basal conditions (r = 0.246; p<0.001), but not during calcitriol treatment.

Plasma phosphate showed only slight changes during calcitriol treatment, whereas the 24 h urinary phosphate excretion increased significantly.

The cAMP/Cr ratio in 24 h urine, an index of parathyroid function, showed normal values in basal conditions: on calcitriol treatment it showed a slightly significant decrease.

Prior to the initiation of treatment serum BGP averaged lower than in a group of age-matched non osteoporotic women (3.8 ng/ml ± 1.1 and 6.8 ng/ml ± 2.0 respectively, p<0.01). One-year of calcitriol therapy promoted a significant increase (4.5 ng/ml ± 1.4, p < 0.001).

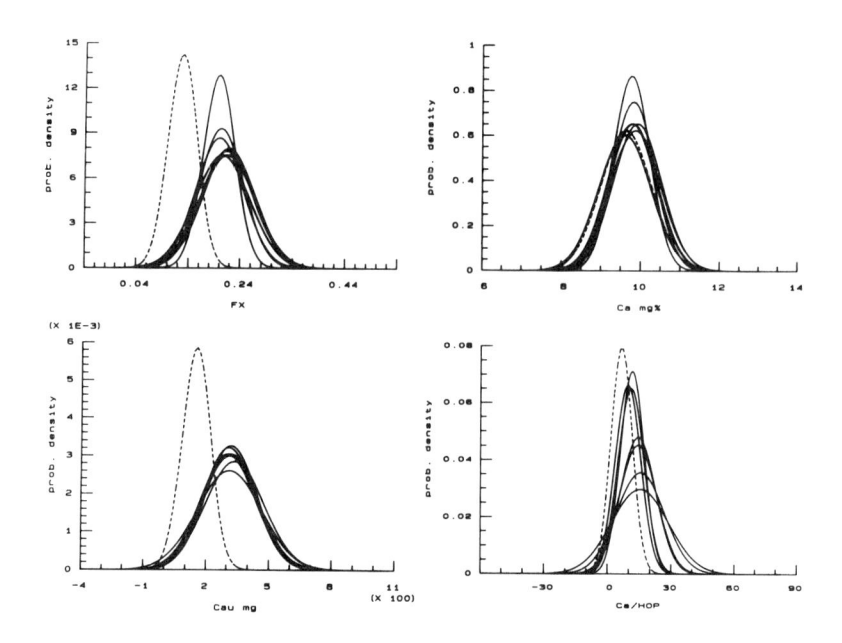

FIG. 2. Changes in intestinal radiocalcium absorption (fx) (p<0.001), plasma calcium (Ca) (p<0.01), 24 h urinary calcium (CaU) (p<0.001) and urinary Ca/HOP (p<0.001), expressed as probability density functions, before and during calcitriol treatment (---- basal values, —— 1-8 years).

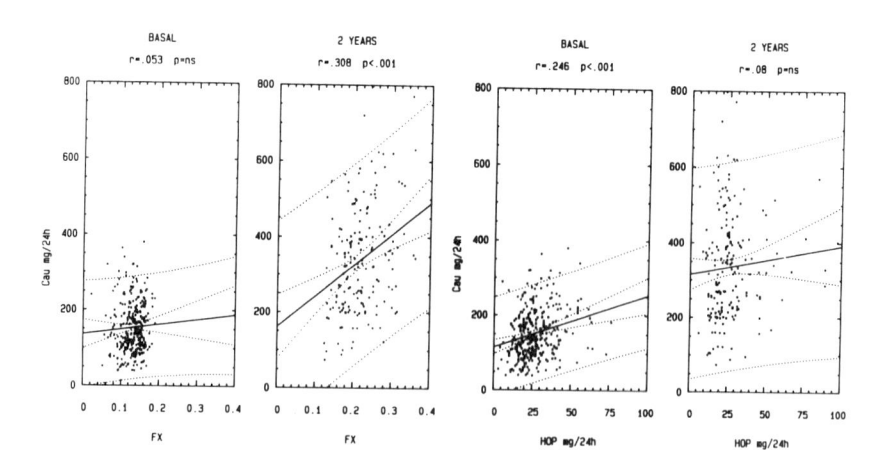

FIG. 3. Correlations of 24 h urinary calcium vs radiocalcium absorption (fx) (left) and 24 h urinary calcium vs 24 h urinary HOP excretion (right) in basal conditions and after 2 years of calcitriol treatment.

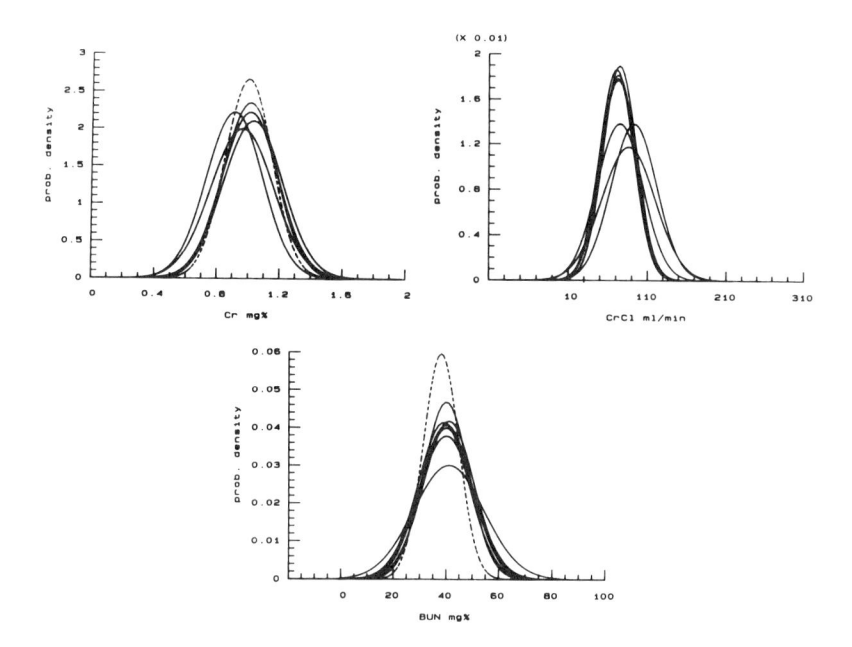

FIG. 4. Changes in serum creatinine (Cr) (n.s.), creatinine clearance (CrCl) (p< 0.05) and blood urea nitrogen (BUN) (n.s.), expressed as probability density functions in postmenopausal osteoporotic patients on long term treatment with calcitriol (---- basal values, —— 1-8 years).

No changes in renal function occurred during long-term calcitriol treatment, as demonstrated by the normal values constantly shown by urine analysis, BUN, plasma creatinine levels and urinary creatinine clearance (Fig. 4). X-ray films demonstrated that no renal stones had developed in the treated patients.

In basal conditions osteoporotic women showed reduced values of TBD (0.910 gr/cm2 ± 0.09 gr/cm2) in comparison to age-matched healthy women (1.05 g/cm2 ± 0.07).

Calcitriol treatment promoted a significant increase in TBD in most of the patients (Figure 5). A decrease exceeding the limits of the variation coefficient was observed in only four patients. The mean percent change was + 1.2 % after 12 months, + 1.48 % after 18 months and + 1.58 % after 24 months. On the contrary in the control group of untreated women a marked reduction in total body density was observed after a one-year period (-1.7%) (Fig. 5).

From a clinical point of view, calcitriol treatment resulted in a consistent and often dramatic relief from pain and improvement of mobility.

The diminution in the occurrence of new, non-traumatic fractures was striking as compared with the period preceding the treatment (Fig. 6): 12.2 fractures/100 patients x year before the initiation of treatment, 2.9

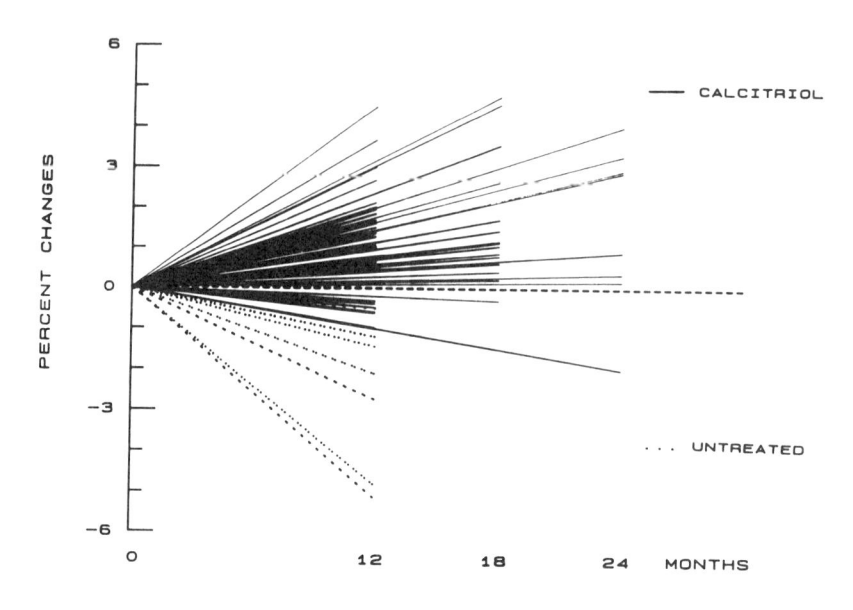

FIG. 5. Percent changes in total body density (TBD) after 12, 18 and 24 months of calcitriol treatment in osteoporotic patients (———) and after 12 months in untreated osteoporotic women (....).

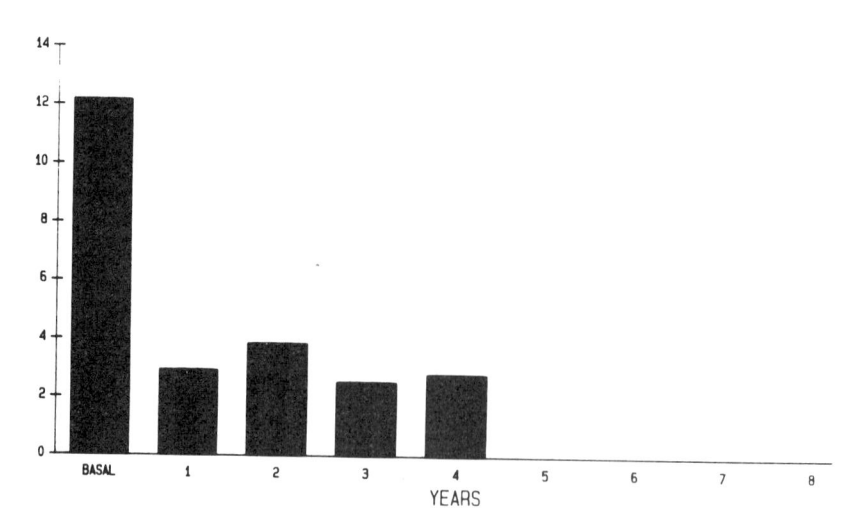

FIG. 6. Occurence of new fractures (fractures/100 patients x year) before and during long-term calcitriol treatment.

fractures/100 patients x year during the first year, 3.8 in the second year, 2.6 in the third year, 2.8 in the fourth year; no new fracture occurred in subsequent years).

DISCUSSION

In the post-menopausal osteoporotic patients of the present study long-term calcitriol treatment produced a prompt and persistent normalization of their depressed intestinal calcium transport. In a placebo-controlled sequential study (24) calcium absorption was found to be lower at the end of the placebo period than in basal conditions.

The hypercalciuria we have observed was not of resorptive origin since the 24 h urinary HOP excretion did not increase throughout the treatment. Moreover, the correlation between urinary calcium and HOP, that was statistically significant in basal conditions, was no longer significant during the treatment. It must be concluded that hypercalciuria was mainly due to the calcitriol effect on the intestinal calcium transport; this was obviously more appreciable after the meals rather than after an overnight fast; so that the low correlation between fasting plasma calcium and 24 h urinary calcium was not surprising.

No patients showed any degree of deterioration of renal function and no renal stones developed during calcitriol treatment. Therefore, it must be recognized that, in spite of a persistent hypercalciuria, the long-term administration of 1 ug/day of calcitriol did not result in any adverse effects on the the kidney and the urinary tract.

It should be stressed that in several trials calcitriol was given in combination with oral calcium, and hypercalcemia with severe hypercalciuria was observed. In our experience, allowing patients to their usual free diet during calcitriol treatment, without calcium supplementation, results in a sufficient utilization of dietary calcium and, at the same time, prevents hypercalcemia.

The decrease in the urinary cAMP/creatinine ratio observed during calcitriol therapy could be accounted for by parathyroid suppression and should therefore be considered a favourable effect in terms of reduction in bone resorption.

The increase in serum BGP produced by calcitriol treatment, showed no correlation with the serum levels of alkaline phosphatase or with urinary HOP excretion. It is likely that the low osteocalcin levels we observed in postmenopausal osteoporotic women, in accordance with Brown et al. (27) were related to an impairment of osteoblast stimulation as a consequence of the reduced endogenous production of 1,25(OH)2D (28).

It is known that calcitriol is a physiological stimulator of BGP synthesis in osteoblasts; our results indicate that in postmenopausal osteoporosis the osteoblasts have not lost their ability to respond to calcitriol.

An exact evaluation of the changes in BMD in longitudinal studies can be hampered by technical difficulties with both single-photon or lumbar dual-photon procedures. In a previous study using single-photon absorptiometry we were able to demonstrate lower basal values in osteoporotic women than in age-matched controls; calcitriol treatment resulted in a statistically significant increase after 12 months of therapy (8,22,24).

The best precision and accuracy in bone mineral content measurements are provided by total body absorptiometry, By this impartial technique we were able to demonstrate an increase in bone mineral density in the majority of our patients.

On the contrary, our untreated patients showed a remarkable loss of bone density.

Nevertheless, in 19 patients treated with calcitriol the change in total body bone density did not exceed the variation coefficient of this technique, so that in these subjects bone mass can be considered to have remained unchanged. However, this cessation of bone loss must be regarded as a "successful therapy" (29), from a practical view point.

The decrease in the occurrence of definite, symptomatic vertebral compression fractures observed in our patients during calcitriol treatment was striking and in agreement with clinical improvement in terms of both pain and mobility.

The compliance of patients was testified by the fact that they diligently came to our department for follow-up analyses. This can be considered a good measure of their compliance and is a confirmation of the beneficial effects of treatment as seen from the point of view of the patients.

In order to test the effects of a treatment an ideal study should be designed in a randomized, double-blind, controlled way. This was not the case of the present trial, due to the following reasons: it is difficult to persuade a woman with osteoporosis to take a placebo (that is a treatment that may have no beneficial effect) for years, and we considered that this would not have been ethically acceptable.

In any case, a real double-blind design was not possible, since it is difficult to disguise the nature of a treatment, at least to the physician, when a drug is so rapidly and clearly effective on parameters such as urinary calcium and intestinal calcium transport.

However, we have recently been able to perform a medium-term, placebo-controlled sequential study in a relatively small group of patients. The result have been reported elsewhere (24).

When dealing with the results of clinical trials concerning calcitriol efficacy in postmenopausal osteoporosis several fundamental factors should be considered: among them the criteria for selection of patients, the dosage administered, the parameters used for evaluation. Adequate sampling size and duration of treatment are also critical elements of clinical trials.

Without this preliminary examination no comparison can be made concerning the results obtained and no conclusion can be drawn as to the efficacy of treatment.

Some papers concerning the management of osteoporosis with calcitriol reported controversial results.

However, in some of these studies the diagnosis of post-menopausal osteoporosis was not established with certainty, so that "old women with back pain" were sometimes included. There are trials in which the participants, instead of being patients with ascertained postmenopausal osteoporosis, were just selected from the 70-year-old female population (30, 31) or were women aged 50-65 who had sustained a fracture of the distal forearm (32).

The majority of the trials did not include a sufficient number of patients or were not prolonged enough for a correct determination of changes in fracture occurrence during calcitriol treatment.

As to the dosage, several Authors administered calcitriol in amounts lower than 0.5 µg per day (mainly 0.25 µg) and generally failed to obtain significant results (33,34); this finding is in complete agreement with our preliminary data showing that such low doses of calcitriol are absolutely ineffective.

As to the criteria for evaluation of efficacy, several studies used the measurement of bone mineral content at the distal forearm, a technique that did not exhibit a uniform response in the hand of the various Authors.

We believe that our work has met all the aforementioned criteria for a reliable assessement of calcitriol efficacy in post-menopausal osteoporosis. Actually, the patients were accurately selected and the study included only women with ascertained post-menopausal osteoporosis; the dose administered was sufficient for eliciting significant changes in mineral metabolism, without side effects; reliable techniques were adopted for evaluation of the effects. Eventually, the number of patients was adequate for a correct estimation of long-term results.

The conclusion we can draw is the following: calcitriol represents a physiological compound that can be given orally at physiological doses without untoward effects; it is biochemically and clinically effective in postmenopausal osteoporosis and inexpensive.

REFERENCES

1. A. Caniggia, C. Gennari, V. Bianchi and R. Guideri, Acta Med. Scand. 173, 613-617 (1963).
2. J.C. Gallagher, B.L. Riggs, J. Eisman, A. Hamstra, S.B. Arnanaud and H.F. DeLuca, J. Clin. Invest. 64, 729-736 (1979).
3. J.C. Gallagher, B.L. Riggs and H.F. DeLuca, J. Clin. Endocr. metab. 51, 1359-1364 (1980).
4. B.L.Riggs, A. Hamstra and H.F. DeLuca, J. Clin. Endocr. Metab. 53, 833-835, (1981).
5. B. Lund, O.H. Sorensen, B. Lund and E. Agner, Hormone metabol. Res. 14, 271-274 (1982).
6. O.H. Sorensen, B.O.Lumholtz, B. Lund, B. Lund, J.L. Hjelmstrand, L. Mosekilde and F. Melsen, J.E. Bishop and A.W. Norman, J. Clin. Endocr. Metab 54, 1258-1261 (1982).
7. J.E. Zervekh, K. Sakhae, K. Glass and CYC Pak, J Clin. Endocr. Metab. 56 410-413 (1983).
8. A. Caniggia, R. Nuti, F. Loré and A. Vattimo, J. Endocr. Invest. 7, 373-378 (1984).
9. F. Loré, R. Nuti, A. Vattimo and A. Caniggia, Hormone metabol. Res. 16 (1984).
10. K.S. Tsai, H. III Heath, R. Kumar and B.L. Riggs, Clin. Res. 32, 411A (1984).
11. K.S. Tsai, H. III Heath, R. Kumar and B.L. Riggs, J. Clin. Invest. 73 1668-1672 (1984).
12. L. Castillo, Y. Tanaka, M.J. Wineland, J.O. Jowesey and H.F. DeLuca, Endocrinology 104, 1598-1601 (1979).
13. C. Christiansen, M.S. Christensen and N.E. Larsen, J. Clin. Endocrinol. Metab. 55, 1124-1130 (1982).
14. A. Caniggia, C. Gennari, G. Borrello, M. Bencini, L. Cesari, C. Poggi and S. Escobar, Brit. Med. J. 4, 30-32 (1970).

15. D.M. Slovik, J.S. Adams, R.M. Neer, M.F. Holick and J.T. Potts Jr., New Engl. J. Med. 305, 372-374 (1981).
16. S.J. Silverberg, E. Shane, R.N. Luz de la Cruz, G.V. Segre, T.L. Clemens and J.P. Bilezikian, N. Engl. J. Med. 320, 277-281 (1989).
17. A. Caniggia and A. Vattimo, Clin. Endocrinol. 11, 99-103 (1979).
18. J.C. Gallagher, C.M. Jerpback, W.S.S. Jee, K.A. Johnson, H.F. DeLuca and B.L. Riggs, Proc. Natn. Acad. Sci. USA 79, 3325-3329 (1982)
19. A. Caniggia, G. Delling, R. Nuti, F. Loré and A. Vattimo, Acta Vitaminol. Enzymol. 6, 117-130 (1984).
20. B.L. Riggs and K.I. Nelson, J. Clin. Endocr. Metab. 61, 457-461 (1985).
21. F. Aloia, A. Vaswani and K. Yeh, Am. J. Med. 84, 401 (1988).
22. A. Caniggia, R. Nuti, F. Loré and A. Vattimo in: Vitamin D: chemical, biochemical and clinical update, A. W. Norman, K. Schaefer, H.G. Grigoleit and V.D. Herrath, eds. (de Gruyter, Berlin 1985) pp 986-95.
23. D.H. Marshall and B.E.C. Nordin, Nature 222, 797 (1969).
24. A. Caniggia, R. Nuti, F. Loré, G. Martini, V. Turchetti and G. Righi in: Vitamin D: molecular, cellular and clinical endocrinology. A.W. Norman, R. Schaefer, H.G. Grigoleit and VD Herrath, eds. (de Gruyter, Berlin 1988), pp 807-816.
25. R. Nuti, G. Righi, G. Martini, V. Turchetti, C. Lepore and A. Caniggia, J. Nucl. Med. All. Sci. 31, 213-221 (1987).
26. C. Scala, Funzioni di densità di probabilità: atlante descrittivo. Lama, Tipi Monotypia Franchi Società Artigiana Tipografica (1985).
27. J.P. Brown, P.D. Delmas, L. Malaval, C. Edouard, M.C. Chapuy and P.J. Meunier, Lancet 1, 1091-1093 (1984).
28. A. Caniggia, R. Nuti, M. Galli, V. Turchetti and G. Righi, Calcif; Tissue Intern. 38, 328-332 (1986).
29. N. Brautbar, Nephron 44, 161-166 (1986).
30. G.F. Jensen, C. Christiansen and I. Transbol, Clin. Endocr. 16 515-524 (1982)
31. G.F. Jensen, B. Meinecke, J. Boesen and I. Transbol, Clin. Orthop. Rel. Res. 192, 215-221 (1985).
32. J.A. Falch, O.R. Odegaard, A.M. Finnanger and I. Matheson, Acta Med. Scand. 221, 199-204 (1987).
33. C. Christiansen, M.S. Christiansen, P. Rodbro, C. Hagen, I. Transbol, Eur. J. Clin. Invest. 11, 305-309 (1981).
34. L. Tjellesen, C. Christiansen and P. Rodbro, Acta Med. Scand. 215, 411-415 (1984).

Benefits/Risks of 1,25-(OH)$_2$D$_3$ in the Treatment of Osteoporosis

John F. Aloia, Ashok Vaswani, and James K. Yeh

Winthrop-University Hospital, Mineola, New York

ABSTRACT

We compared 1,25-(OH)$_2$D$_3$ with placebo in the treatment of postmenopausal osteoporosis in a double-blind, randomized, parallel clinical trial of 24 months duration. The protocol was designed to achieve maximal doses of 1,25-(OH)$_2$D$_3$ because of the hypothesis that bone formation would be stimulated. The study was completed by 15 patients who received placebo and 12 patients who received 1,25-(OH)$_2$D$_3$. The treatment group had positive slopes (compared with negative slopes for the placebo group) for total body calcium, bone mineral content of the radius, bone mineral density of the lumbar spine, and radiographic absorptiometry of the middle phalanges. Biochemical measurements suggested that 1,25-(OH)$_2$D$_3$ administration increased bone mineral density by decreasing bone resorption but not by increasing bone formation.

Hypercalciuria occurred in all subjects treated and generally preceded hypercalcemia by about 2 weeks. A decrease in creatinine clearance was observed in two patients taking calcitriol, one of whom had nephrolithiasis on sonography. Calcitriol is effective in preventing bone loss, but must be used with caution.

INTRODUCTION

A decrease in the level of calcitriol has been implicated in the pathogenesis of postmenopausal osteoporosis. Lower circulating levels of calcitriol have been found in women with the crush fracture syndrome when compared with age-matched controls [1]. Women with osteoporosis have an impaired ability to synthesize calcitriol in response to parathyroid hormone infusion [2]. There is a decline in circulating levels of calcitriol following menopause which is accompanied by a decrease in calcium absorption; furthermore, administration of either estrogen or calcitriol to postmenopausal women increases circulating levels of calcitriol to the normal range and restores calcium absorption to premenopausal levels [3,4].

In addition to its classic effect on intestinal calcium absorption, it has been suggested that calcitriol may stimulate osteoblastic activity directly. These combined effects led to the hypothesis that calcitriol may be useful in the treatment of postmenopausal osteoporosis. Indeed, a number of studies concerning treatment of osteoporosis with calcitriol have been reported [4-8]. Unfortunately, the findings from these studies have been divergent, with some reports suggesting that calcitriol is useful whereas others found no benefit. In this manuscript we describe a 24 month, double-blind, randomized, parallel trial comparing calcitriol to placebo in the treatment of postmenopausal osteoporosis. The protocol was designed to maximize serum levels of calcitriol in the hope that a dramatic improvement in bone mass could be obtained through stimulation of osteoblast activity. It was recognized that in order to accomplish this goal hypercalciuria and hypercalcemia would occur. Consequently, the women in the study were monitored frequently for these events, as well as for deterioration in renal function.

MATERIALS AND METHODS

Protocol

A. Recruitment phase. Women between the ages of 50 and 80 years with postmenopausal osteoporosis were recruited to participate in the study. Osteoporosis was diagnosed by the presence of at least one non-traumatic vertebral compression fracture. The women were otherwise healthy and had no disorder known to influence bone metabolism.

B. Titration phase. On entry into the study, each patient was given 400 IU of vitamin D daily which was continued in both groups throughout the study. Calcium intake was assessed by the use of a three day diet history. The patients were instructed in a 1000 mg calcium intake. Following the baseline measurements, all patients were started on 2 capsules per day, one before breakfast and the second before dinner. The capsules contained either 0.25 mcg of calcitriol or matching placebo. The stepwise escalation in dose that was permitted was as follows: after two weeks to two capsules twice daily, after four weeks to three capsules twice daily, and after six weeks to the maximum of four capsules twice daily (2 mcg daily). The investigator was also given the option of stepwise escalation of one instead of two capsules every two weeks. As indicated earlier, the objective of the titration phase was to maximize circulating levels of calcitriol. For the purposes of this study, 24-hour urinary calcium excretion greater than 400 mg was taken as an indication for modifying calcium intake or the dosage schedule. When this level was exceeded, dietary calcium intake was lowered. If lowering the dietary calcium intake was ineffective in reducing urinary calcium excretion, the dosage of drug was decreased. Significant hypercalcemia was defined as serum levels greater than 11.6 mg/dl. Whenever this occured the drug was temporarily discontinued. Following resumption of normocalcemia, the dose would later be initiated at one capsule daily. Informed written consent was obtained from each patient.

C. Continuation phase. Following completion of 24 months of study, the code was broken. All participants were invited to continue in an open study to assess long term safety. Eighteen patients agreed to continue in this study, six who previously received calcitriol and twelve who previously received placebo. At the completion of this phase of the study, it was decided to perform renal sonograms on each patient. Fourteen patients agreed to have sonography performed.

Methods

A. Bone mineral measurements. Each of the bone mineral measurements were performed at baseline and every six months using techniques that have been described previously [8-11]. Total body calcium provides a measure of calcium balance in a free living population. This measurement was performed at the Brookhaven National Laboratory facility by total body neutron activation analysis and whole body counting. Bone density of the distal radius (8 cm site) was measured by single photon absorptiometry using a Norland Instruments (Ft. Atkinson, Wisconsin) single photon absorptiometer with an ^{125}I source. Bone density of the lumbar spine (L2-L4) was measured using dual photon absorptiometry with a ^{153}Gd source (Lunar Instruments, DP$_3$, Madison, Wisconsin). Radiographic absorptiometry of the second, third and fourth middle phalanges of the left hand was performed using scanning with an optical densitometer for detection of bone edges.

B. <u>Biochemical determinations</u>. Urinary hydroxyproline was determined by a modification of the method of Prockop and Udenfriend [12]. Vitamin D metabolites were measured by the technique of Eisman et al [13]. PTH radioimmunoassay was performed using a Diagnostic System Laboratory radioimmunoassay kit. Calcium was measured on an atomic absorption spectrometer. Serum samples were collected after an overnight fast. Following completion of the study it was decided to measure serum levels of osteocalcin [14]. Samples were available on 11 patients in the treatment group for the following time limits: baseline, three, six, nine, and twelve months. All samples were assayed simultaneously.

C. <u>Radiography</u>. Radiographs were interpreted by the Brookhaven National Laboratory radiologists to determine eligibility for inclusion in the study [15]. Subsequently, the fracture incidence was determined by analysis of pretreatment and the annual radiographs of the thoracolumbar spine by one physician who was unaware of whether the patients were receiving placebo or calcitriol.

D. <u>Bone biopsy</u>. A transiliac bone biopsy was performed under local anesthesia using a Bordier trephine. Double tetracycline labeling was utilized; the biopsies were performed at baseline and upon completion of the study [15]. All patients had baseline biopsies. Repeat biopsies were performed on 12 patients in the placebo group and 12 patients in the calcitriol group. All biopsies were interpreted by one physician who was unaware of the treatment received by the patients.

E. <u>Statistical analyses</u>. The individual slopes for each of the bone mineral measurements were computed and expressed as %/year. Each data point was expressed as the difference from the mean of all of the individual values. The slopes of the calcitriol and control groups were then compared by a student t-test to determine if calcitriol was more effective than placebo. Since our hypothesis was unidirectional, a one tailed t-test was used. Unless otherwise stated, the data presented in this manuscript are for the subjects that completed the 24 months of the study. A multivariate analysis of variance was also carried out using each of the four different bone mineral measurements (weighted appropriately and expressed as an annual rate of change) as criteria. The biochemical data that were obtained each six months were analyzed with one way analysis of variance using repeated measurements.

RESULTS

A. <u>Subjects</u>. The mean age of the placebo group was 64.9 $\pm$ 1.7 (SE) years and the calcitriol group was 64.1 $\pm$ 1.5 (SE) years. Other clinical characteristics such as age at menopause, and number of children were similar for the two groups. Seven patients dropped out of the study. The reasons for the dropouts were not complications of therapy as far as could be determined.

B. **Bone mineral measurements.** There were no significant differences between the two groups in their baseline bone mineral measurements. The mean change in the bone mineral content of the radius for the calcitriol group was 1.26%/year as contrasted with a change of -1.63%/year for the placebo group (P<.01) (Fig. 1). There was no loss of bone density of the spine in the calcitriol group whereas a loss of 4.3%/year was observed in the placebo group (P<.05). The same findings were observed in overall calcium balance assessed by total body calcium measurement, where the calcitriol group increased by .96%/year and the placebo group had a reduction of .73%/year (P<.05). The radiographic absorptiometry measurements yielded the following slopes: .98%/year for the calcitriol group and -1.39%/year for the placebo group (P<.03).

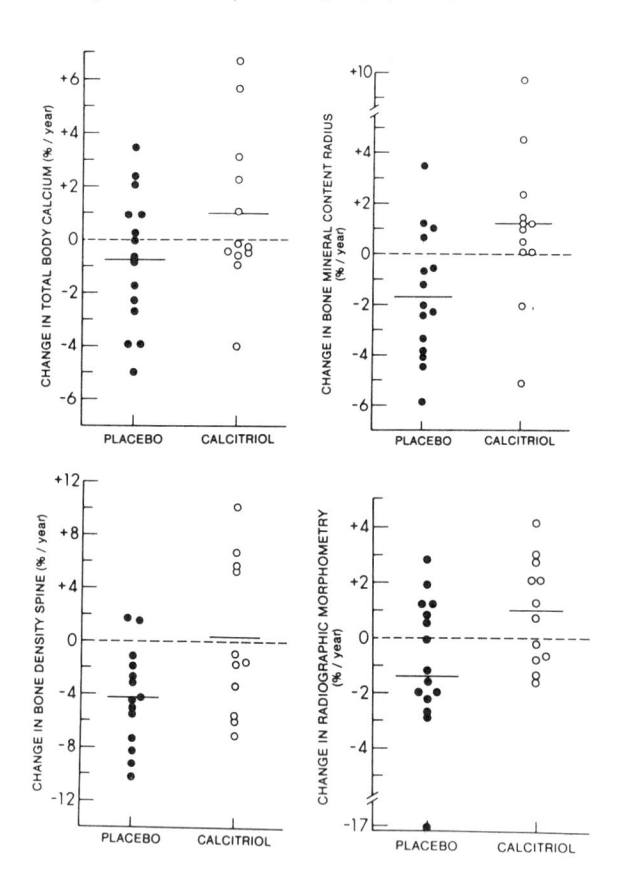

FIG. 1. Bone mineral measurements as expressed as percent per year for each subject who completed the 24 months of study.

B. **Biochemical measurements.** There were no significant baseline differences between two groups in the biochemical variables. None of the patients had 25-(OH) vitamin D levels indicative of vitamin D deficiency. Urinary calcium excretion was higher than 250 mg per 24 hours in 3 patients in the calcitriol treatment group. Significant changes in the biochemical indices were confined to the treatment group as follows: urinary calcium increased, (F=4.18, P<.01) and there was a decrease in urinary hydroxyproline (F=2.64, P<.05) and in serum alkaline phosphatase (F=2.65, P<.05) (Fig. 2). An increase in serum 1,25-(OH)$_2$D levels was observed. Mean monthly values are plotted in Figure 3. The higher levels of serum

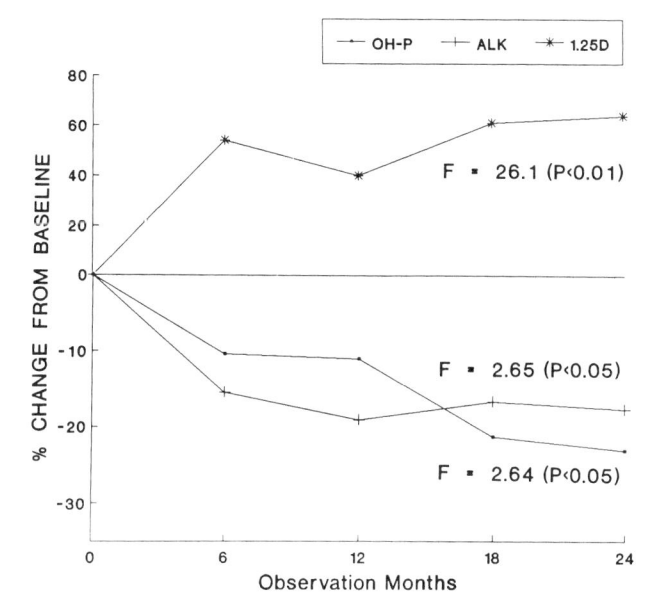

Fig. 2. The changes in serum 1,25-(OH)$_2$D, alkaline phosphatase and urinary hydroxyproline following treatment.

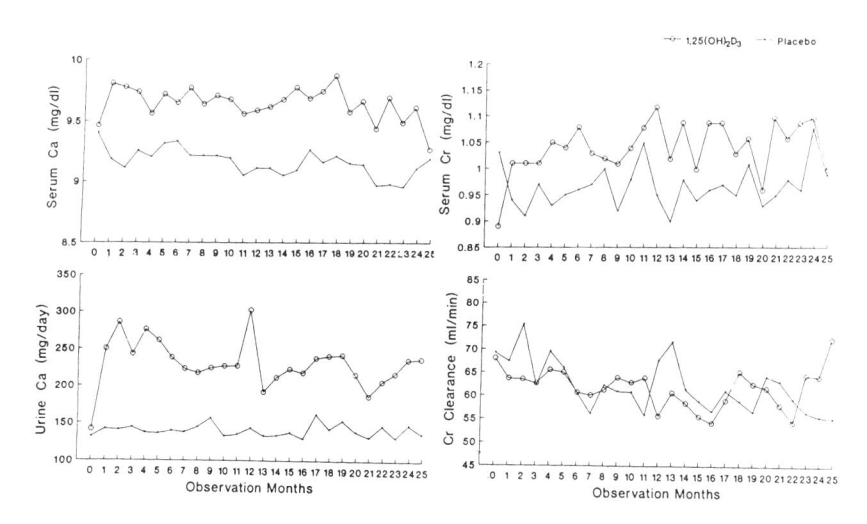

FIG. 3. Values at monthly intervals for serum calcium and creatinine, urine calcium and creatinine clearance.

calcium and creatinine and of urinary calcium excretion in the treatment group are apparent. The creatinine clearance was not significantly different in the 2 groups. There was no change in serum osteocalcin levels. Mean (+ SE) values for serum osteocalcin (ng/ml) were as follows: baseline: 9.04 + 1.6; three months: 11.0 + 0.91; six months: 11.5 + 2.7; nine months: 8.94 + 1.3; and 12 months: 8.95 + 1.3 (F=0.38). There were no significant changes in mean PTH levels in either group.

C. Bone biopsies. The trabecular bone volume was below 20% of the marrow space as would be expected in osteoporotic patients. There was no evidence for osteomalacia on the pretreatment biopsy specimens. There were no significant changes between the two groups or within each group following treatment (t test).

D. Fracture incidence. There were more fractures in the placebo group at baseline (66[range, one to 10]) than in the treatment group (32[range, one to 7]). The mean number of compression fractures for the placebo and calcitriol groups were 3.2 + 0.6 (SE) and 2.5 + 0.4 (SE), respectively. During the 24 months of the study, ten new fractures occurred in five of the palcebo treated patients and six new fractures occurred in three of the calcitriol treated patients. Thus, the fracture rate (per 1000 patient-years) was 333 for the placebo group and 250 for the calcitriol group. The difference in fracture incidence between the two groups was not statistically significant.

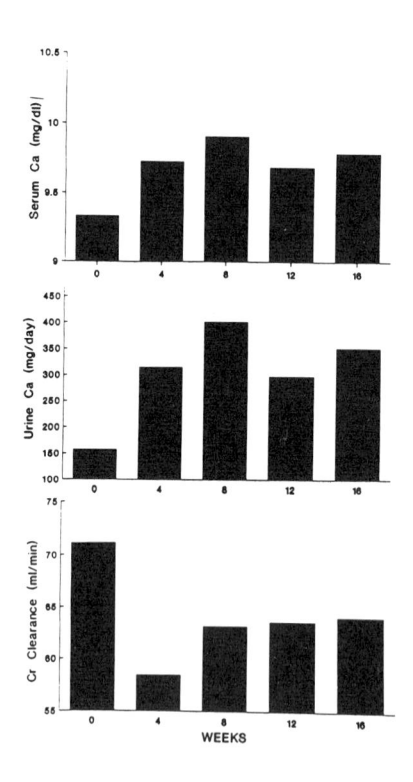

FIG 4. Baseline and monthly mean values during titration phase.

E. <u>Dosage and complications</u>. The mean dose of calcitriol was 0.8 mcg/day. It was necessary to lower dietary calcium by 250 to 500 mg/day in most patients because of persistent hypercalciuria. The dosage in the titration phase ranged from 1 to 2 mcg/day before a reduction in dosage was necessary. The daily dose of calcitriol following titration was 0.5 to .75 mcg for 8 subjects with four subjects taking 1 to 1.25 mcg/day. After dietary modification, the serum calcium levels generally returned to the normal range but nevertheless remained higher than the values in the control subjects (Fig. 3). Hypercalciuria usually preceded the development of hypercalcemia by about two weeks. During the titration phase, hypercalcemia occurred in 11 of the 12 subjects receiving calcitriol.

To further evaluate short term toxicity with higher doses of calcitriol, the data of the titration phase was pooled for those individuals in the blinded phase of the study and those who were started on calcitriol during the continuation phase of the study (n=23). These data are presented in Fig. 4. Calcium excretion increased considerably. There was a drop in creatinine clearance following one month of therapy. The creatinine clearance subsequently returned towards baseline but did not attain baseline levels even one month after the titration phase was complete. Statistical analysis revealed that this change in creatinine clearance was not significantly different from baseline. The increase in serum and urinary calcium was statistically significant (F=2.68, P<.05 and F=14.7, P<.001, respectively).

The maximal elevation in serum calcium was seen in one subject who was given a thiazide diuretic for hypertension by her physician. This occurred during dose titration in the continuation phase of the study. The values for this patient are depicted in Figure 5. She was treated with intravenous saline therapy along with discontinuation of the calcitriol and the thiazide

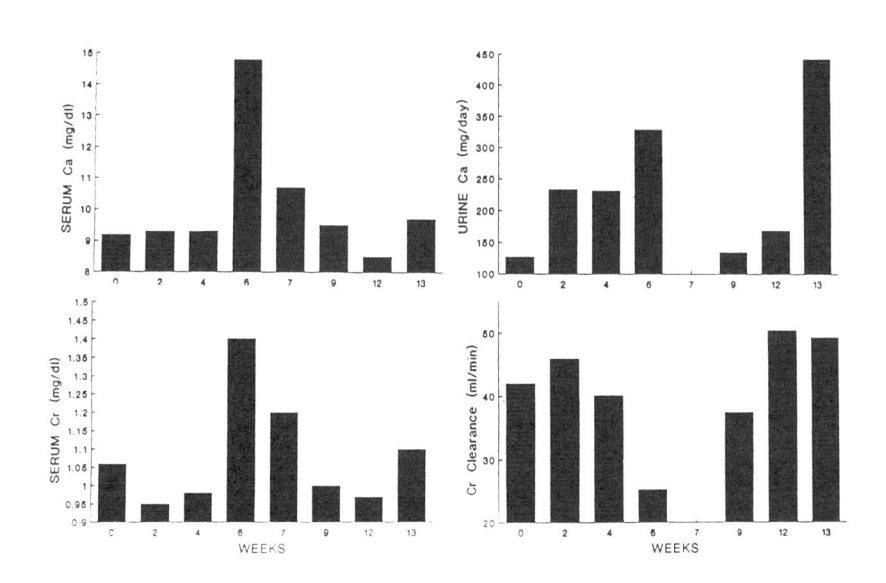

FIG 5. Changes in response to treatment during development of hypercalcemia.

diuretic in order to bring hypercalcemia under control. This patient experienced a decline in creatinine clearance during the titration phase. One other patient experienced a persistent reduction in creatinine clearance following calcitriol therapy.

The sonogram studies revealed a stone in one patient. This patient had taken calcitriol for 31 months. She had experienced nine episodes of hypercalcemia (five during the first two years) and had hypercalciuria at baseline. There was no evidence of nephrocalcinosis on the sonograms.

DISCUSSION

Our study demonstrates that calcitriol used in a manner to maximize serum levels of $1,25-(OH)_2D_3$ is effective in the prevention of bone loss in women with postmenopausal osteoporosis. Calcium balance (as measured by total body calcium) was positive in the group treated with calcitriol and was negative in the placebo group. Similar findings were observed in the density of the radius and metacarpals confirming that the calcium is deposited in bone rather than in extra-skeletal tissues. The density of the spine decreased in the placebo group whereas it did not change in the treatment group. The multivariate analysis of variance showed a significant treatment effect. However, the increase in bone mass that was observed for the treatment group was modest and similar to values that have been observed with other types of antiresorptive therapy.

Several earlier studies concerning treatment of postmenopausal osteoporosis with calcitriol have been reported but few of these measured bone mass or bone density. Caniggia et al [16] studied calcitriol treatment in both an open and double-blinded protocol. They observed a statistically insignificant increase in bone density of the radius in a group treated with 0.5 mcg of calcitriol per day. On the other hand, Jensen et al [5] treated 70 year old women with calcitriol or estrogen-gestagen and noted that the bone mineral content of the radius increased in the group treated with estrogen-gestagen but remained unchanged or decreased with calcitriol therapy.

Ours was a single center study which was also conducted at two other sites using similar protocols. Recently, one center (Seattle) published its results and concluded that $1,25-(OH)_2D_3$ therapy is not effective in osteoporosis [17]. The lower mean dose of $1,25-(OH)_2D_3$ in the Seattle study (only 0.43 mcg/day) suggests that either a different protocol was followed for dose adjustment or their patients were more sensitive to calcitriol. Moreover, the control group in the Seattle study did not lose bone mass. Previous reports suggest that osteoporotic women receiving 1000 mg of calcium per day will generally experience bone loss. Thus, we favor some peculiarity of the patient population, dosage adjustment or technical factors in the Seattle study to explain the divergent findings between the two sites. At the third site (Creighton) that conducted a similar protocol, the dose titration was identical to the one we used (mean dose 0.68 mcg/day). This group also found statistically significant higher levels of total body bone mineral, although the other measurements of bone mineral were not significant [18]. In addition, the Omaha group observed a reduction in levels of serum alkaline phosphatase and urinary hydroxyproline excretion similar to our findings. Similar findings concerning efficacy in the two sites supports the conclusion that calcitriol can prevent bone loss.

The mechanism of action whereby calcitriol produced positive calcium balance appears to be a reduction in bone resorption (evidenced by reduced urinary hydroxyproline) accompanied by an increase in calcium absorption.

It is possible that bone resorption decreased as a result of reduced PTH secretion following an increase in serum calcium. There was no evidence for an increase in bone formation from the histomorphometric analyses or from the serum alkaline phosphatase or osteocalcin levels.

The changes that may have occured in bone remodeling are of too small a magnitude to have been detected in a population of this size with a technique having the measurement reproducability of histomorphometry. The lack of change in the bone biopsy measurements does indicate, however, that treatment with calcitriol does not produce the dramatic changes in bone remodeling that would be necessary to restore the skeleton to a non-osteoporotic state. Moreover, since the efficacy phase of this study was not carried out for a prolonged period of time, it is not known whether calcitriol treatment will produce a sustained increment in bone mass or whether there will be a "plateau effect" as has been observed with other drugs that reduce bone remodeling such as calcitonin or estrogen.

In the current study there were fewer new fractures in the treatment group compared with the number in the control group at the end of the 24 months of treatment. The number of new fractures in the calcitriol group when compared with other reports of fracture rate suggests a beneficial effect of treatment [19]. However, we are reluctant to emphasize this finding because of the small number of new fractures observed over a short time period in a limited patient sample and because the differences were not statistically significant.

Concomitant prescription (or self administration) of calcium supplements could result in marked hypercalciuria at the dosage used in this study. The marked hypercalcemia we observed in the one patient in the current study following prescription of a thiazide diuretic by another physician underscores the possible hypercalcemic effects of treatment with calcitriol. It is evident that drug interactions must be considered continuously and that frequent monitoring of serum calcium, as well as urinary calcium excretion is necessary in any patient treated with this drug.

The results of the dose titration phase of this study was presented in detail to illustrate the effects of hypercalcemia resulting from $1,25-(OH)_2D_3$ ingestion. Renal function, as measured by creatinine clearance, declines following the development of hypercalcemia. It is unknown whether the kidney stone that we observed in one patient was due to calcitriol administration since the patient did not have a baseline sonogram. Although we could not find a relationship between creatinine clearance and other variables throughout the 24 month study period, and there were no significant differences in creatinine clearance between groups, the finding of reduced creatinine clearance in two patients should lead us to be cautious concerning the use of calcitriol in high doses.

In conclusion, calcitriol treatment reduces bone loss in women with postmenopausal osteoporosis by increasing intestinal calcium absorption and reducing bone resorption. We found no evidence for calcitriol having an effect on bone formation. The development of hypercalciuria and hypercalcemia is dose related whereas an increase in calcium absorption can be attained with lower doses than used in the current study. Further studies of efficacy and safety with lower doses of calcitriol would be of interest. Moreover, the side effects we observed were in part due to the oral route of administration, i.e. absorptive hypercalciuira resulted from the intestinal passage of calcitriol. It is likely that higher levels of serum calcitriol could be achieved using a parenteral route of administration without the side effects that we observed. Alternately, administration of this drug at bedtime (during fasting) might also achieve higher blood levels without producing absorptive hypercalciuria. Further studies achieving similar or higher serum levels of calcitriol through other routes of administration would be of interest.

REFERENCES

1. J.C. Gallagher, B.L. Riggs, J. Eisman, et al. J Clin Invest 64, 729 (1979).
2. D.M. Slovick, J.S. Adams, R.M. Nier, M.F. Huick and J.T. Potts, Jr., N Engl J Med 305, 372 (1981).
3. A.G. Need, M. Horowitz, J.C. Philcox and B.E.C. Nordin, Miner Electrolyte Metab 11, 35 (1985).
4. B.J. Lund, O.H. Sorenson, B. Lund and E. Agner, Horm Metab Res 14, 271 (1982).
5. G.F. Jensen, C. Christiansen and I. Transbol, Clin Endocrinol (Oxf) 16, 515 (1982).
6. B.L. Riggs and K. Nelson. J Clin Endocrinol Metab 61, 457 (1985).
7. J.C. Gallagher, C.M. Jerpbak, W.S.S. Jee, K.A. Johnson, H.F. DeLuca and B.L. Riggs. Proc Natl Acad Sci USA, 79, 3325 (1982).
8. J.R. Cameron, R.B. Mazess and J.A. Sorenson, Invest Radiol 3. 141 (1968).
9. M. Madsen, Invest Radiol 12, 185 (1977).
10. C. Colbert, R.S. Bachtell in: Non-invasive Measurements of Bone Mass and their Clinical Application, S. Cohn, ed. (CRC Press, Boca Raton, Florida 1981) pp. 51-84.
11. S.H. Cohn, K.K. Sukla, C.S. Dombrowski and R.G. Fairchild, J Nucl Med 13, 487 (1972).
12. D.J. Prockop and S. Udenfriend, Anal Biochem 1, 228 (1970).
13. J.A. Eisman, A.J. Hanstra, B.E. Kream, et al. Arch Biochem Biophys 176, 235 (1976).
14. P.V. Hauschka, J. Frenkel, R. DeMuth and C.M. Gundberg, J Biol Chem 258, 176 (1983).
15. C. Elias, R.P. Heaney and R.R. Recker, Calcif Tissue Int 37: 6, (1985).
16. A. Caniggia, R. Nuti, M. Galli, F. Lore, V. Turchetti and R.A. Righi, Calcif Tisue Int 38, 328 (1986).
17. S.M. Ott and C.H. Chesnut III, Ann Intern Med 110, 267 (1989).
18. J.C. Gallagher, D. Goldgar and J. O'Neill, in: Vitamin D, Molelcular, Cellular and Clinical Endocrinology, A.W. Norman, K. Schaefer, H.G. Grigoleit and B. Herrath, eds. (Walter de Gruyter & Co, Berlin, Germany 1988) pp. 836.
19. B.L. Riggs, E. Seeman, S.F. Hodgson, et al, N Engl J Med 306, 446 (1982).

Long Term Use of 1α(OH)D3 in Involutional Osteoporosis

H. Orimo and M. Shiraki

Department of Geriatrics, Faculty of Medicine, University of Tokyo, Tokyo, Japan

INTRODUCTION

Involutional osteoporosis is a syndrome of decreased bone mass affecting postmenopausal women and older people, which causes bone to be more susceptible to fractures.

Among many factors involved in the pathogenesis of this morbid state, deficiency of vitamin D and/or calcitonin (CT) has been suggested to play some role.

Plasma 25(OH)D level is usually normal (1,2) and plasma 1,25(OH)2D level is reported to be lower in patients with involutional osteoporosis (3,4,5). On the other hand, normal levels of 1,25(OH)2D in involutional osteoporosis are also reported (6,7).

Gut absorption of Ca is decreased in involutional osteoporosis and this is probably related to the decreased serum levels of 1,25(OH)2D.

In view of these data, 1α(OH)D3 has been tried in the treatment of involutional osteoporosis. Treatment of involutional osteoporosis with 1α(OH)D3 was first reported by Peacock et al (8) who found increased gut absorption of Ca and increased bone resorption in senile osteoporosis following treatment with 1α(OH)D3.

Furthermore, Lund et al (9) and Lindholm et al (1) reported the improvement of low back pain and the increase in bone mass in senile osteoporosis following treatment with 1α(OH)D3. We had previously shown by the double blind study that bone mineral density of 2nd metacarpal bone was significantly greater in 1α(OH)D3 treated patients than in control patients (11).

Furthermore, we have recently shown that the treatment with 1α(OH)D3 was effective not only in preventing the loss of radial mineral content (measured by single photon absorptiometry (]2), but also effective in reducing the occurrence of vertebral crush fractures in senile osteoporosis (13).

The purpose of the present study is to clarify the role of vitamin D in the pathogenesis of involutional osteoporosis and furthermore to examine the long term therapeutic effect of 1α(OH)D3 in this state.

I. Role of active Vit D metabolites in the pathogenesis of involutional osteoporosis.

To examine the possible role of active Vit D metabolites in the pathogenesis of involutional osteoporosis, serum levels of 25(OH)D, 24,25(OH)2D, 1,25(OH)2D,PTH and CT were measured in 61 female osteoporotic subjects with the mean age of 74.5±6.4 years.

Radial mineral density in each subject was measured by single photon absorptiometry and the presence or absence of vertebral fractures were also evaluated. Female osteoporotics were divided into 2 groups, group 1: subjects with lower serum 1,25(OH)2D levels (≦40 pg/ml), n=26, Group 11: subjects with higher serum 1,25(OH)2D levels (>40 pg/ml), n=35 and various parameters were compared in these 2 groups.

No significant difference was found in age, body weight, body height, body mass index, years after menopause, serum levels of Ca, Pi, alkaline phosphatase, BUN, Cr, urinary Ca/Cr, and Pi/Cr between these 2 groups.

Serum levels of C-PTH was significantly higher in the low 1,25(OH)2D group than in the higher 1,25(OH)2D group. On the other hand, there was no significant difference in serum levels of 25(OH)2D, 24,25(OH)2D, CT and urinary r-Gla protein between these 2 groups (Table 1).

Vertebral fractures are significantly more common in lower 1,25(OH)2D group than in higher 1,25(OH)2D group, while no difference was found in RMD between these 2 groups. (Table 2) In Summary, 1) Vertebral fractures were more common in osteoporotic females with lower serum levels of 1,25(OH)2D than in those with higher levels of 1,25(OH)2D. 2) Osteoporotic females with lower serum levels of 1,25(OH)2D are associated with high serum levels of C-PTH.

Table 1 Back ground data of the subjects

1,25(OH)D	$\leq$ 40 Pg/ml	40 pg/ml<	Statistics
No. of cases	28	17	
Age (y.o.)	71.6 ± 1.3	73.3 ± 1.6	NS
Initial RMD (g/cm^2)	0.51 ± 0.02	0.47 ± 0.02	NS
Body weight (kg)	49.2 ± 1.5	49.0 ± 2.3	NS
BUN (mg/dl)	18.7 ± 0.7	17.5 ± 0.8	NS
Creatinine (mg/dl)	0.90 ± 0.03	0.87 ± 0.03	NS
Ca (mg/dl)	9.1 ± 0.1	9.2 ± 0.1	NS
P (mg/dl)	3.6 ± 0.1	3.6 ± 0.1	NS
Al-p (IU)	142.3 ± 6.3	156.9 ± 10.2	NS
1,25(OH)$_2$D (pg/ml)	26.8 ± 1.8	50.7 ± 2.0	p<0.01
24,25(OH)$_2$D (ng/ml)	1.4 ± 0.1	1.4 ± 0.2	NS
25(OH)D (ng/ml)	20.6 ± 1.2	22.4 ± 1.8	NS
PTH (ng/ml)	0.43 ± 0.03	0.35 ± 0.03	p<0.10
U-Gla (n mole/mg·Cr)	81.6 ± 4.3	78.1 ± 3.9	NS
U-Ca/Cr	0.09 ± 0.01	0.11 ± 0.02	NS
U-P/Cr	0.61 ± 0.10	0.48 ± 0.03	NS

(Mean ± S.E.)

Table 2 RMD and fracture rate in female osteoporotics with lower or higher serum level of 1,25(OH)$_2$D

values: Mean ± S.E.

		Low ≤ 40 pg/mℓ	High 40 pg/mℓ <	
		26	35	
R M D (g/cm^2)		0.47 ± 0.02	0.45 ± 0.02	N.S.
Fracture	−	10 cases	23 cases	χ^2 = 4.46
	+	16 cases	12 cases	P < 0.01

II. Long term therapeutic effect of 1α-OH-D$_3$ in involutional osteoporosis

Twenty female osteoporotic subjects (mean age of 74.3±1.6) and twenty female osteoporotic subjects treated with 1α-OH-D$_3$ (0.5-1.0μg/day) for more than 3 years (mean age of 74.6±1.4 yrs) were selected from 86 osteoporotic subjects (59 control subjects and 27 1α-OH-D$_3$ treated subjects) by the matched pair method.

Percent changes in the proximal radial mineral density (RMD) measured by single photon absorptiometry were compared between control and 1α-OH-D$_3$ treated groups. Subsequently, fracture incidence was compared between these 2 groups.

Background data of the subjects are summarized in Table 3.

There was no significant difference as for age, observation period, initial RMD, serum levels of alkaline phosphatase, BUN, Cr, 1,25(OH)$_2$D, 24,25(OH)$_2$D, 25(OH)D, PTH, Ca, P, u-Ca/Cr, u-P/Cr and u-Gla protein between these 2 groups.

Percent decrease of RMD was significantly greater in control group than in 1α-OH-D$_3$ treated group at 1, 2, 3 and 4 years during the observation period. (Fig. 1)

There was a transient increase of RMD during 2 years treatment with 1α-OH-D$_3$ followed by a plateau during the subsequent period.

Fracture incidence in both of these 2 groups are shown in Fig. 2.

Incidence of new vertebral fractures appeared to be less in 1α-OH-D$_3$ group than in control group, but this difference was not statistically significant. Changes in serum level of Ca, BUN, creatinine and alkaline phosphatase are shown in Fig. 3. Serum level of alkaline phosphatase was significantly lower in 1α-OH-D$_3$ group than in control group, while no significant change in serum Ca, BUN and creatinine was observed between these 2 groups. In summary, these results clearly demonstrated that administration of 1α-OH-D$_3$ significantly prevented the age related loss of bone mass in female osteoporotic patients.

III. Adverse effects of 1α(OH)D$_3$ in osteoporotic patients

During these 6 years 7405 osteoporotic patients were treated with 1α(OH)$_2$D$_3$. Dose of 1α(OH)D$_3$ given to the patients ranged from 0.5 μg/day (16%) to 1 μg/day (67%) and the most of the patients treated were above the age of 60 years (93%). The details of the adverse effects were shown in Table 4. Adverse effects of 1α(OH)$_2$D$_3$ were found in 1.35%. Hypercalcemia (S.Ca>11mg/dl) was found 0.39% and increase of BUN was found in 0.76%, but no kidney stone was found. These data suggest that 1α(OH)D$_3$ is a safe drug for the treatment of senile osteoporosis.

Table 3 Background data of the subjects

		control	1α(OH)D$_3$	Statistics
No. of Patients		20	20	
Age	(y.o.)	74.3 ± 1.6	74.6 ± 1.4	NS
observation period	(years)	4.1 ± 0.2	4.2 ± 0.2	NS
initial BMD	(g/cm^2)	0.45 ± 0.01	0.43 ± 0.02	NS
Ca	(mg/dℓ)	9.1 ± 0.1	9.1 ± 0.1	NS
P	(mg/dℓ)	3.6 ± 0.1	3.4 ± 0.1	NS
Aℓ-P	(IU)	140.0 ± 6.1	158.2 ± 11.5	NS
BuN	(mg/dℓ)	18.3 ± 1.0	18.6 ± 0.8	NS
Cr	(mg/dℓ)	0.91 ± 0.04	0.94 ± 0.04	NS
U-Ca/Cr		0.10 ± 0.02	0.13 ± 0.04	NS
U-P/Cr		0.49 ± 0.04	0.50 ± 0.05	NS
U-Gla	(n mole/mg·Cr)	73.5 ± 5.9	71.6 ± 4.8	NS
1-25(OH)$_2$D$_3$	(pg/mℓ)	32.6 ± 4.8	35.9 ± 5.2	NS
24-25(OH)$_2$D$_3$	(ng/mℓ)	1.7 ± 0.2	1.7 ± 0.3	NS
25(OH)D$_3$	(ng/mℓ)	22.9 ± 2.5	21.5 ± 2.8	NS
PTH	(ng/mℓ)	0.37 ± 0.07	0.39 ± 0.03	NS

Mean ± SE

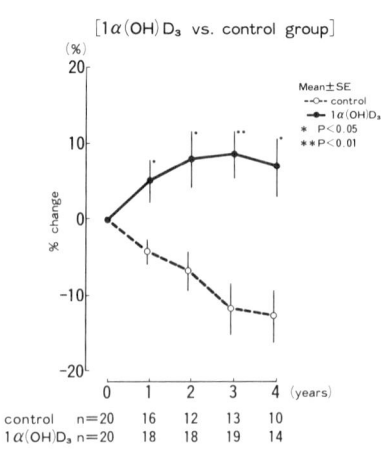

Fig. 1 % change of radial mineral density in involutional osteoporosis

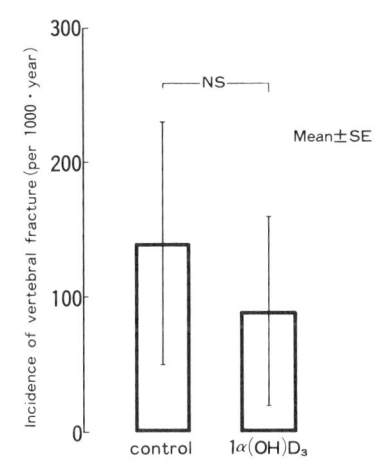

Fig. 2 Incidence of vertebral fracture

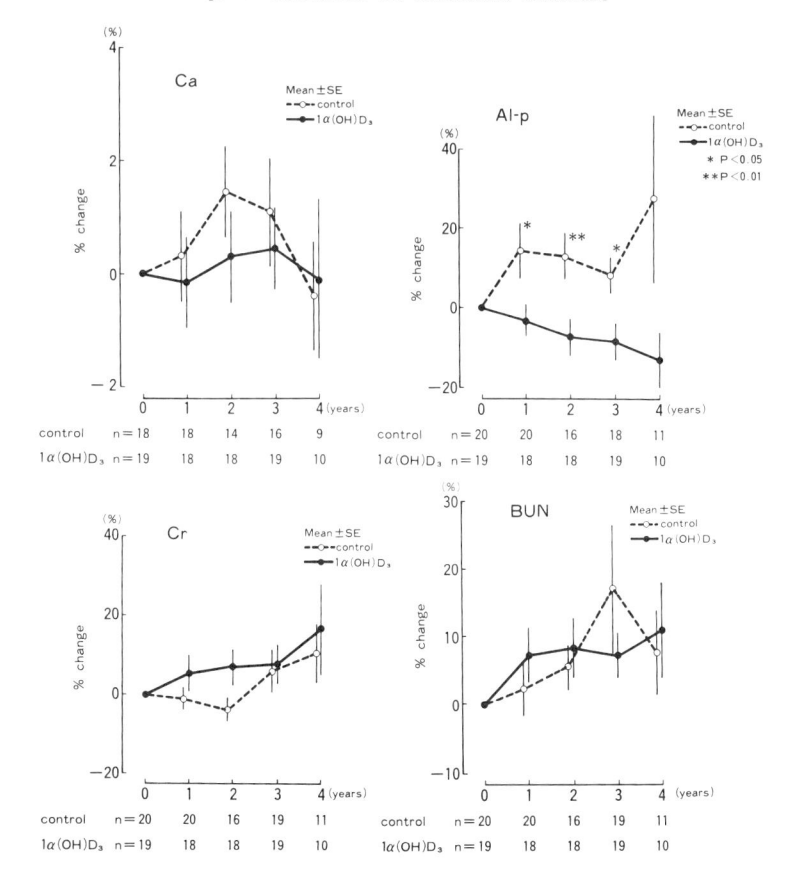

Fig. 3 % change of serum parameters in involutional osteoporotics [1α(OH)D$_3$ vs. control group]

Table 4 Adverse effects and hypercalcemia found in 7,405 osteoporotic patients treated with 1α(OH)D$_3$ during 6 years

1. Adverse effects		No. of events	occurrence(%)
Gastro intestinal system	Loss of appetite	6	0.08
	Nausea	9	0.12
	Vomiting	1	0.01
	Stomach discomfort	7	0.09
	Abdominal discomfort	1	0.01
	Oral cavity dryness	1	0.01
	Stomachache	5	0.07
	Constipation	4	0.05
	Diarrhea	2	0.03
	Oral cavity discomfort	1	0.01
	Abdominal pain	2	0.03
	Stomatitis	1	0.01
	No. of pts.*	36	0.49
Psycho-nerous system	Dizziness	1	0.01
	Tension acceleration	2	0.03
	Palpitation	1	0.01
	Decrease in memory	1	0.01
	No. of pts.	5	0.07
Cardiovascular system	Increase of blood pressure	1	0.01
	Arrhythmia	1	0.01
	No. of pts.*	2	0.03
Liver-bile duct system	Increase of serum GOT	13	0.18
	Increase of serum GPT	11	0.15
	Increase of serum γ-GTP	8	0.11
	No. of pts.*	21	0.28
Metabolism nutrition	Increase of serum LDH	6	0.08
	Gout	1	0.01
	Increase of serum uric acid	1	0.01
	No. of pts.	7	0.09
Hematology	Decrease of RBC	1	0.01
	Decrease of hemoglobin	1	0.01
	Decrease of hematocrit	1	0.01
	increase of platelet	1	0.01
	No. of pts.*	2	0.03
Skin	Itching	3	0.04
	Eruption	5	0.07
	No. of pts.	8	0.11
Eye		0	0
Urinary system	Increase of BUN	19	0.26
	Increase of serum creatinine	3	0.04
	Ureteral stone	0	0.
	No. of pts*	19	0.26
General whole body disturbance	Facial redness	2	0.03
	Edema	1	0.01
	Facial edema	1	0.01
		4	0.05
	Total events	125/7,405	1.69
Total of patients* with adverse effects		100/7,405	1.35

* : Patients were overlapping

| 2. Hypercalcemia** | | 29/7,405 | 0.39 |

** : Serum Ca level > 11.0mg/dl

1) Gallagher, J.C., Riggs, B.L., Eisman, J., Hamstra, A., Amaud, S.B., and DeLuca, H.F. (1979): J. Clin. Invest., 64:729-736
2) Nordin, B.E.C., Peacock, M., Crilly, R.G., and Marshall, D.H. (1979): Calcium absorption and plasma 1,25(OH)2D levels in postmenopausal osteoporosis. In: Vitamin D, Basic Research and Its Clinical Application.
3) Aloia, J.F., Cohn, S.H., Vaswani, A., Yeh, J.K., and Ellis, K. (1985): Am. J. Med. 78:95-100.
4) Lore, F., Nuti, R., Vattimo, A., and Caniggia, A. (1984): Horm. Metab. Res., 16:58
5) Lund, B., Sorensen, O.H., Lund, B., and Agner, E. (1982): Horm. Metab. Res., 14:271-274.
6) Christiansen, C., and Rodbro, P. (1984): Calcif. Tissue Int., 36:19-24.
7) Francis, R.M., Peacock, M., Taylor, G.A., Storer, J.H., and Nordin, B.E.C. (1984): Clin. Sci., 66· 103-107.
8) Peacock, M. Lancet 1974: I: 385-389
9) Lund B. Lancet 1975: II: 1168-1171
10) Lindholm, J.S. Vitamin D, basic research and its clinical application In: Norman AW et al. ed. Berlin, New York, Walter de Gruyter, 1979: 115
11) Orimo, H., Inoue, T., Fujita, T., Itami, V., Vitamin D., Chemical, biochemical and clinical endocrinology of Ca metabolism. In "Norman A.W. et al. eds. Berlin, New York, Walter de Grayter, 1982: 1239
12) Shiraki, M., Orimo, H., Ito, H., Akiguchi, I., Nakao, J., Takehashi, R., and Inshizuka, S., Endocrinol. Japon. 1985: 32(2), 305-315
13) Orimo, H., Shiraki, M., Hayashi, T. and Nakamura, T., Bone and Mineral, 1987:3, 47-52

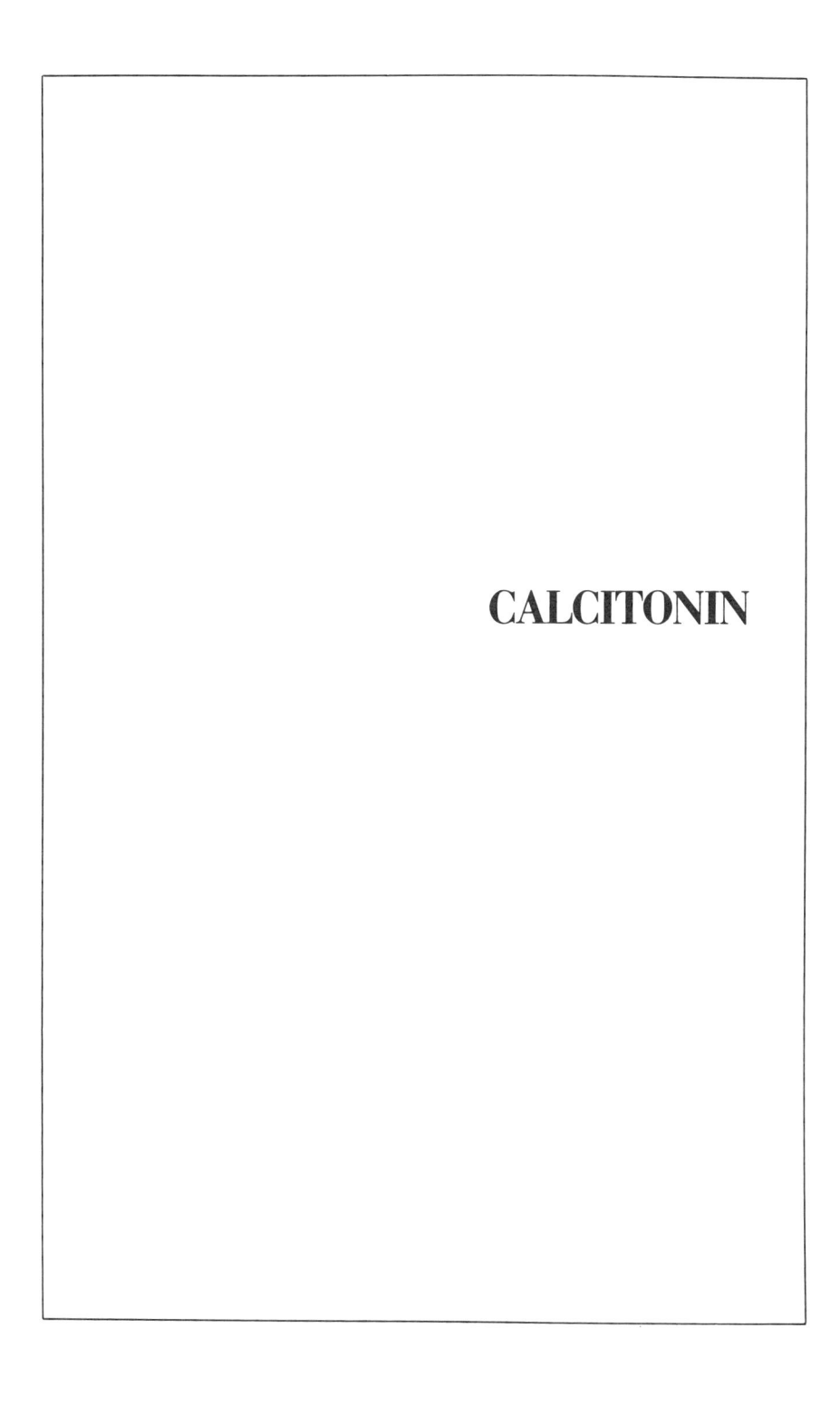

CALCITONIN

Calcitonin: Some Recent Developments

Iain MacIntyre and Mone Zaidi

Endocrine Unit, Department of Chemical Pathology, Royal Postgraduate Medical School, London, U.K.

ABSTRACT

   The modes of osteoclastic activity are summarized, and the mechanism of action of calcitonin discussed. Evidence is provided which shows that at least two second messengers are involved in calcitonin action on the osteoclast. Reliable immunoassays need to be shown to be in agreement with bioassays, and two-site assays based on monoclonal antibodies are to be preferred. A patient with complete calcitonin deficiency and severe osteoporosis is described. The calcitonin deficiency may be due to the gene defect which was identified. This case supports at least a permissive role for calcitonin in the development of osteoporosis. As might be predicted from this study, calcitonin prevents postmenopausal bone loss. Calcitonin is likely to be widely used in the prevention and treatment of osteoporosis.

INTRODUCTION

   Over the last few years it has become clear how calcitonin acts at a cellular level. This new knowledge will help to guide the development of rational use of the peptide in clinical medicine.

   It appears likely that the rather tedious controversies related to assay of the hormone in plasma are likely to be resolved in the near future. Two-site monoclonal radiometric assays are now available and combined with sensitive bioassays applicable to plasma should resolve the differences of interpretation which have impeded progress in the field. In addition to discussing these two areas briefly below, we shall summarize some of the evidence that indicates that lower calcitonin levels are at least a permissive factor in the development of osteoporosis.

The Function of the Osteoclast

   The osteoclast resorbs bone by a complex of interacting effects many of which are essential for resorption but insufficient in themselves. The actions of the osteoclast which are essential to resorptive activity can be listed as follows:

i)   <u>Cell motility</u>. This includes ruffling of the cell membrane, granule movement, and maintenance of cell area. Abolition of any of these can prevent bone resorption [1,2].

ii) <u>Secretory activity</u>. After sealing itself peripherally to the bone surface the osteoclast secretes acid, enzymes and probably free radicals at the interface with the bone surface. Again, we know that prevention of any one of these activities can completely prevent bone resorption [3].

For example, inhibition of secreted acid phosphatase by molybdate abolishes bone resorption, as do specific antibodies directed against acid phosphatase (Figures 1 and 2). It is interesting that it is possible that the phosphatase-inhibiting effects of the diphosphonates may be an important part of their effect in preventing bone resorption [3].

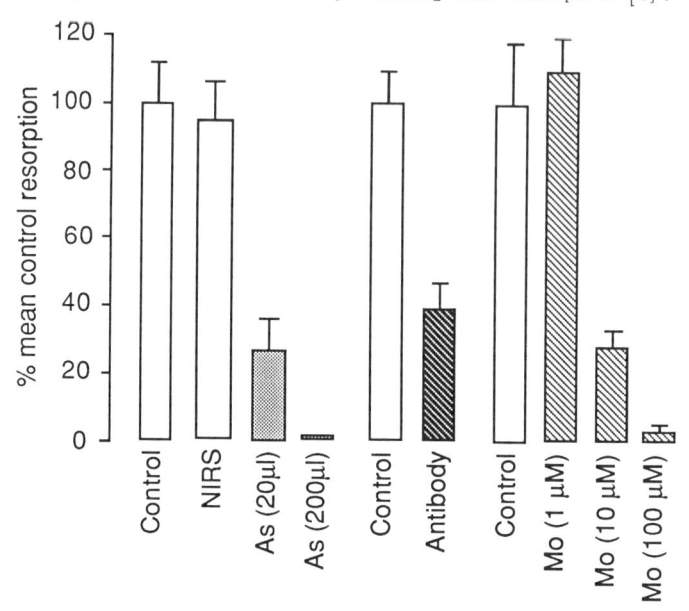

FIG. 1. Effect of anti-porcine uteroferrin (As) (20 µl and 200 µl), affinity-purified antibody (Antibody; 60 g/ml) and molybdate ions (Mo; 1, 10 and 100 µM) on the area of bone resorbed by isolated rat osteoclasts, expressed as a percentage of mean control resorption. NIRS: non-immune rabbit serum.

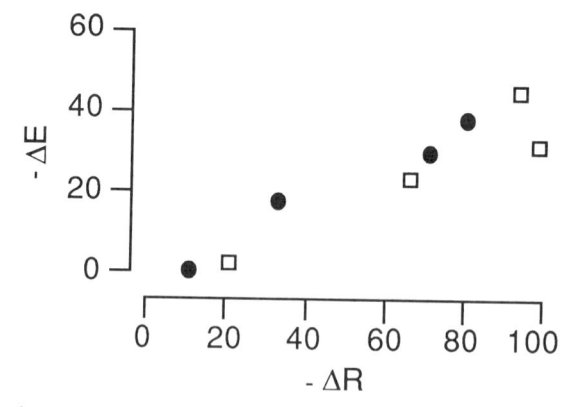

FIG. 2. Correlation between the percentage fall in measured resorption (per bone slice) ($-\Delta R$) and the percentage fall in supernatant enzyme concentration ($-\Delta E$) using affinity-purified anti-porcine uteroferrin antibody (closed circles) and molybdate ions (open squares).

The Mode of Action of Calcitonin

After interaction with the abundant specific receptors on the osteoclast surface [4], calcitonin has the following effects:

i) Cell motility. Here calcitonin has two quite separate effects. First, it rapidly abolishes ruffling of the cell membrane and granule movement (the 'Q' effect). Second, calcitonin causes a marked diminution

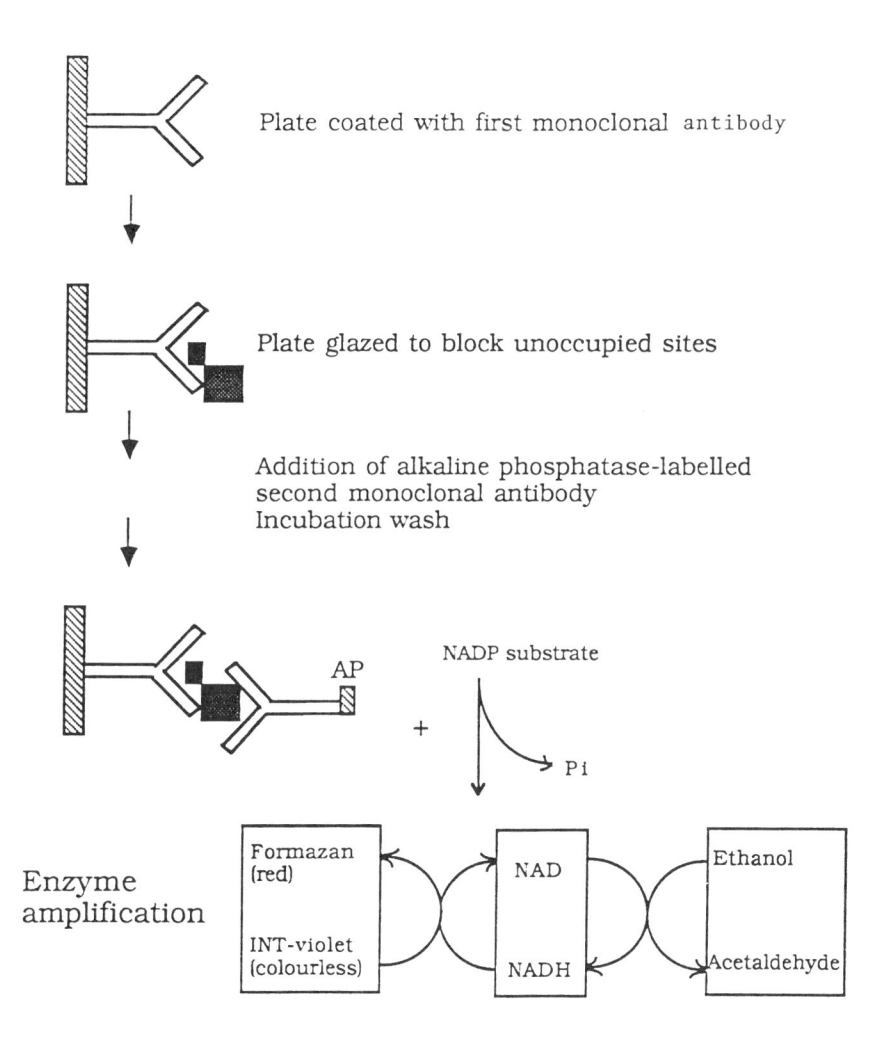

FIG. 3. Diagrammatic representation of a two-site enzyme immunoassay for human calcitonin (hCT) utilising monoclonal antibodies recognizing two different epitopes located along the hCT molecule and an enzyme amplification system which facilitates signal detection.

in cell area which may proceed to the production of a very contracted form ('R' effect). Prevention of either one of these two separate actions of calcitonin on motility abolishes its effect in preventing bone resorption. We now know that more than one second messenger must be involved [5]. Thus, although cyclic AMP can mimic the 'Q' effect, it does not produce the 'R' effect and this must be produced by a different second messenger still to be identified.

ii) Secretory activity. Calcitonin markedly diminishes or abolishes enzyme secretion (for example, acid phosphatase) [6] and probably also inhibits acid and free-radical production. The second messenger involved in these actions on osteoclast secretion remains to be identified. However, this effect of calcitonin is certainly an important part of its inhibitory activity. The potency of calcitonin is probably explained by its multiple effects in abolishing several activities, each one of which is essential for bone resorption.

Assay of plasma calcitonin

The limitations in specificity and sensitivity of conventional radioimmunoassays are too well known to need enumeration here, but many of these difficulties can be overcome using a two-site double monoclonal antibody radiometric assay. One satisfactory type has recently been described [7] (Figure 3). When this highly sensitive and specific assay is combined with the sensitive bioassays devised in collaboration with Chambers and applied to plasma [8], it becomes quite clear that plasma calcitonin circulates in several quite distinct forms. More than one of these is highly active biologically (Figure 4; [8]). It is very important that standard assays based on monoclonal antibodies and accompanied by sensitive bioassays are widely adopted so that the obscurities produced by unsatisfactory assays can be removed.

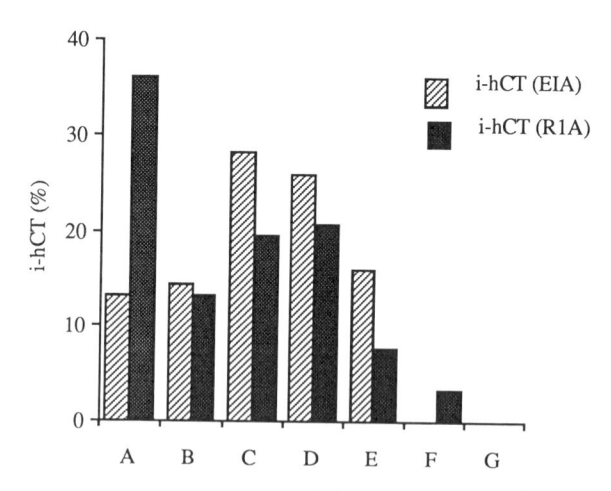

FIG. 4. Comparison of the percentage of immunoreactive calcitonin (i-hCT) in the various peaks pooled from fractions obtained after gel filtration chromatography of plasma of medullary thyroid carcinoma patients using enzyme-immunometric assay and radioimmunoassay. E is the peak coeluting with monomeric human calcitonin and A is the void volume peak: both peaks are biologically active as assessed by the osteoclast-resorption based biological assay.

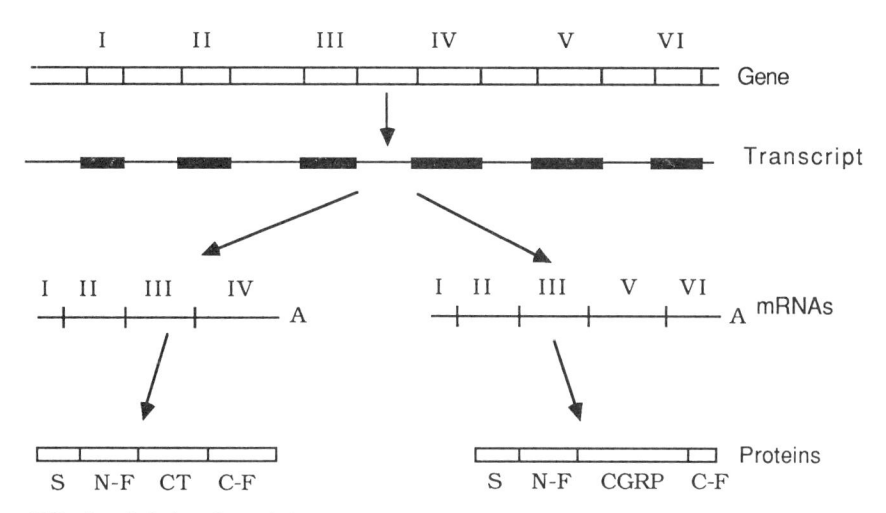

FIG. 5. Calcitonin-calcitonin gene related peptide gene. Numbers refer to exons of gene. S = Signal peptide, N-F = amino terminal flanking peptide, CT = calcitonin, C-F = carboxy terminal flanking peptide, and CGRP = calcitonin gene related peptide.

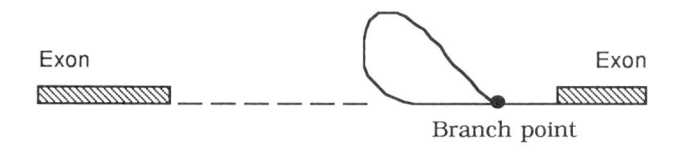

FIG. 6. Formation of looped structure during maturation of messenger RNA precursors. First step in eliminating intervening sequence is cleavage after first exon and looping back to branch point.

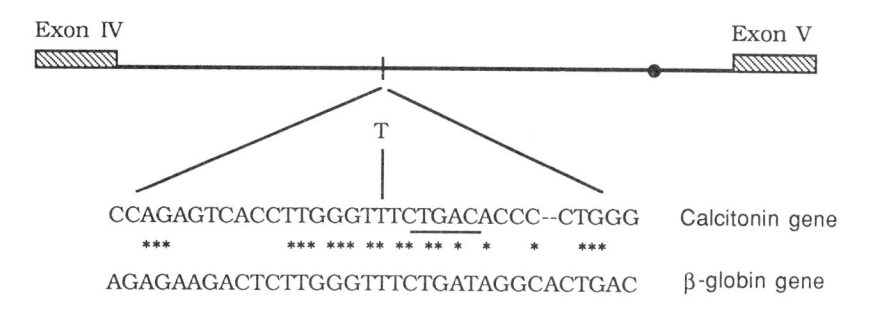

FIG. 7. Altered calcitonin gene sequence from patient with osteoporosis. Sequence from intervening sequence between exons IV and V shows single base insertion, which is next to consensus sequence for formation of branch point (CTGAC (underlined)) and has homology with more extensive sequence from branch point in the β globin gene. Asterisks show identical residues in calcitonin and β globin genes.

Calcitonin and Osteoporosis

It is our view that the fall in plasma calcitonin which we observe after the menopause and which is reversed by oestrogen is likely to be at least a permissive factor for the development of osteoporosis. It is of course, quite unlikely that this is the only important factor. However, it is important to note that complete deficiency of calcitonin can be associated with severe osteoporosis. We have recently described such a case [9]. This was a young boy in whom calcitonin was completely absent from the plasma, and was associated with severe osteoporosis. The patient's gene encoded normal calcitonin and precursor polypeptides of calcitonin gene-related peptide; the only abnormality found was a single base insertion in the intron separating exons IV and V of the gene. It seems possible that this single change was responsible for the patient's calcitonin deficiency. One possibility is that the altered sequence has the properties of a branch point, forcing an abortive splice precluding the production of calcitonin (Figures 5-7).

Certainly this case is consistent with an important role for calcitonin in the aetiology of osteoporosis, even if that role is not more than permissive. Our findings do, however, suggest that the therapy of osteoporosis with calcitonin is rational and that at least arrest of the disease may be anticipated.

Calcitonin in the Prevention of Postmenopausal Bone Loss

The administration of calcitonin to the calcitonin-deficient patient just described resulted in arrest of the disease. For this reason we expected that administration of calcitonin to postmenopausal women, in whom calcitonin levels are generally low, should arrest or even partially reverse the rapid postmenopausal bone loss. This was found to be the case. Appropriate calcitonin dosage was as effective as oestrogen in arresting bone loss; in addition, there is clear evidence of a dose-related effect [10] (Figures 8,9; Table 1).

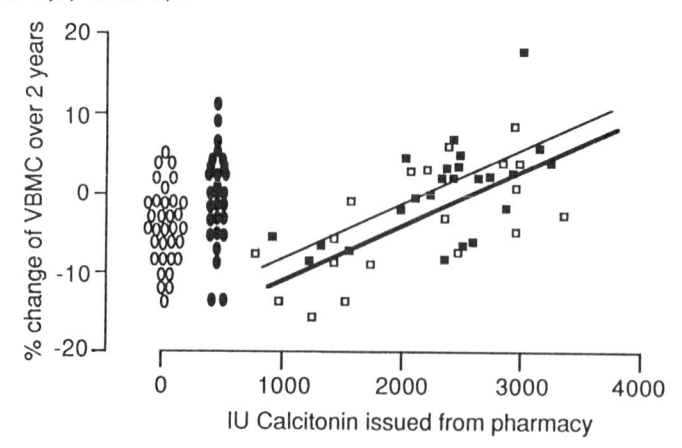

FIG. 8. Relationship of percentage annual change in vertebral bone mineral content (VBMC) in each of two years of study to IU of calcitonin issued from the pharmacy. (□), Patients receiving calcitonin (CT) alone; (■), patients receiving a combination of CT plus oestradiol/progesterone; (○), placebo group; ( ), patients receiving oestradiol/progesterone alone, (●). The fitted lines refer to the patients on combination therapy (light line) and calcitonin alone (heavy line).

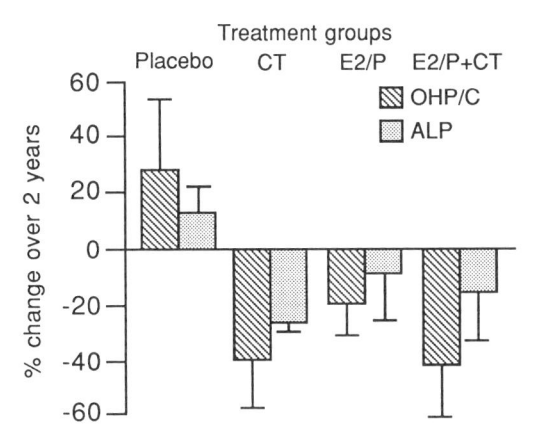

FIG. 9. Percentage change over 2 years in plasma bone-specific alkaline phosphatase (ALP) and urinary hydroxyproline (OHP/C) (mmol/mmol creatinine).

We anticipate that calcitonin will become widely used in the prevention and treatment of osteoporosis provided that appropriate means of administration can be developed. Administration by injection as used in our study [10] is quite impractical as a preventive or long-term therapeutic measure.

TABLE 1

Percentage change of VBMC over 2 years

Group	Treatment (n)	% Change in VBMC Mean (SEM)
1	Placebo (17)	-10.20 (1.20)
2	CT compliers (4)*	-2.75 (4.43)
	CT non-compliers (6)	-11.42 (2.25)
3	E2/P (15)	-3.85 (2.30)
4	E2/P + CT (11)	-3.10 (2.09)
2 + 4	CT compliers (11)*	-1.16 (2.13)
2 + 4	CT non-compliers (10)	-10.76 (1.72)

* Compliers in the calcitonin (CT) group were taken as patients receiving more than 50 IU calcitonin/week.

SUMMARY

1. Gel filtration chromatography shows that immunoreactive calcitonin circulates in at least 5 forms, of which 3 are biologically active. The major biological activity in plasma may not circulate as the 'monomer' form.

2. Discrepant claims about the effects of oestrogen and about the levels of calcitonin in osteoporosis are unlikely to be reconciled until improved assays correlating with biological activity are in general use.

3. Complete absence of calcitonin was associated with severe osteoporosis in one young subject. Replacement therapy prevented further progress of the disease.

4. Calcitonin prevents postmenopausal bone loss and arrests, or partly reverses, established osteoporosis. It seems likely that the hormone will play an important role in the prevention and treatment of this common condition.

Acknowledgements

The authors acknowledge the support of ISF (IM), Bartos Foundation (IM), Arthritis & Rheumatism Council (MZ) and Research into Ageing (IM).

REFERENCES

1. T.J. Chambers, and C.J. Magnus. J. Pathol. 136, 27 (1982).
2. T.J. Chambers, and A. Moore. J. Clin. Endocrinol. Metab. 57, 819 (1983).
3. M. Zaidi, B.S. Moonga, and D.W. Moss. Biochem. Biophys. Res. Commun. 159, 68 (1989).
4. G.C. Nicholson, J.M. Moseley, P.M. Sexton, P.A.O. Mendelsohn, and T.J. Martin. J. Clin. Invest. 78, 355 (1986).
5. M. Zaidi, H.K. Datta, A. Patchell, G. Abeyasekera, and I. MacIntyre. Submitted to J. Cell Biology (1989).
6. T.J. Chambers, K. Fuller, J.A. Darby. J. Cell Physiol. 132, 90 (1987).
7. R. Seth, P. Motte, A. Kehely, S.J. Wimalawansa, C.H. Self, D. Bellet, C. Bohuon, and I. MacIntyre. J. Endocrinology 119, 351 (1988).
8. M. Zaidi, T.J. Chambers, A. Patchell, R.E. Gaines Das, and I. MacIntyre. Clin. Chem. in press (1989).
9. M. Alevizaki, J.C. Stevenson, S.I. Girgis, I. MacIntyre, and S. Legon. Brit. Med. J. 298, 1215 (1989).
10. I. MacIntyre, J.C. Stevenson, M.I. Whitehead, S.J. Wimalawansa, L.M. Banks, and M.J.R. Healy. Lancet 1, 900 (1988).

Secretion, Metabolism, and Action of Endogenous Calcitonin in Human Beings

Hunter Heath III and Robert D. Tiegs

Endocrine Research Unit, Division of Endocrinology, Metabolism, and Internal Medicine, Mayo Clinic and Foundation, Rochester, Minnesota

ABSTRACT

Calcitonin (CT)[*] is only one of several products of the CT gene, but the one most possibly tied to effects on systemic bone and calcium (Ca) metabolism. CT is primarily secreted by the C-cells of the thyroid gland under control of ambient ionic Ca levels. The basal CT secretion rate approximates 22 ng/d·kg^{-1} in women and 59 ng/d·kg^{-1} in men. The metabolic clearance rate for human CT in man is 5-10 ml/min·kg^{-1}, declining with age. CT is degraded to some extent by circulating peptidases, but is primarily taken up by the kidney, filtered, degraded by peritubular cells, and excreted as free amino acids. Lesser amounts of CT are taken up by the liver, bone, and other tissues, but the kidney is the major site of degradation. While the pharmacologic actions of CT are well-established, the physiologic role of CT in man remains uncertain, and there is no clearly-defined CT deficiency syndrome.

INTRODUCTION

CT was discovered about 30 years ago, but the nature of its complex gene has been known for less than 10. Human CT is but one product of a gene that also produces a carboxyl-associated peptide known as katacalcin or PDN-21, a separate neuropeptide named calcitonin gene-related peptide (CGRP), and possibly others [1-3]. In man, CT and PDN-21 are co-secreted [4,5], whereas there appears to be a reciprocal relationship between synthesis and secretion of CT and CGRP [6]. The "choice" between CGRP and CT production occurs through alternative processing of mRNA [6]. There is presently no evidence that the various CT gene products affect one another's biological activity, although CT itself may feed back to inhibit its release from the C-cell [e.g., 7]. CGRP has weak effects on skeletal tissue in vitro, and PDN-21 has none [8-10], whereas the pharmacologic effects of CT on bone and systemic Ca handling are well-described [11]. Therefore, this review will focus primarily only on secretion, metabolism, and--briefly--action of human CT in man.

STRUCTURE OF CT

Mature secreted human CT is a 32-amino acid peptide distinguished by a disulfide link between residues 1 and 7, forming an amino-terminal ring structure, and by prolinamide at position 32 [11]. Destroying or removing either the ring or the C-terminal amide structure enormously reduces the bioactivity of CT.

Copyright 1990 by Elsevier Science Publishing Co., Inc.
Osteoporosis: Physiological Basis, Assessment, and Treatment
Hector F. DeLuca and Richard Mazess, Editors

SECRETION OF CT

CT-like immunoreactivity has been found in several sites, but the only clearly-established source of circulating CT is the thyroidal C-cell or parafollicular cell. Thyroidectomy and radioiodine treatment virtually abolish CT secretory capacity [12]. The major form of CT secreted in response to simulation is monomeric CT [13]. In the peripheral circulation several immunochemically heterogeneous forms of CT are found in plasma of patients with CT-secreting medullary thyroid carcinoma [13], and possibly in normal persons [14]. While a large number of factors can stimulate CT secretion in vitro, extracellular Ca ion is the dominant regulator of CT release in vivo [15,16].

Concentrations of CT in plasma are highest in infancy and decline rapidly through early childhood [17], but change little if at all thoughout adult life [12]. Many groups have verified our original observation [12,18] that men of all ages have substantially higher basal plasma CT concentrations and CT responses to secretagogues than do women. Some groups have suggested that CT secretion is estrogen-sensitive [19,20], but we [21] and others [22,23] have been unable to verify this finding. Similarly, we and others found no evidence for decrease of plasma CT levels after menopause [12,22].

EFFECT OF CT IMMUNOCHEMICAL HETEROGENEITY ON MEASUREMENT OF THE PEPTIDE AND ASSESSMENT OF METABOLISM

As stated above, immunoreactive CT in blood is heterogeneous, consisting of material co-eluting with authentic CT monomer, and other forms of larger apparent molecular weight [13,24]. Chromatography under denaturing conditions reduces the apparent heterogeneity somewhat, but larger forms persist, suggesting that dimeric, polymeric, or precursor forms of CT may be secreted. Monomeric CT added to plasma or infused into patients elutes from chromatographic columns as a single peak [13,24], so the multiple endogenous forms are not the result of CT "sticking" together. Therefore, measurements of CT by conventional RIA in plasma include multiple species of related peptides [25], and not just the peptide of primary interest, monomeric CT. The biologic activity of circulating CT seems to reside primarily in the monomeric form [26], so measurement of that form would seem to be most useful for physiologic studies [25].

As expected from the foregoing, early assays for CT based on simple RIAs yielded much higher values for apparent CT concentrations--as high as 1,000 pg/ml--than did later assays [27]. In particular, immunoaffinity purification and silica cartridge extraction assays suggest that normal concentrations of CT in human plasma are quite low, perhaps less than 10 pg/ml (3 pmol/L) [12,25,28]. Calculations of secretion and metabolic clearance rates (SRs and MCRs) for CT include the basal CT concentration, so obtaining an accurate CT value is important. SR values, especially, derived with various techniques differ in expected ways because of this (see below).

SITES OF CT UPTAKE AND METABOLISM

The major target organs for CT are thought to be the bone (specifically, the osteoclast) and the kidney. Infused radiolabeled CT (biologically-active and -inactive alike) appears primarily in renal cortical tissue [29-32]. The peptide appears to be almost completely filtered, then reabsorbed and rapidly degraded by peritubular cells to constituent amino acids [30,32,33]. Only a small portion of infused CT appears intact in urine [29,30]. Lesser amounts of CT are taken up by bone and liver. In addition to organ-specific degradation, CT can be cleaved in plasma by circulating peptidases [34,35]. CT apparently binds to mature osteoclasts, but not to normal osteoblasts; it is not known if osteoclasts metabolize CT.

ESTIMATED SECRETION AND METABOLIC CLEARANCE RATES FOR CT

MCRs for CT have been estimated by infusing radiolabeled heterologous species bioinactive peptides, radiolabeled biologically-active heterologous species and human peptides, and unlabeled animal and human CTs. Levels of peptide in the blood have been estimated by gamma counting, conventional whole-plasma RIA, and RIA after silica extraction and concentration to measure only monomeric CT. Only some of the available data can be summarized here.

Infusion of porcine CT to constant concentrations in humans yielded an MCR of 14.5 ± 0.8 ml/min·kg^{-1} [36], similar to the value of 13.0 ± 0.7 ml/min·kg^{-1} obtained in pigs [37]. Radioiodinated, non-bioactive human CT infusion gave an apparent MCR of about 2.2 ml/min·kg^{-1} [38]. Kanis, et al. [39] infused human CT in normal volunteers for 2-24 hours, and calculated the MCR to be 854 ± 66 (SE) L/d; at 70 kg body weight, the MCR would be about 8.5 ml/min kg^{-1}. Huwyler, et al. [40] infused unlabeled human CT to volunteers arriving at an MCR of 8.4 ± 1.1 ml/min kg^{-1}. We infused human CT to constant concentration after a priming dose in "young" (21-30 yr) and "old" (54-70 yr) men and women [12]. Most other studies either have found no effect of age or sex, or did not seek one [37-41]. For our "young" group, the MCR was about 9 ml/min kg^{-1}, and in the older one, 6 ml/min·kg^{-1}, in fairly good agreement with the results of Kanis [40] and Huwyler [41]. There were no significant differences between the sexes for MCR. Whether we used whole-plasma or extracted CT values for calculation had little impact on calculated MCRs, because steady-state CT levels during infusion were similar. More recently, Reginster, et al. [42] carried out 2 hour infusions of human CT in 9 pre- and 16 post-menopausal women (11 with osteoporosis) and reported MCRs in L/24 hrs. Assuming (as they did for other studies) an average body weight of 65 kg, their MCR values averaged about 3.2 - 4.5 ml/min·kg^{-1}, somewhat lower than values derived by others [12, 39-41] for reasons not addressed by the authors. However, on balance, the nature of infused material and the measurement technique employed do not appear to have major influence on calculated MCR for CT in humans. Calculated secretion rates are a different story.

Kanis, et al. [30] infused unlabeled human CT, and measured basal and infused CT values with a RIA that gave an average basal CT concentration of 130 pg/ml (20% undetectable). Normal values in their assay ran as high as 980 pg/ml, far higher than is generally accepted today [27]. Because of this high basal CT level, the calculated SR for CT was 124 ± 24 ug/d, or approximately 1771 ng/day·kg^{-1}. In contrast, in addition to our conventional RIA, we used an assay system essentially specific for monomeric CT [25], which gave a normal value for CT of 2.4 ± 0.1 pg/ml in women, and 4.8 ± 0.3 pg/ml in men [12]. When we infused CT, we derived SRs of 22 ± 3 ng/day·kg^{-1} in women, and 59 ± 6 ng/day·kg^{-1} in men, far less than the value calculated by Kanis. Reginster, et al. [42] infused unlabeled human CT for 2 hours without a priming dose, and used a RIA on whole plasma that gave normal values in women as high as 119 pg/ml. Expectedly, they derived SRs in healthy women far higher than ours, or 300-475 ng/day·kg^{-1}. For our study, SRs calculated with extractable basal and infused steady-state CT values were only 8-20% of those calculated from our whole-plasma CT data. This difference was almost completely attributable to the lower basal values obtained by the silica extraction method.

Thus, there is good agreement among investigators about the MCR for CT in man, but recent data suggest that the actual SR for CT is considerably lower than suggested on the basis of studies using less specific CT RIAs. In addition, the difference in plasma CT levels between the sexes is primarily a result of lower SR in women, rather than enhanced clearance.

There is very little information about possible controls for CT metabolism. We examined MCR for human CT infused into dogs during acute "calcium clamp" at high and low Ca levels, and found no change [41]. Chronic hypercalcemia reduced MCR, but subsequent acute variations of plasma Ca did not further change MCR. Thus, renal clearance and degradation of CT apparently is not regulated by ambient Ca.

ACTIONS OF CT IN HUMANS

The pharmacologic properties of CT have mainly been studied using salmon or eel CT in mammals and animal tissues, but the structures, receptor binding characteristics, and bioactivities of teleost CTs are so different from those of mammalian CTs that one must question the relevance of those findings to normal physiology. In contrast, there are few studies clearly documenting any biological effects of human CT in humans at physiological concentrations. In vitro, human CT at near-physiologic concentrations will inhibit resorptive activity of rat and rabbit osteoclasts [43], but this again represents a cross-species experiment. A critical look at the literature shows no convincing evidence for a CT-deficiency syndrome in thyroidectomized persons whose CT secretory reserve is shown to be abolished. One study showed small reductions of bone mineral density in thyroidectomized people [44], but the same group found no increased rate of bone loss in similar patients [45]. Of course, there are alternative explanations for these findings besides CT deficiency, including effects of antecedent disease, osteolytic effects of therapeutic L-thyroxine, and selection bias. We found no evidence of spinal or appendicular bone loss after thyroidectomy for benign disease [46]. Some groups have reported reduced Ca-stimulated CT plasma levels in patients with hip fracture [47], postmenopausal osteoporosis [48,49], and mixed cases of osteoporosis [50]. However, we and others have been unable to document CT deficiency in osteoporotic patients [51-53]. Similarly, chronic CT excess in patients with medullary thyroid carcinoma is not associated with increased bone mass [52,54]. Reginster, et al. [42] recently reported that basal whole-plasma immunoreactive CT levels were low in postmenopausal women, and positively related to serum estrogen levels. Furthermore, they stated that CT PR was significantly reduced in postmenopausally osteoporotic women. Therefore, they thought low CT levels to be "determining factors in the pathogenesis of postmenopausal osteoporosis" [42]. This provocative claim must be interpreted in light of problems with the study, including uncertainty as to substances measured by their RIA, etc. Undoubtedly, their report will spark additional research, but the published record is sobering if not discouraging. We are forced to conclude that the true role of CT in adult human physiology remains unknown.

SUMMARY

While a great deal is known about the synthesis, secretion, metabolism, and pharmacologic actions of CT in man, its role in adult physiology is obscure and controversial. It remains possible that CT is important at some point in fetal or neonatal development, or that it has actions unrelated to systemic bone or calcium metabolism. However, these uncertainties in no way reduce the very real importance of CT in various forms for therapy of Paget's disease of bone, hypercalcemia of malignancy, and possibly accelerated osteoporosis.

ACKNOWLEDGMENTS

The work from our own laboratory cited here would not have been possible without the contributions of numerous Research Associates, Research Fellows, and research technologists over the last 15 years; particular gratitude is due Drs. G.W. Sizemore and C.D. Arnaud, whose generosity, guidance, and support at the beginning made it all possible. Work from Dr. Heath's laboratory has been supported by various NIH grants over the years, and the work cited here was supported in particular by grants RR-585, AM-19607, AM-27440, and DK-38855.

REFERENCES

1. A. Ali-Rachedi, I.M. Varndell, P. Facer, C.J. Hillyard, R.K. Craig, I. MacIntyre, and J.M. Polak, J. Clin. Endocrinol. Metab. 57, 680-682 (1983).
2. M.R. Edbrooke, D. Parker, J.H. McVey, J.H. Riley, G.D. Sorenson, O.S. Pettengill, and R.K. Craig, EMBO J. 4, 715-724 (1985).
3. P.H. Steenbergh, J.W.M. Hoppener, J. Zandberg, A. Visser, C.J.M. Lips and H.S. Jansz, FEBS Lett. 209, 97-103 (1986).
4. W. Woloszczuk, H. Schuh, J. Kovarik, J. Clin. Chem. Clin. Biochem. 24, 451-455 (1986)
5. D.L. Hurley, H.H. Katz, R.D. Tiegs, M.S. Calvo, J.R. Barta, and H. Heath III, J. Clin. Endocrinol. Metab. 66, 640-644 (1988)
6. M.I. Sabate, L.S. Stolarsky, J.M. Polak, S.R. Bloom, I. M. Varndell, M.A. Ghatei, M. Evans, and M.G. Rosenfeld, J. Biol. Chem. 260, 2589-2592 (1985)
7. A.L. Orme and J.T. Pento, Proc. Soc. Exp. Biol. Med. 151, 110-112 (1976)
8. I. Yamamoto, N. Kitamura, J. Aoki, C. Shigeno, M. Hino, K. Asonuma, K. Torizuka, N. Fujii, A. Otakea, and H. Yajima, Calcif. Tis. Int. 38, 339-341 (1986)
9. S.M. D'Souza, I. MacIntyre, S.I. Girgis, and G.R. Mundy, Endocrinology 119, 58-61 (1986)
10. B. A. Roos, J. A. Fischer, W. Pignat, C. B. Alander, and L.G. Raisz, Endocrinol. 118, 46-51 (1986)
11. L.A. Austin and H. Heath III, N. Engl. J. Med. 304, 269-278 (1981)
12. R.D. Tiegs, J. J. Body, J.M. Barta, and H. Heath III, J. Bone Min. Res. 1, 339-349 (1986)
13. H. Heath III and G.W. Sizemore, J. Lab. Clin. Med. 93, 390-401 (1979)
14. S.I. Girgis, C. McMartin, and I. MacIntyre, J. Endocrinol. 83, 55-56 (1979)
15. L.A. Austin, H. Heath III, and V.L.W. Go, J. Clin. Invest. 64, 1721-1724 (1979)
16. J.J. Body, P.E. Cryer, K.P. Offord, and H. Heath III, J. Clin. Invest. 71, 572-578 (1983)
17. G.L. Klein, E.L. Wadlington, E.D. Collins, B.D. Catherwood, L.J. Deftos, Calcif. Tis. Int. 36, 635-638 (1984)
18. H. Heath III and G.W. Sizemore, J. Clin. Invest. 60, 1135-1140 (1977)
19. M.L. Delorme, Y. Digioia, J. Fandard, R. Merceron, J.Y. Raymond, H.P. Klotz, Annales d'Endocrinologie (Paris) 37, 503-504 (1976)
20. J.C. Stevenson, G. Abeyasekara, C.J. Hillyard, K-G Phang, I. MacIntyre, S. Campbell, G. Lane, P.T. Townsend, O. Young, and M.I. Whitehead, Eur. J. Clin. Invest. 13, 481-487 (1983)
21. D.L. Hurley, R.D. Tiegs, J. Barta, K. Laakso, and H. Heath III, J. Bone Min. Res. 4, 89-95 (1989)
22. O. Tørring, E. Bucht, and H.E. Sjöberg, Horm. Metab. Res. 17, 536-539 (1985)
23. P. Selby and M. Peacock, Clin. Endocrinol. 25, 543-547 (1986)
24. F.R. Singer and J.F. Habener, Biochem. Biophys. Res. Comm. 61, 710-716 (1974)
25. J.J. Body, and H. Heath III, J. Clin. Endocrinol. Metab. 57, 897-903 (1983)
26. D.R. Wright, E.F. Voelkel, K.M. Sides, J.E. Tice, and A.H. Tashjian, Jr., Clin. Res. 25, 404A (1977)
27. H. Heath III, J.J. Body, and J. Fox, Biomed. Pharmacother. 38, 241-245 (1984)
28. J.G. Parthemore and L.J. Deftos, J. Clin. Invest. 56, 835-841 (1975)
29. F. Singer, J.F. Habener, E. Greene, P. Godin, J.T. Potts, Jr., Nature 237, 269-270 (1972)
30. M.B. Clark, C.C. Williams, B.M. Nathanson, R.E. Horton, H.I. Glass, and G.V. Foster, J. Endocrinol. 61, 199-210 (1974)
31. P.J. Scarpace, W.F. Neuman, and L.G. Raisz, Endocrinol. 100, 1260-1267 (1977)
32. P.J. Scarpace, J.G. Parthemore, and L.J. Deftos, Endocrinol. 103, 128-132 (1978)
33. R.E. Simmons, J.T. Hjelle, C. Mahoney, L.J. Deftos, W. Lisker, P. Kato and R.

Rabkin, Am. J. Physiol. 254, F593-F600 (1988)
34. J.F. Habener, F.R. Singer, L.J. Deftos, and J.T. Potts, Jr., Endocrinol. 90, 952-960 (1972)
35. S.B. Baylin, T.H. Hsu, and G.V. Foster, Endocrinology 94, 214A, (1974)
36. B.L. Riggs, C.D. Arnaud, R.S. Goldsmith, W.F. Taylor, J.T. McCall, and A.D. Sessler, J. Clin. Endocrinol. Metab. 33, 115-127 (1971)
37. P.B. Greenberg, T.J. Martin, R.A. Melick, P. Jablonski, and J.McK. Watts, J. Endocr. 54, 125-135 (1972)
38. R. Ardaillou, P. Sizonenko, A. Meyrier, G. Vallee, C. Beaugas, J. Clin. Invest. 49, 2345-2352 (1970)
39. J.A. Kanis, G. Heynen, T. Cundy, F. Cornet, A. Paterson, and R.G.G. Russell, Clin. Sci. 63, 145-152 (1982)
40. R. Huwyler, W. Born, E.E. Ohnhaus, and J.A. Fischer, Am. J. Physiol. 236, E15-E19, (1979)
41. J. Fox and H. Heath III, Horm. Metab. Res. 16, 46-49 (1982)
42. J.Y. Reginster, R. Deroisy, A. Albert, D. Denis, M.P.Lecart, J. Collette, and P. Franchimont, J. Clin. Invest. 83:1073-1077 (1989)
43. T.J. Chambers, J.C. Chambers, J. Symonds, and J.A. Darby, J. Clin. Endocrinol. Metab. 63, 1080 (1986)
44. M.T. McDermott, G.S. Kidd, P. Blue, V. Ghaed, F.D. Hofeldt, J. Clin. Endocrinol. Metab. 56, 936-939 (1983)
45. M.T. McDermott, F.D. Hofeldt, G.S. Kidd, J. Bone Min. Res. 1(suppl. 1):352(A) (1986)
46. D.L. Hurley, R.D. Tiegs, H.W. Wahner, H. Heath III, N. Engl. J. Med. 317, 537-541 (1987)
47. J.C. Stevenson, P.R. Allen, G. Abeyasekera, and P.A. Hill, Europ. J. Clin. Invest. 16, 357-360 (1986)
48. H. McA. Taggart, C.H. Chesnut, J.L. Ivey, D.J. Baylink, K. Sisom, M.B. Huber, B.A. Roos, Lancet 1:475-478 (1982)
49. J. Zseli, J. Szucs, K. Steczek, M. Szathmari, E. Kollin, C. Horvath, M. Gvoth, I. Hollo, Horm. Metab. Res. 17, 696-697 (1985)
50. G. Milhaud, M. Benezech-Lefevre, and M.S. Moukhtar, Biomedicine 29, 272-276 (1978)
51. J. Leggate, E. Farish, C.D. Fletcher, W. McIntosh, D.M. Hart, and J.M. Sommerville, Clin. Endocrinol. 20, 85-92 (1984)
52. R.D. Tiegs, J.J. Body, H.W. Wahner, J. Barta, B.L. Riggs, H. Heath III, N. Engl. J.Med. 312, 1097-1100 (1985)
53. Beringer, T.R.O., J. Ardill, and H. McA. Taggart, Calcif. Tiss. Int. 39, 300-303 (1986)
54. K.E.W. Melvin, A.H. Tashjian, Jr., and P. Bordier, in Clinical Aspects of Metabolic Bone Disease (Excerpta Medica, Amsterdam 1973) pp. 193-200.

```
*Abbreviations used:  CT = calcitonin; CGRP - calcitonin related peptide;
PDN-21 = calcitonin gene related peptide with neural activity; RIA =
radio immune assay; MCR = metabolic clearance rate; SR = secretion rate;
PR = production rate.
```

Use of Calcitonin in the Treatment of Postmenopausal Osteoporosis

Charles Nagant de Deuxchaisnes

The Arthritis Unit, University of Louvain in Brussels, St-Luc University Hospital, Brussels, Belgium

ABSTRACT

The anti-osteoclastic activity of calcitonin will find its best place in the prevention (primary or secondary) of bone loss, especially since it can be used intranasally. It is more effective in doing so at the axial rather than at the appendicular skeleton. There are no data as yet concerning its relative efficacy on the hip area. If calcitonin is to be used to restore the bone mass which has been lost, the gain to be expected is rather small and transient. Exception to this rule may be a site-specific action on the spine when bone turnover is elevated, and where a substantial, although probably transient, gain can be expected. Perhaps a better response can be anticipated with intermittent therapy, or with sequential therapy (phosphate continuously, and calcitonin discontinuously), or with coherence therapy. More data are needed to document this, as well as to resolve the questions raised by long-term administration of the nasal spray. Are the receptors on the osteoclasts going to remain sensitive ? Is their down-regulation going to be a limiting factor ? Are there neutralizing antibodies going to appear ? Will the nasal mucosa retain its permeability ? Much work needs to be accomplished before these questions can be answered.

INTRODUCTION

Postmenopausal osteoporosis (PMOP) results from an imbalance between osteoblastic bone formation and osteoclastic bone resorption. Any agent that can effectively counteract the latter, is liable to reduce the gap between bone resorption and bone formation. The result of such therapy will be an increase in bone mass which might be expected to be more or less transient because of the coupling phenomenon, i.e. bone formation decreasing more or less in proportion to the decrease of bone resorption, after a period of time when filling in of the remodeling spaces takes place.

Any agent which has anti-osteoclastic activity will achieve this, be it estrogens, progestogens of the 19 nortestosterone family, or bisphosphonates. Calcitonin (CT) deserves a special place in this group, because of the conspicuous absence of systemic and skeletal harmful side effects. In the rat, the osteoclasts contain specific CT receptors of high affinity in great numbers, several millions per cell [1]. This is not so in the chicken [2] where they can only be demonstrated either in animals fed several weeks a diet deficient in calcium and vitamin D [3] so as to decrease the high circulating levels of calcitonin, or in freshly isolated osteoclasts from vitamin D-deficient chicks, using a non-enzymatic method [4]. In ordinary circumstances, neither salmon calcitonin (sCT) nor chicken calcitonin (cCT) can inhibit chick osteoclasts [5]. Some have hypothesized that there is receptor lability in the chick [6]. Human osteoclasts behave in an intermediate manner. At doses of 1 ng/ml to 1 μg/ml, human calcitonin (hCT) was shown to cause a 70 % inhibition of bone resorption by human osteoclasts over a 24 h period, without showing any apparent effect on the morphology or motility of either fetal or adult osteoclasts [7]. This is in contradistinction to the behavior of rat osteoclasts whose resorbing action is almost completely abolished by as low a concentration as 1 pg/ml of CT, while motility and cytoplasmic spreading is also completely inhibited [8], an action which is so specific that it can be used as a bioassay for CT [9]. This shows that human fetal osteoclasts are less sensitive to CT than neonatal rat osteoclasts in that high concentrations of the hormone do not completely eliminate bone resorption. This is not only of academic interest, but also means that the conclusions of experiments conducted in the rat may not necessarily be extrapolated as such to humans. They merely show what can be achieved in a model which is maximally responsive. One example is the prevention of experimental osteoporosis induced by a combination of immobilization and ovariectomy in the rat at a dosage of 1 U/kg of (Asu^{1,7})-eel CT [10].

Exactly how CT acts on the osteoclasts is being investigated. There is notably a CT-mediated cAMP production by the osteoclasts [11], as well as a CT-mediated decline in cell acidity [6]. There is thus a direct action of CT on bone resorption that has been known for a long time [12]. It also opposes the resorptive action of PTH, as was recently reemphasized in a new bone resorption system in vitro utilizing vertebral bone from neonatal mouse [13], a model that may be more pertinent to the problem of PMOP since it involves vertebral bone. Whether CT also has a beneficial action on bone formation is uncertain, although it has been shown recently that sCT was able to increase calvarial cell proliferation in embryonic chickens, and bone matrix synthesis in intact calvariae and tibiae [14].

How can this anti-bone-resorptive agent be utilized in PMOP ? There are mainly two situations to be considered : the prevention (primary, secondary) of osteoporosis (prophylactic therapy) and the cure of osteoporosis, once it is established (restorative therapy). It is more desirable to prevent PMOP rather than to have to cure it. The former goal can and has been achieved, notably by estro-progestogens, while the latter is more hazardous and the results are often unsatisfactory.

The future of CT therapy is mainly in the prevention of PMOP, and yet most of the studies up until now have been performed in established PMOP. This is essentially because until recently, CT has been administered parenterally, so that it was only conceivable to give it to patients affected by a disease. Moreover, since CT has an excellent action on pain [15], which is part of the syndrome, motivating patients in accepting parenteral therapy has not been a problem as a rule.

Now that a nasal spray is available, the emphasis is shifting towards prevention, where CT is a most promising drug, certainly in those women who have contra-indications for the use of estro-progestogens, who tolerate them poorly or who do not wish to take them.

We first demonstrated the activity of the nasal spray in April-May 1983 in healthy volunteers in a double-blind trial with 2 doses of sCT and a placebo, versus an IM injection of sCT. The results were reported at the 1984 Calcitonin Conference held in Milan, and published in the Proceedings of that Conference [16]. They can also be found in a later paper [17]. It was shown that the spray was absorbed by the nasal mucosa. How much exactly is absorbed is not known. CT is a natriuretic hormone. If we compare the urinary output of sodium, which may or may not be the right thing to do, after the administration of 100 U sCT as an IM injection to the same dose administered as a nasal spray, the action of the latter was of the order of 20 % as compared to the IM administration [16,17].

In reviewing the available data, due consideration will be given to the differential action of calcitonin on the axial and the appendicular skeleton. Indeed in preliminary studies, where we followed patients with Paget's disease of bone while they were receiving 50 U of sCT three times weekly to twice daily, there was a tendency towards better conservation of bone mineral content (BMC) at distal radius, with a sizeable trabecular compartment, than at midshaft radius, consisting of almost purely cortical bone [18,19]

Prophylactic therapy

The only study with parenteral calcitonin on patients recruited at a menopause clinic has been conducted by MacIntyre et al. [20] using hCT. It was intended to administer subcutaneously 0.1 mg (20 U) thrice weekly for a period of 2 years (6240 U total). As could be anticipated in these healthy patients compliance was rather poor, but could be estimated retrospectively by studying the pharmacy records. 10 patients out of 15 finished the trial, 4 being compliers as defined by taking more than 50 U/week and 6 noncompliers. Vertebral mineral bone density (VBMD) was followed by quantitative computed tomography (QCT). In 2 years the compliers lost 2.57 % and the noncompliers 11.42 %. From the figure produced in their paper, it can be deduced that to maintain *ad integrum* VBMD, it was needed to administer 6000 U *in toto*, i.e. 60 U/week, the very dose which the authors initially anticipated to provide. It should be noticed that this study only concerns purely trabecular bone.

The nasal spray was used in a non double-blind, but controlled and randomized study, using 50 U/day and measuring lumbar bone mineral density (L-BMD) by dual photon absorptiometry (DPA). Bone loss did not occur in the treated group while the non treated group lost 3.16 % in one year [21]. No measurements of the appendicular skeleton were made in this trial . In a double-blind study versus placebo, Overgaard et al. [22] used 100 U/day during 12 mo. The L-BMD was stabilized, but no effect was seen at the forearm (distal and proximal forearm), as measured by single photon absorptiometry (SPA). We used 50 U/d in a double-blind study versus placebo in an entirely different model, i.e. soon after oophorectomy, and found no effect either on the axial or on the appendicular skeleton [23]. When we realized that the bone mass was diminishing in every patient, we multiplied the active substance and the placebo by a factor of four, thus providing in the active treatment group 200 U/d during the second year of the trial. This abolished the bone loss at the axial skeleton in the treated group, but not in the placebo group, while the loss in the appendicular skeleton continued unabated.

Many double-blind trials with the nasal spray are being conducted. More data are needed to know the exact dosage required to counteract axial bone loss, and especially what dosage will be required to counteract appendicular bone loss. The latter is important insofar that it may be predictive of the conservation of the cortical compartment of bone. Hip fractures, which are on the increase [24] and represent soaring costs to the society as well as a dreadful event for the individual, have been considered to represent mainly a cortical fracture. Although more trabecular than cortical bone is lost in the hip with aging, the hip fracture patient looses significantly more hip cortical bone than age-matched controls [25,26,27] and has less cortical bone elsewhere [28,29,30]. Recently though, it has been calculated that the deficit of trabecular bone in a hip fracture group was twice that of cortical bone in the hip [31]. Another recent study on cadaveric femur specimens [32] also emphazised the importance of the trabecular bone density. In contradistinction, another study showed that the mechanical strength of the femoral neck correlated better with the BMD of the femoral shaft ($r = 0.74$) than with the Singh index ($r = 0.50$) [33]. Clearly both compartments are important. Trials with the more precise dual-energy X-ray technology with analysis of the hip area and its different components are badly needed. If the hip only requires what is needed for lumbar spine bone preservation, intranasal sCT will be regarded as "the" alternative to estro-progestogens in the future, not only because of its lack of toxicity, but also because, unlike bisphosphonates, it does not remain trapped in the bone lattice, which may be of importance in these groups of women with an ever-expanding life expectancy. Needless to say if CT is effective in the primary prevention of bone loss during the postmenopausal period of rapid bone loss, it will *a fortiori* be effective in the secondary prevention of bone loss once osteoporosis as a disease has occurred (i.e. osteopenia plus fractures). Comparing osteoporotics longitudinally (admittedly treated with small supplements of calcium) and normal postmenopausal women, Aloia et al. [34] found that the osteoporotics lost less bone than postmenopausal women. These findings have been confirmed by Pacifici et al. [35]. Thus the bone loss once osteoporosis is established is not necessarily very rapid and if primary prevention is effective, no problem is anticipated in achieving secondary prevention with the same dosage.

Restorative therapy

Once the fracture threshold has been crossed and fractures have occurred, the purpose is to restore entirely or partly what has been lost, if this can be achieved without too many side effects. Once vertebral crush fractures occur, L-BMD is 30 to 35 % lower than in adult normal women, and about 14 % lower, as compared to age-matched controls, some of whom must be in a "prefracture" state, both differences being highly significant [31]. For those who believe that there is a correlation between L-BMD and fractures, for which there seems to be a consensus and for which there is even recent evidence on a prospective basis [36], it may be necessary and sufficient to fill in the gap between those who fracture and those who do not. This would be so if it can be achieved without losing bone quality. It has been shown, for example, that when feeding massive doses of fluoride without calcium supplements to pigs, the bone strength does not reflect the increase in bone mineral [37]. So if increasing L-BMD is not *per se* a guarantee of improved strength, it has not yet been convincingly shown that, without increasing BMD, bone strength could be significantly improved.

It is therefore important to review the available evidence on the ability of CT to increase bone mass, especially in the absence of convincing data on fracture rate. It would be too long to review all the data, some of which date back as long as three decades ago [38,39]. Exhaustive reviews on this subject have been published [40,41,42].

We shall first review what is available in terms of total body calcium (TBCa) performed by total body calcium neutron activation analysis (TBC-NAA). The first study (uncontrolled) provided 100 U/d + 1.0 g Ca to 12 patients, and compared this to another group of 13 patients receiving 50 U + 1.0 g Ca thrice weekly. The first group increased its TBCa after one year by 4 %, the second group by 1 % [43]. The same team did another (controlled) study in 26 male veterans randomized into three groups : 10 patients received multivitamins, 7 received multivitamins + Ca supplements (1.0 g/d), and 9 received the same plus 100 U/d of sCT. This last group had a non significant increase of 0.4 % after 1 year and a non significant increase of 2.7 % after 2 years [44]. They divided the CT-treated patients from both studies into responders and nonresponders, without providing evidence of a bimodal distribution. Half of the patients in both studies were responders. They speculated that the responders were those with the greatest difference between rates of bone resorption and bone formation and with the highest rates of skeletal turnover, but could not prove this. The CT group had significantly less new vertebral events than the other groups. Zanzi et al. [45] provided another study with TBC-NAA on 24 patients with PMOP randomly allocated to a group receiving 100 U/d sCT (n=10) plus Ca supplements and a control group (n=14) receiving only the Ca supplements. Maximum increase in the CT group occurred at 12 mo. (+ 5.2 %), while the control group had lost 1 %. After 24 mo. of therapy, the gain in the CT group had dropped to 2.1 %, whereas the loss in the control group was 2.1 %. The difference between both groups was statistically significant. There were no significant changes at the appendicular skeleton.

The largest controlled trial was performed by Gruber et al. [46] who studied 45 patients, of whom 24 were given 100 U sCT + 1.2 g calcium carbonate and 400 U vitamin D daily for a period of two years. There was a significant increase from baseline (+ 2 %) after 18 mo. but none after 24 mo. , while in the control group there was a significant decrease at both 18 and 24 mo. No effect was seen on midshaft or on distal radius. There were more vertebral fractures in the treated than in the control group, but the difference failed to reach statistical significance. On histomorphometric analysis of bone biopsies there was a significant decrease of both the eroded surface and the mineral apposition rate, showing a slowing down of bone turnover.

Other studies have been performed by Aloia et al. [47]. In the first study 13 patients were given 100 U four times/wk + 1.0 g Ca for 24 mo., with a significant increase in TBCa of 1.33 %/yr. Once more the peak was achieved after 18 mo., with a subsequent trend towards a decrease. No significant change was noticed in the appendicular skeleton. It has been shown in the rat that chronic infusions of CT were able to increase 1,25(OH)2D3 production [48]. This could not be confirmed in humans, at least not in this study. Aloia et al. [49] performed another study in 7 patients using intermittent therapy, 100 U/d every other day for 3 mo. , with a therapy free interval of 5 mo., repeating the sequence three times. The TBCa fell 0.45 %/yr (NS). Clearly, this is not enough CT to affect the bone mass.

The conclusion from this is that CT in high dosages, as measured by TBC-NAA, consistently produced a transient moderate increase in TBCa. Longer studies should be performed to see whether this gain can be maintained. TBCa takes into account both the cortical bone mass (80 %) and the trabecular bone mass (20 %). PMOP leading to crush fractures is characterized by predominant trabecular bone loss [50]. In this regard, Riggs et al. [51] demonstrated that the Z-score in patients with vertebral crush fractures was - 1.92 ± 0.98 ($p < 0.001$) at the lumbar spine, and - 1.03 ± 1.11 ($p < 0.001$) at midshaft radius, thus confirming a predominant but not elective trabecular bone loss in these patients with the so called type I osteoporosis. To best approach this phenomenon, L-BMC or L-BMD should be studied by DPA, while the appendicular skeleton should be followed preferably by SPA. There are many studies on this topic, but the different techniques and modes of expression often preclude adequate comparisons, especially useful when several dosages and different schemes of administration have to be compared. Many data have been gathered by the Siena group, and will be discussed here, while making one exception for the first double-blind trial, which was performed by Mazzuoli et al. [52] who found an increase at distal radius, as measured by DPA, of 13 % in the group (n = 16) treated for one year by 100 U every other day, while the placebo group (n = 16) had an average decrease of 4 %. These results have sofar not been reproduced, and the magnitude of the changes observed is rather unexpected.

Gennari et al. [53], comparing one group of patients (n = 15) receiving 100 U/d sCT + 1.0 g Ca to one group (n = 15) receiving 100 U every other day + 1.0 g Ca, and one group (n = 15) receiving only 1.0 g/d Ca each for 12 mo., found an increase of 8.5 % in L-BMC in the first group, and an increase of 4.0 % in the second group, while the third group lost 4.0 %, with all changes being significant. The same trend was seen at the femoral diaphysis with a gain of 2.5 % and 1.2 % respectively on the high and on the low dose of CT. Thus, the gain at both scanning sites was clearly dose-dependent. However, if the treatment is pursued longer than 12 mo. (50-100 U/d), the gain at the lumbar spine is lost [54]. Intermittent therapy (3 mo. on, 3 mo. off) at the same dosages has a more prolonged action [54], but the same phenomenon of wearing off occurs.

A crucial paper from the same group appeared recently [55], where the patients were divided into high bone turnover osteoporosis (HTOP) and normal bone turnover (NTOP), as assessed by measurement of whole body retention (WBR) of ^{99m}Tc-methylene diphosphonate. The dose of sCT used was 50 U every other day. The increase in L-BMC was 7.4 % (p < 0.05) in one year, while there was a decrease of 3.0 % (p < 0.05) at femoral diaphysis. 32 % of these patients had HTOP and they gained 22.4 % in L-BMC over 12 mo., while they gained 1.9 % (NS) at the femoral diaphysis. In the 68 % of patients with NTOP, the gain in L-BMC was not significant (+ 0.3 % in 12 mo.), while the loss of BMC at the femoral diaphysis was 5.3 % in 12 mo. (p < 0.05). For the first time, it was possible to distinguish the responders from the nonresponders. WBR correlated with osteocalcin (r=0.60, p<0.001) and the hydroxyproline/creatinine ratio in the urine (r=0.65, p<0.001). Osteocalcin and the hydroxyproline/creatinine ratio were elevated by a factor of 1.8 - 2.0 in HTOP as compared with NTOP. Thus, it can be anticipated which patients are going to benefit from a course of CT and which patients are not, and this almost on an individual basis. Benefit will be striking for the lumbar spine but not for the cortical bone at midshaft femur. One might have wished to have had more information within the framework of this most elegant study : what is going to happen the second (or the third) year of administration (although one might anticipate from previous results what would happen), and, second, what would have been the result on hip-BMD measurements, which the available technique did not allow to measure. The same study should be repeated with the precise modern methods, and their sophisticated hip software programs. This study probably accounts for the responders and nonresponders in the earlier studies [43,44] and shows that the hypothesis of Wallach et al. [43], which was mentioned earlier, was correct. What prospects does this study offer ? Perhaps CT should be continued until the parameters of high bone turnover have normalized. Despite a significant decrease, this was not yet achieved after 12 mo., and perhaps CT should be resumed whenever they become elevated again, should this occur.

It is interesting to compare what the same group has achieved with estrogen [56] with the same methodology. Conjugated equine estrogens were given for 12 mo. at a fairly high dose (1.25 mg/d) in a double-blind placebo controlled trial over 12 mo. The patients under estrogens (n=11) had an increase in L-BMD of 8.3 % at 12 mo., while the increase at the femoral diaphysis was 2.6 %, both reaching the level of significance. Thus 1.25 mg daily of conjugated estrogens achieved at the lumbar spine the same result as CT at a dosage of 50 U every other day [55], while at the femoral shaft apparently 100 U/d (an increase by a factor of four) is required to obtain the same result [53].

Calcitonin has also been used as a nasal spray in a double-blind, placebo-controlled study [57], using 200 U/d + 0.5 g Ca during 12 mo. There was no significant gain or loss at the lumbar spine, neither in the treatment group (n = 17) nor in the placebo group (n = 20). There were no significant changes either at proximal forearm, or at distal forearm in the treatment group, while there was a significant decrease at the two scanning sites in the placebo group. The results when comparing the groups were statistically significant at proximal forearm in favor of calcitonin. Since there was neither increase nor decrease with the nasal spray at any site, this study shows that at this dosage the nasal spray is the perfect drug for secondary prevention, all the more so that there was a significant difference at a scanning site where cortical bone is predominant, and that the biochemical markers of bone turnover were significantly affected. Goldmann et al. [58] performed a similar study (although not double-blind) opposing one group (n = 22) receiving 200 U/d nasal spray + 1.0 g Ca to one group (n = 22) receiving 1.0 g Ca only for a period of 15 mo. The method of evaluation was completely different using low dose QCT at the distal radius and distal tibia. There was no difference between both groups taken as a whole. However, if one considers fast-bone losers (n = 5) prior to therapy, the bone loss in these patients was significantly affected by the nasal spray. Here again, there also seems to be a clue for predicting what patients are going to benefit more from secondary prevention.

There are other ways to administer calcitonin parenterally. The sequential therapy consisting of continuous phosphate administration (1.5 g/d of elemental phosphorus), able to induce secondary hyperparathyroidism, used as an activator at the level of the bone remodeling units, whereupon sCT is administered, 50 U/d subcutaneously during 5 days every third week. This regimen has met with success whenever it has been evaluated, usually only by histomorphometric analysis [59,60]. The increase in trabecular bone volume was found to have resulted from a reduction of bone resorption associated with stimulation of bone formation along the trabecular bone surface [61]. This increase in bone volume did not occur at the expense of the appendicular skeleton [62].

Attempts have also been made to combine CT with another hormone, i.e. growth hormone (GH). However, the combined therapy was not more effective on the gain at the lumbar spine (1.68 %/yr versus 1.33 %/yr) for CT alone, but furthermore had a deleterious effect on cortical bone mass [47]. Another attempt was made to use CT and GH in sequence in a coherence therapy using the frostian concept of ADFR. Human GH 7 IU/d administered subcutaneously for 2 mo. was used as an activator, followed by sCT 100 every other day for a period of 3 mo. in the role of a depressor, whereafter a free interval was maintained for another 3 mo. The sequence GH-CT-rest was repeated for a total of three cycles, thus taking 24 mo. The coherence treatment group (n = 7) was compared to a similar group (n = 7) without GH. In the ADFR group, the gain in TBCa was of 2.3 %/yr (p < 0.05), while there was no gain in the group with intermittent CT administration. The difference between the two groups, however, was not statistically significant. Once again, the appendicular skeleton remained unaffected. The interest of this study was that there was no plateauing of the response. Unfortunately only three cycles of therapy could be followed because of the reports of possible toxicity of human GH. The latter is now available from recombinant DNA technology, whereas the GH used in the study was extracted from human pituitary glands.

In conclusion, CT therapy of established PMOP at first sight is of limited value because of the self limited nature of the gain in bone mass, when anti-bone-resorptive agents (or anti-resorbers) are given. This is due to the very nature of the life cycle in the bone remodeling unit (BMU) and the inherent concept of bone remodeling transients. When bone resorption is inhibited, bone formation remains unchanged, until the existing remodeling space is filled, after which it also declines reaching a new equilibrium between bone resorption and bone formation. The modest transient increase in bone mass is due to this transient remodeling asynchrony, whereafter bone loss may resume at a rate similar to or less than that previously. The studies with CT are too short to evaluate the rate of bone loss once the new steady equilibrium has been achieved. Since the gain is proportional to the gap between bone formation and bone resorption, it is therefore logical that a substantial gain can be achieved in those patients with high bone turnover in that area of the skeleton where bone turnover is the highest, i.e. the spine with its predominant trabecular compartment. Since PMOP is characterized essentially by vertebral crush fractures, it may be worthwhile to treat this selected group of patients with CT during a period of 12-18 mo., and perhaps to repeat this after a therapy-free interval. In these cases (perhaps up to one third of the cases of PMOP), it may be useful to fill in the remodeling spaces because they are so abundant. This is a site-specific therapy with little side effects. If this statement could also be made of the hip area for which we badly need accurate measurements of BMD under these circumstances, this would considerably reinforce the indication of CT therapy in selected cases. It must be stressed that in the case of vertebral crush fractures, the decrease in hip BMD is identical to or more pronounced than that of the lumbar spine [31].

Because of its very nature, the self limited increase of bone mass is not restricted to CT, but extends to all "anti-resorbers". The same trend has been recently suggested for a very powerful anti-resorber, the bisphosphonate disodium pamidronate (APD) when given orally uninterruptedly, admittedly in another model, i.e. glucocorticoid osteoporosis [63]. To overcome this, other schemes of administration must be used, like for example the sequential therapy with continuous phosphate and intermittent CT, or some kind of coherence therapy, whose modalities are always very difficult to define.

Another problem of CT is down regulation of the receptors. That this exists has been elegantly shown by Gibbs and Peacock [64], by injecting 100 U sCT subcutaneously in patients with osteoporosis, and following the drop in Ca x P (molar product). This drop at the first injection was 0.56 ± 0.08. When the second injection was performed two days later, the drop was only 0.16 ± 0.08, but when it was performed four days later it was 0.52 ± 0.13, and when the interval was seven days, it became 0.92 ± 0.01. The authors concluded that the tolerance to CT can be avoided, and that in a therapeutic regimen in osteoporosis, sCT should be given every 7 days. The feasibility of this therapeutic regimen has not been tested, but the results of daily CT administration compared to the administration of CT every other day are in favor of the former regimen. Giving CT every other day may not be a long enough time interval to avoid down regulation, and under those circumstances the total dose provided may be the predominant factor. On the other hand, giving CT once or twice weekly might not provide enough active susbtance. Avoidance of down regulation may explain that intermittent therapy is more effective than continuous therapy [54].

If there is an inherent difficulty in gaining substantial bone mass with CT, there should be no problem in maintaining bone mass, i.e. in insuring primary and secondary prevention of bone loss, especially since the advent of a nasal spray. There are two additional problems which remain to be solved. The first one is that of neutralizing antibodies, which have arisen on reexposure to sCT in certain patients with Paget's disease [65]. The second is that of the persisting permeability of the nasal mucosa to CT when administered for prolonged periods of time, a problem which was also raised in a study of Paget's disease of bone [66]. If it can be shown that patients on continuous nasal spray of sCT maintain, in their vast majority, at least the lumbar bone mass for protracted periods of time (several years), as estrogens do, then the problems of permeability, antibody production, down regulation of the receptors (or even a modification of the receptors) are no more than of academic interest. Perhaps intermittent administration of nasal spray might resolve some of these problems, as well as that of compliance and of the economic cost. If it could be shown that each time the nasal spray is resumed the vertebral bone mass which has been lost during the interruption can be regained by the filling in of the remodeling spaces, then ultimately the bone mass might remain constant. This, however, remains to be demonstrated.

REFERENCES

1. G.C. Nicholson, J.M. Moseley, P.M. Sexton, F.A.O. Mendelsohn, and T.J. Martin, J.Clin. Invest. 78, 355-360 (1986).
2. G.C. Nicholson, J.M. Moseley, P.M. Sexton, and T.J. Martin, J. Bone Min. Res. 2, 53-59 (1987).
3. E.C. Eliam, M. Basle, A. Bouizar, J. Bielakoff, M. Moukhtar, and M.C. de Vernejoul, J. Endocrinol. 119, 243-248 (1988).
4. B.R. Rifkin, J.M. Auszmann, A.P. Kleckner, A.T. Vernillo, and A.S. Fine, Life Sci. 42, 799-804 (1988).
5. D.W. Dempster, R.J. Murrills, W.R. Horbert, and T.R. Arnett, J. Bone Min. Res. 2, 443-456 (1987).
6. S.J. Hunter, H. Schraer, and C.V. Gay, J. Bone Min. Res. 3, 297-303 (1988).
7. R.J. Murrills, E. Shane, R. Lindsay, and D.W. Dempster, J. Bone Min. Res. 4, 259-268 (1989).
8. T.J. Chambers and C.J. Magnus, J. Pathol. 136, 27-40 (1982).

9. T.J. Chambers, J.C. Chambers, J. Symonds, and J.A. Darby, J. Clin. Endocrinol. Metab. 63, 1080-1085 (1986).
10. T. Hayashi, T. Yanamuro, H. Okumuro, R. Kasai, and K. Tada, Bone 10, 25-28 (1989).
11. M.E. Holtrop, L.G. Raisz, and H.A. Simmons, J. Cell Biol. 60, 346-355 (1974).
12. J. Friedman and L.G. Raisz, Science 150, 1465-1467 (1965).
13. P.T. Stewart and P.H. Stern, Calcif. Tissue Int. 40, 21-26 (1987).
14. J.R. Farley, N.M. Tarbaux, S.L. Hall, T.A. Linkhart, and D.J. Baylink, Endocrinology 123, 159-167 (1988).
15. C. Gennari and D. Agnusdei, Curr. Ther. Res. 44, 712-722 (1988).
16. C. Nagant de Deuxchaisnes, J.P. Devogelaer, J.P. Huaux, J.P. Dufour, G, Depresseux, and W. Esselinckx in : Calcitonin 1984, A Pecile, ed. (Elsevier Science Publisher BV, Amsterdam 1985) pp. 329-343.
17. C. Nagant de Deuxchaisnes, J.P. Devogelaer, J.P. Huaux, et al., Clin. Orthop. 217, 56-71 (1987).
18. C. Nagant de Deuxchaisnes, Triangle 22, 103-128 (1983).
19. C. Nagant de Deuxchaisnes and J.P. Devogelaer, Clin. Rheum. Dis. 12, 559-635 (1986).
20. I. MacIntyre, J.C. Stevenson, M.I. Whitehead, S.J. Wimalawansa, L.M. Banks, and M.J.R. Healy, Lancet 1, 900-901 (1988).
21. J.Y. Reginster, D. Denis, A. Albert, et al., Lancet 2, 1481-1483 (1987).
22. K. Overgaard, B.J. Riis, and C. Christiansen, J. Bone Min. Res. 3 (suppl. 1) S162 (1988).
23. J.P. Devogelaer, C. Nagant de Deuxchaisnes, C. Lecart, J. Donnez, and K. Thomas, J. Bone Min. Res. 3 (suppl. 1), S162 (1988).
24. C. Nagant de Deuxchaisnes and J.P. Devogelaer, Calcif. Tissue Int 42, 201-203 (1988).
25. N. Fredensborg and B.E. Nilsson, Acta Radiol. Scand. 18, 492-496 (1977).
26. H. Bohr and O. Schaadt, Calcif. Tissue Int. 37, 340-344 (1985).
27. B.E.C. Nordin, R.G. Crilly, and D.A. Smith in : Metabolic Bone and Stone Disease, B.E.C. Nordin, ed. (Churchill Livingstone, London 1984) pp. 1-70.
28. R. Wootton, P.J. Brereton, M.B. Clark, et al., Clin. Sci. 57, 93-101 (1979).
29. A. Horsman, B.E.C. Nordin, J. Aaron, and D.H. Marshall in : Osteoporosis. Recent Advances in Pathogenesis and Treatment, H.F. DeLuca, H.M. Frost, W.S.S. Jee and C.C. Johnston Jr, eds. (University Park Press, Baltimore 1981) pp. 175-184.
30. G.F. Jensen, C. Christiansen, J. Boesen, V. Hegedüs, and I. Transbol, Clin. Orthop. 166, 75-81 (1982).
31. R.B. Mazess, H. Barden, M. Ettinger, E. Schultz, J. Bone Min. Res. 3, 13-18 (1988).
32. A. Alho, T. Husby, and A. Hoiseth, Clin. Orthop. 227, 292-297 (1988).
33. O. Delaere, A. Dhem, and R. Bourgois, Arch. Orthop. Trauma Surg. 108, 72-75 (1989).
34. J.F. Aloia, P. Ross, A. Vaswani, I. Zanzi, and S.H. Cohn, Am. J. Physiol. 242, E82-E86 (1982).
35. R. Pacifici, N. Susman, P.L. Carr, S.J. Birge, and L.V. Avioli, J. Clin. Endocrinol. Metab. 64, 209-214 (1987).
36. P.D. Ross, R.D. Wasnich, and J.M. Vogel, J. Bone Min. Res. 3, 1-11 (1988).
37. L. Mosekilde, J. Kragstrup, and A. Richards, Calcif. Tissue Int. 40, 318-322 (1987).
38. D. Hioco, P. Bordier, L. Miravet, H. Denys, and S. Tun-Chot in : Calcitonin 1969, S. Taylor and G. Foster, eds. (William Heinemann Medical Books Ltd, London 1970) pp. 514-522.

39. A. Caniggia, C. Gennari, M. Bencini, L. Cesari, and G. Borrello, Clin. Sci. 38, 397-407 (1970).
40. A.M. Parfitt, Triangle 22, 91-102 (1983).
41. M.T. McDermott and G.S. Kidd, Endocr. Rev. 8, 377-390 (1987).
42. L.V. Avioli, Ann. Chir. Gynaecol. 77, 224-228 (1988).
43. S. Wallach, S.H. Cohn, H.L. Atkins, et al., Curr. Ther. Res. 22, 556-572 (1977).
44. R. Agrawal, S. Wallach, S. Cohn, et al. in : Calcitonin 1980, A. Pecile ed. (Excerpta Medica, Amsterdam 1981) pp. 237-246.
45. I. Zanzi, K. Thompson, and S.H. Cohn in : Hormonal Control of Calcium Metabolism, D.V. Cohn, R.V. Talmage and J.L. Matthews, eds. (Excerpta Medica, Amsterdam 1981) p. 400.
46. H.E. Gruber, J.L. Ivey, D.J. Baylink, et al., Metabolism 33, 295-303 (1984).
47. J.F. Aloia, A. Vaswani, A. Kapoor, J.K. Yeh, and S.H. Cohn, Metabolism 34, 124-129 (1985).
48. P. Jaeger, W. Jones, T.L. Clemens, and J.P. Hayslett, J. Clin. Invest. 78, 456-461 (1986).
49. J.F. Aloia, A. Vaswani, P.J. Meunier, et al., Calcif. Tissue Int. 40, 253-259 (1987).
50. C.C. Johnston, J. Norton, M.R.A. Khairi, et al., J. Clin. Endocrinol. Metab. 61, 551-556 (1985).
51. B.L. Riggs, H.W. Wahner, E. Seeman, et al., J. Clin. Invest. 70, 716-723 (1982).
52. G.F. Mazzuoli, M. Passeri, C. Gennari, et al., Calcif. Tissue Int. 38, 3-8 (1986).
53. C. Gennari, S.M. Chierichetti, S. Bigazzi, et al., Curr. Ther. Res. 38, 455-464 (1985).
54. C. Gennari, M. Montagnani, P. Nardi, F. Zacchei, S. Bigazzi, and C. Cepollaro in : Osteoporosis 1987, C. Christiansen, J.S. Johansen and B.J. Riis, eds. (Norhaven A/S, Viborg 1987) pp. 919-921.
55. R. Civitelli, S. Gonnelli, F. Zacchei, et al., Clin. Invest. 82, 1268-1274 (1988).
56. R. Civitelli, D. Agnusdei, P. Nardi, F. Zacchei, L.V. Avioli, and C. Gennari, Calcif. Tissue Int. 42, 77-86 (1988).
57. K. Overgaard, B.J. Riis, C. Christiansen, J. Podenphant, J.S. Johansen, Clin. Endocrinol. 30, 435-442 (1989).
58. A.R. Goldmann, M.A. Dambacher, F. Levy, P. Rüegsegger, K. Schmid, D. Welzel, J. Bone Min. Res. 3 (suppl. 1), S163 (1988).
59. H. Rasmussen, P. Bordier, P. Marie, et al., Metab. Bone Dis. Rel. Res. 2, 107-111 (1980).
60. C. Alexandre, D. Chappard, F. Caulin, A. Bertrand, S. Palle, and G. Riffat, Calcif. Tissue Int. 42, 345-350 (1988).
61. P.J. Marie and F. Caulin, Bone 7, 17-22 (1986).
62. D. Kuntz, P. Marie, M. Berthel, and F. Caulin, Int. J. Clin. Pharm. Res. 6, 157-162 (1986).
63. I.R. Reid, S.W. Heap, A.R. King, and H.K. Ibbertson, Lancet 2, 1144 (1988).
64. C.J. Gibbs and M. Peacock, Bone 7, 309 (1986).
65. F. Levy, R. Muff, S. Dotti-Sigrist, M.A. Dambacher, and J.A. Fischer, J. Clin. Endocrinol. Metab. 67, 541-545 (1988).
66. F.R. Singer, R. Villanueva, K. Ginger, Calcif. Tissue Int. 44 (suppl.), S-87 (N32)(1989).

Intranasal Calcitonin for Prevention and Treatment of Osteoporosis

Kirsten Overgaard, Bente Juel Riis, and Claus Christiansen

Department of Clinical Chemistry, Glostrup Hospital, Denmark

INTRODUCTION

Osteoporosis may be regarded as a condition with a decreased amount of bony tissue per unit volume of bone and an increased susceptibility to fracture. However, factors other than a mere decrease in the amount of bone may be determinant for the occurrence of fractures. Osteoporotic fractures most often occur in the forearm, spine, and hip, but an osteoporotic person will fracture any bone more easily than a non-osteoporotic counterpart.

Epidemiology of osteoporosis - magnitude of the problem

Mankind took a long time to number the first billion inhabitants up to the year 1850. Then the population growth started to accelerate: the next billion was reached within 80 years, in 1930; the third was reached within 30 years, in 1961; and the fourth within only 15 years, in 1976. The United Nations estimates that the world population will continue to grow for another 110 years and is expected to stabilize at 10.5 billion by the end of the 21st century. Ninety-five per cent of this future growth in global population will occur in the developing countries of the world. In 1980 about 26% of mankind were living in the developed countries; by the end of the 21st century only 13% will live in the developed countries.

In addition to these changes, the 21st century will show a dramatic increase in life expectancy at birth, and the marked differences that exist today between developed and developing countries will gradually disappear. It is thus estimated that by 2025 the global life expectancy will be as high as 70 years. The rapidly increasing life expectancy will further significantly alter the age structure of the population. The number of people aged 60 and above in the developing countries is expected to double between 1975 and 2025, and the global population of elderly people is expected to reach 1100 millions within the next 40 years, with more than 70% living in the developing countries by 2025. In terms of osteoporosis, this means that by the year 2000 almost 24% of the global population will consist of women aged 45 and over. They will constitute 39% of the population in the developed countries, and approach 20% in the developing countries (1). The problems of ageing, especially in women, are thus not restricted to Western societies.

Copyright 1990 by Elsevier Science Publishing Co., Inc.
Osteoporosis: Physiological Basis, Assessment, and Treatment
Hector F. DeLuca and Richard Mazess, Editors

Osteoporosis and associated fractures are common in the West, especially among elderly white women. In the United States alone, the total cost of osteoporosis and osteoporotic fractures is estimated to be between 6 and 8 billion dollars (2,3). In addition to enormous economic costs, these fractures cause considerable disability and many premature deaths.

Fractures of the hip are associated with more deaths, greater disability, and heavier medical costs than all other osteoporotic fractures combined. The prevalence of hip fractures is about 2.5% in a population of 70-year old women (4) (Fig. 1), but thereafter increases twofold every five years. In the United States about 210,000 hip fractures are sustained every year. After age 50, the incidence rate rises dramatically with age, and at all ages after 50 the incidence rate in the United States, is about twice as high for white women as for white men. Seventy-five to 80 per cent of all hip fractures affect women, and almost 50 per cent occur in persons who are 80 years of age or older (5). The consequences of hip fracture are often severe. The average length of stay in hospital is about three weeks, and patients with hip fractures thus occupy more hospital beds than patients with any other disease. In the first year after the fracture, the mortality rate is about 12-20 % higher than in persons of the same age (6). Those who survive hip fractures often suffer permanent disability and dependency.

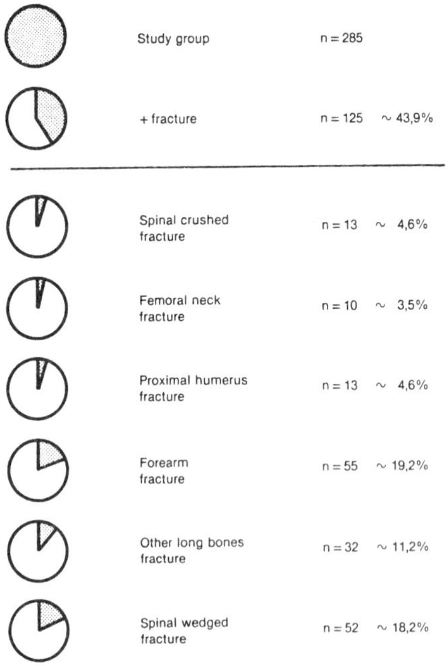

◯	Study group	n = 285	
◔	+ fracture	n = 125	~ 43,9%
◷	Spinal crushed fracture	n = 13	~ 4,6%
◷	Femoral neck fracture	n = 10	~ 3,5%
◷	Proximal humerus fracture	n = 13	~ 4,6%
◔	Forearm fracture	n = 55	~ 19,2%
◔	Other long bones fracture	n = 32	~ 11,2%
◔	Spinal wedged fracture	n = 52	~ 18,2%

Figure 1.
Distribution of fracture attributable to osteoporosis in 70-year-old women.
(Copyright C Christiansen, used with permission).

Although other osteoporotic fractures are less severe than hip fracture, they do constitute a problem. Colles' fracture is the commonest in white women in the United States and Northern Europe up to age 75, when the frequency is surpassed by hip fracture. Colles' fracture is, of course, rarely fatal, but nevertheless about 20% necessitate hospitalization (6).

The epidemiology of vertebral fracture is more obscure than that of the other fractures. In fact, vertebral fractures are often not diagnosed and treated. One Danish survey found that 6-4% of 70-year-old women had complete compression fractures, and an additional 18% had partial deformities of at least one vertebra (4) (Fig. 1). By the age of 80 most white women have had at least one partial deformity of the spine (6). Vertebral fractures cause acute pain, which will last for a couple of months and often gradually turn into chronic pain. Although vertebral fractures only rarely result in hospitalization, the quality of life for such women is seriously impaired.

All the data outlined above originate from Western societies and mostly concern Caucasians. Few data are available on other races and virtually none at all from the developing countries.

The physiological action of calcitonin

The only target organ of proved physiological significance for calcitonin is the skeleton. Calcitonin does indeed have an action on the kidney, but its effects in elevating the excretion of sodium, water, and calcium are unlikely to be of physiological importance. Calcitonin does, however, have an effect on the proximal straight tubule. Here it enhances the activity of the 1 alpha-hydroxylase enzyme to increase production of 1,25-dihydroxycholecalciferol from its substrate 25-hydroxycholecalciferol, but its main action is certainly on the skeleton. Calcitonin rapidly inhibits osteoclast activity, so that the plasma concentrations of calcium fall if the bone turnover is high. Administration to normal adults produces very little change in plasma calcium, but in the presence of Paget's disease, where bone tureover is increased it may produce marked hypocalcaemia. Calcitonin also has a more chronic action on the number of osteoclast. This is seen best when calcitonin is used therapeutically in Paget's disease. After some months of therapy, the number of osteoclasts in affected bone is greatly diminished, which suggests that their production from the osteoclast precursor has been inhibited (7).

Soon after calcitonin became available for clinical and laboratory investigation it was found to reduce bone resorption (8,9). Since osteoporosis was (and is) widely believed to be a disorder characterized mainly by increased bone resorption, it seemed logical to try treatment with calcitonin, and many such clinical trials are still in progress. Workers have more recently proposed that the age-related decline in calcitonin secretion may play a role in the pathogenesis of age-related bone loss, a concept that appears to provide an additional rationale for the use of calcitonin not only in the treatment, but also in the prevention, of osteoporosis.

Calcitonin for prevention of postmenopausal bone loss and osteoporosis

Oestrogen is generally accepted as effective in the prophylaxis of postmenopausal bone loss (10,11) (Fig. 2) and osteoporosis (3,4). This effect may partly be mediated through calcitonin, as elevated plasma concentrations of calcitonin have been found in subjects receiving oestrogen therapy (12,13). Not all studies, however, have been able to reproduce this relation between calcitonin and oestrogen (14,15).

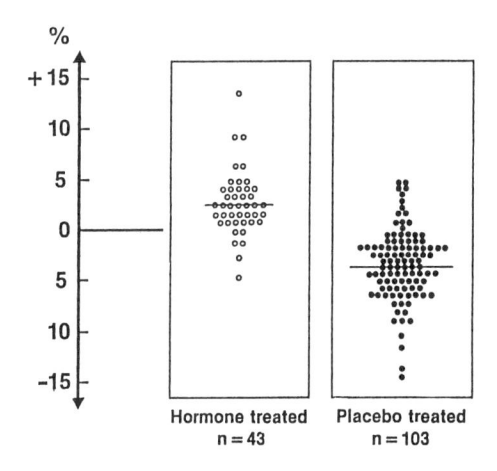

Figure 2.
Bone mineral content in the forearms expressed as percentage per 2 years, calculated from slopes of individual regression lines.
(Copyright C Christiansen, used with permission).

Calcitonin has until recently only been available as an injectable preparation. Because of the inconvenience of frequent administrations, calcitonin injections would not be acceptable to many asymptomatic, apparently healthy persons, even if it were shown to be effective. But the recent development of an intranasal spray form has extended the therapeutic potential to include preventive objectives.

Two published studies have demonstrated that calcitonin both injectable (16) and as a nasal spray (17) is effective for prevention of early postmenopausal bone loss. A recent double-blind study from our group has supported these findings. Thirty-nine healthy, early postmenopausal women were treated for 2 years with a daily intranasal administration of 100 IU of salmon calcitonin. All participants further received a daily supplement of 500 mg calcium.

The results demonstrated that this treatment regimen stopped bone loss in the lumbar spine (measured by dual photon absorptiometry), but not in the forearms (single photon absorptiometry). This study therefore raises the question whether the effect of calcitonin is limited to trabecular bone with a relatively high bone turnover, or whether a somewhat higher dose would affect areas of the skeleton with a relatively high content of cortical bone (like the forearms).

Calcitonin for treatment of established osteoporosis
This will be discussed under two headings: first, the use of calcitonin alone with or without a calcium supplement, and second, the use of calcitonin in combination with other agents.

a) Calcitonin alone (with or without calcium): The first clinical studies used porcine calcitonin and ran for only 2 to 8 weeks, but they showed a reduction in the kinetic and biochemical indices of resorption and formation and an improvement in calcium balance, most probably the result of depression of activation (18,19). Given over longer periods (4 to 6 months), porcine calcitonin produced either no effect at all (20,21) or biochemical and histological evidence of secondary hyperparathyroidism (22). Salmon calcitonin has been studied for longer periods and seems more promising. When given in a dose of 100 units/day for 12 to 15 months, it was no more effective than calcium alone, with or without vitamin D (23), but in that study, the change in bone mass was only estimated in iliac biopsy specimens. In an uncontrolled study, 25 patients treated with salmon calcitonin 100 units daily and a calcium supplement of 1 g daily for 10 to 29 months gained about 3% in total body calcium, as measured by neutron activation, urinary hydroxyproline and kinetic measurements of bone turnover were persistently depressed (24). In a subsequent controlled study solely with men, the same investigators again observed a 3% increase in total body calcium after calcitonin and calcium, and they also found a suggestive decline in the vertebral fracture rate. There were no significant changes in the control group receiving calcium alone (25). In both studies the patients were divided into responders and non-responders, but no evidence was presented that the response was bimodally rather than normally distributed. Moreover no baseline measurement was useful in predicting the response, contrary to the earlier (and still reasonable) suggestion that calcitonin would be most effective in patients with increased bone remodelling (19). Caniggia suggested that two patterns of response could be observed: a rapid response in patients with high remodelling, mainly due to the direct resorption-suppressing activity of calcitonin, and a slow response in patients with low remodelling, due to secondary hyperparathyroidism, increased calcitriol synthesis and consequent increase in intestinal absorption of calcium (26).

The largest controlled trial with salmon calcitonin involved 50 patients randomly assigned to two groups, who were well matched with respect to age, height, number of fractures, total body calcium, and dietary calcium intake (27). Both groups received 1.2 g of elemental calcium and 400 units of vitamin D daily, and the treatment group received in addition 100 units of salmon calcitonin daily. Total body calcium increased significantly in the treated group during the first year, whereas it fell in the control group. Changes occuring during the second year of treatment were interpreted by the investigators as indicating the emergence of resistance to calcitonin, either on the basis of antibody development or receptor down-regulation. However, there was no significant difference between the last three measurements in either the treated or the control group, so that the results are equally consistent with the attainment of a plateau response after an initial increase which was the outcome of a reduction in the reversible mineral deficit brought about by the reduction in the activation frequency.

A very large number of studies on calcitonin treatment of osteoporosis have been published during the last few years. The first published double-blind study (28) showed that injection of 100 IU salmon calcitonin given on alternate days day produced an increase of 13% in forearm bone mineral after 1 year of treatment.

A recent double-blind study carried out by our group demonstrated for the first time that nasal administration of salmon calcitonin is also effective in the treatment of postmenopausal osteoporosis.

Fourty women with moderate osteoporosis (forearm fracture) entered and 37 completed a one-year double-blind placebo-controlled study of the effect of nasal calcitonin (200 IU daily) on bone and calcium metabolism. In the calcitonin group, the bone mass measured in the forearm (Fig. 3) (single photon absorptiometry) and in the spine and total body (dual photon absorptiometry) showed a small increase, whereas the bone mass in the control group decreased about 2%/year ($p<0.01$). Biochemical estimates of bone formation (serum alkaline phosphatase, pBGP) and bone resorption (FU Calcium/ Cr) showed a significant decrease in the calcitonin group, but were virtually unchanged in the control group. The nasal administration form produced no metabolic, vascular, or gastrointestinal side effects, nor was there any local

p(α)	0.0102	0.0022	0.0038	0.0110
p(β)				

p(α)	0.0037	0.2444	0.2052	0.1758
p(β)		0.4336	0.4201	0.5350

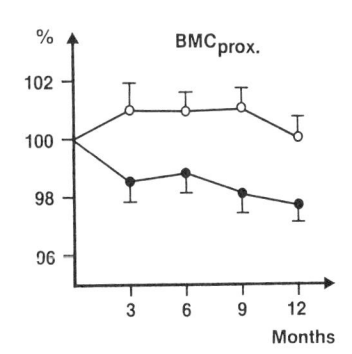

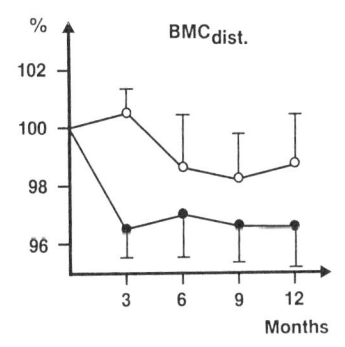

Figure 3.
Bone mineral content in the proximal (BMCprox) and distal (BMCdist) parts of the forearms during treatment with nasal calcitonin (o) (200 IU daily) or placebo (●). The levels of significance between the two groups are shown at the top.
(Clinical Endocrinol 1989, in press; with permission).

irritation. We concluded from the study that nasal calcitonin is a potential treatment for prevention of further bone loss in women with moderate osteoporosis 10-15 years after the menopause.

b) Combination therapy: Because suppression of bone resorption alone will never restore bone mass to normal, it would seem logical to combine calcitonin with an agent that increase bone formation. In a controlled study (29), a combination of salmon calcitonin and human growth hormone, however, seemed to have a deleterious effect on cortical bone mass, whereas calcitonin alone was effective in producing an increment in bone mass. A large-scale trial of low-dose calcitonin in combination with calcitriol is in progress (30), and encouraging results on radial bone mineral content are reported.
More promising is the combination of calcitonin with phosphate supplements, an idea that originated from several sources. Phosphate infusion prevents the adverse effect of parathyroid hormone on the calcium and phosphate balance in the rat (31), and the increase in urinary calcium and phosphate and the fall in plasma phosphate in some human subjects are possible adverse effects of calcitonin for which phosphate supplements appear a logical countermeasure (19). Phosphate may also stimulate the secretion of parathyroid hormone and thus function as an indirect activator of skeletal remodelling, as well as promoting some aspects of osteoblast function and bone formation.

In a double-blind controlled study, the combination of intermittent calcitonin 50 units given daily for 5 days every three weeks with continuous oral phosphate 1.5 g/day significantly increased bone-forming surfaces and trabecular bone volume in iliac bone biopsies, compared with calcitonin alone, phosphate alone, or no treatment (33,34). Cortical bone in the radius measured by photon absorptiometry remained constant in the combination group but declined significantly in the other groups (33). The patient samples were too small to permit measurement of fracture rates, but the results were sufficiently encouraging to justify a larger controlled study of longer duration using fracture rate as the end point.

REFERENCES

1. E. Diczfalusy in: The Climacteric in Perspective, M. Notelovitz and P. van Keep, eds. (Parthenon Publishing 1984) pp. 1-15.
2. W.A. Peck, E. Barrett-Connor, J.A. Buckwalter, R.D. Grambrell, B.H. Hahn, R.S. Paffenbarger, J.T. Potts Jr., R.S. Rivlin, G.A. Rodan, P.H. Stern, B. Warden, B.N.W. Weissman, G.D. Whedon, and J.J. Wildgen, JAMA 252, 799-802 (1984).
3. C.D. Arnaud, C. Christiansen, S.R. Cummings, H.A. Fleisch, C. Gennari, J.A. Kanis, J.G.G. Ledingham, I. MacIntyre, T.J. Martin, W.A. Peck, P. Riis, G. Samsioe, and L.E. Shulman, Br. Med. J. 295, 914-915 (1987).
4. C.F. Jensen, C. Christiansen, J. Boesen, V. Hegedüs, I. Transbøl, Clin. Orthop. Rel. Res. 166, 75-81 (1982).
5. S.R. Cummings, J.L. Kelsey, M.C. Nevitt, and K.J. O'Doud, Epidemiol. Rev. 7, 178-208 (1985).
6. J.S. Jensen and E. Tøndevold, Acta Orthop. Scand. 50, 161-167 (1979).
7. I. MacIntyre, Triangle 22, 69-74 (1983).
8. J. Friedman and L.G. Raisz, Science 150, 1465-1467 (1965).
9. J.J. Reynolds and J.T. Dingle, Calcif. Tissue Res. 4, 339-349 (1970).
10. R. Lindsay, D.M. Hart, J.M. Aitken, E.B. Macdonald, J.B. Anderson, and A.E. Clarke, Lancet i, 1038-1041 (1976).
11. C. Christiansen, M.S. Christensen, P. McNair, C. Hagen, K.-E. Stocklund, and I. Transbøl, Eur. J. Clin. Invest. 10, 273-279 (1980).
12. B. Ettinger, H.K. Genant, and C.E. Cann, Ann. Int. Med. 102, 319-324 (1985).
13. D.P. Kiel, D.T. Felson, J.J. Anderson, P.W.F. Wilson, and M.A. Moskowitz, N. Engl. J. Med. 317, 1169-1174 (1987).
14. J.C. Stevenson, G. Abeyasekera, C.J. Hillyard, K.-G. Phang, I. MacIntyre, S. Campbell, G. Lane, P.T. Townsend, O. Young, and M.I. Whitehead, Eur. J. Clin. Invest. 13, 481-487 (1983).
15. C. Greenberg, S.C. Kukreja, E.N. Bowser, G.K. Hargis, W.J. Henderson, and G.A. Williams, Endocrinology 118, 2594-2598 (1986).
16. I. McIntyre, J.C. Stevenson, M.I. Whitehead, S.J. Wimalawansa, L.M. Bants, and M.J.R. Healy, Lancet i, 900-902 (1988).
17. J.Y. Reginster, D. Denis, A. Albert, R. Deroisy, M.P. Lecart, M.A. Fontaine, P. Lambelin, and P. Franchimont, Lancet ii, 1481-1483 (1987).
18. A. Caniggia, C. Gennari, M. Bencini, L. Cesari, and G. Borrello, Clin. Sci. 38, 397-407 (1970).
19. D. Hioco, P. Bordier, L. Miravet, H. Denys, S. Tun-Chot in: Calcitonin 1969. Proceedings of the Second International Symposium, S. Taylor and G. Foster, eds. (Springer-Verlag, New York 1970) pp. 514-522.
20. P. Brown, C.G. Thin, D.N.S. Malone, P. Roscoe, and J.A. Strong, Scot. Med. J. 15, 207-212 (1970).

21. R.A. Melick, T.J. Martin, and E. Storey, Aust. NZJ Med. 3, 285-289, (1973).
22. J. Jowsey, B.L. Riggs, R.S. Goldsmith, P.J. Kelly, and C.D. Arnaud, J. Clin. Endocrinol. 33, 752-758 (1971).
23. J. Jowsey, B.L. Riggs, P.J. Kelly, and D.L. Hoffman, J. Clin. Endocrinol. Metab. 47, 633-639 (1978).
24. S. Wallach, S.H. Cohn, H.L. Atkins, K.J. Ellis, R. Kohberger, J.F. Aloia, and I. Zanzi, Curr. Ther. Res. 22, 556-572 (1977).
25. R. Agrawal, S. Wallach, S. Chon, M. Tessier, R. Verch, M. Hussain, and I. Zanzi in: Calcitonin 1980. Chemistry, Physiology, Pharmacology and Clinical Aspects, A. Pecile, ed. (Excerpta Medica, Amsterdam 1981).
26. A. Caniggia, F. Lore, R. Nuti, A. Vattimo, in: Calcitonin 1980. Chemistry, Physiology, Pharmacology and Clinical Aspects, A. Pecile, ed. (Excerpta Medica, Amsterdam 1981).
27. H.E. Gruber, J.L. Ivey, D.J. Baylink, M. Matthews, W.B. Nelp, K. Sisom, and C.H. Chesnut III, Metabolism 33, 295-303 (1984).
28. G.F. Mazzuoli, M. Passeri, C. Gennari, S. Minisola, R. Antonelli, C. Voltorta, E. Palummeri, G.F. Cervellin, S. Gonnelli, and G. Francini, Calcif. Tissue Int. 38, 3-8 (1986).
29. J.F. Aloia, A. Vaswani, A. Kapoor, J.K. Yeh, and S.H. Cohn, Metabolism 34, 124-129 (1985).
30. P. Vigo, E. Corghi, P. Favini, R. Girardello, S. Ortolani, and E.E. Polli, N. Engl. J. Med. 305, 1469 (1981).
31. M.M. Pechet, E. Bobadilla, E.L. Carroll, and R.H. Hesse, Am. J. Med. 43, 696-710 (1967).
32. H. Rasmussen and P.J. Bordier in: The Physiological and Cellular Basis of Metabolic Bone Disease (Williams and Wilkins, Baltimore 1974).
33. P.J. Marie, H. Rasmussen, D. Kuntz, and F. Caulin, Calcif. Tissue Int. 35, A 11 (1983).
34. H. Rasmussen, P. Bordier, P. Marie, L. Auquier, J.B. Eisinger, D. Kuntz, F. Caulin, B. Argemi, J. Gueris, and A. Julien, Metab. Bone Dis. Rel. Res. 2, 107-111 (1980).

Calcitonin and Bone Pain

C. Gennari, D. Agnusdei, and S. Gonnelli

Institute of Clinical Methodology, University of Siena, Siena, Italy

ABSTRACT

   Bone pain is the most common symptom in osteoporotic patients. To date there is mounting evidence that calcitonin significantly reduces bone pain in osteoporosis, and that the analgesic effect can be evident as soon as the second week of treatment. The limitations to the use of calcitonin, that are parenteral administration and side effects, can now be overcome by the availability of the new nasal spray preparation. At present, controlled studies have demonstrated the analgesic activity of calcitonin given by nasal spray in patients with vertebral crush fractures and bone pain. The mechanism for the analgesic effect of calcitonin is yet to be clarified. In animals and man it has been demonstrated that the i.v. infusion of calcitonin determines a parallel and dose-dependent increase in circulating beta-endorfin and ACTH, which indicates a common origin in the pituitary gland. Recently, a significant beta-endorphin increase after salmon calcitonin nasal spray has been demonstrated in man. Given that nasal mucosa is close to the hypotalamic area regulating pain, these findings suggest a central direct effect of calcitonin nasal spray.

INTRODUCTION

   Bone pain is a symptom which frequently accompanies bone disease characterized by excessive bone resorption, such as Paget's bone disease, metastatic bone disease and osteoporotic syndromes. The mechanism of bone pain remains poorly understood. The periosteum is certainly painsensitive, whereas the cortex and bone marrow are considered to be insensitive. It is well known that bone pain occurs from activation of free nerve endings: the nerve endings in bone can be activated by both mechanical and chemical stimulation. The hypothesis of mechanical genesis of bone pain can be justified when weight bearing is implicated. The chemical hypothesis for pain generation relates to the presence of humoral factors, as in the case of prostaglandins in bone metastases.
   Calcitonin has been widely employed in the treatment of Paget's disease of bone where the hormone exerts its beneficial effect by inhibiting bone resorption. Since the first therapeutic application in this disorder, it has been evident that calcitonin could be effective in relieving bone pain as well. Relief of bone pain was first associated with an improvement of bone lesions. It soon became evident, however, that in many cases pain relief occurred prior to any modifications of the biochemical indexes of bone disease. Moreover, this analgesic effect induced by calcitonin

administration in Paget's disease was maintained even when resistance to calcitonin therapy developed. These observations led to speculation that calcitonin could have an analgesic effect, independent of its classic action on bone. The concept that the analgesic potency of calcitonin is not restricted to bone pain has been confirmed by studies demonstrating a good or even dramatic pain relief in headache (1) and in postoperative soft tissue pain (2).

Since all the clinical manifestations of osteoporosis are a direct or indirect consequence of fracture, it is obvious that bone pain is the most common symptom in osteoporotic patients. To date there is mounting evidence that calcitonin significantly reduces bone pain in osteoporosis. Clinical trials in postmenopausal osteoporotic patients using calcitonin at doses ranging from 25-200 MRC units per day, and for periods spanning 1 to 19 months, have documented clinical improvement in pain and disability in 60-100 percent of the subjects treated with calcitonin (3). The analgesic effect can be evident as soon as the second week of treatment (Fig.1), and it increases with the lenght of treatment. These observations should be considered supportive of the potential symptomatic improvement to be offered by calcitonin treatment of the osteoporotic syndrome.

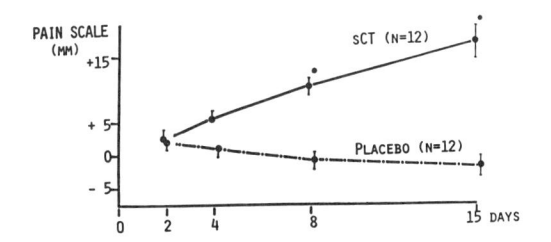

Fig.1. Analgesic effect of salmon calcitonin (100 I.U. daily by i.m. injection) in postmenopausal osteoporotic patients with bone pain. Pain was measured by a visual analogue scale, and pain relief was calculated by subtracting the after-treatment pain score from the initial pain score.

POSSIBLE MECHANISM OF THE ANALGESIC EFFECT OF CALCITONIN

The mechanism for the analgesic effect of calcitonin is yet to be clarified. Many hypotheses have been proposed:
(a) the calcitonin-induced hypocalcemia could per se reduce the pain threshold by modifying the sensitivity of some pain mediator-receptor interactions (4);
(b) on the basis of some results obtained from animal studies, it has been suggested that calcitonin may reduce the local synthesis of pain humoral factors in tissues, such as prostaglandins (5);
(c) the presence of calcitonin-binding sites in the central nervous system (6), coupled with the demonstration that intracerebroventricular administration of calcitonin to rats enhances the pain threshold (7),

led to speculation that calcitonin could directly act on the central regulatory mechanism of pain;
(d) since some similarities have been observed between morphine and calcitonin-induced analgesia, it has been hypothesized that the analgesic effect of calcitonin might be mediated by the endogenous opiate system, in particular by an increase of betaendorphin synthesis (8).

Some clinical studies have demonstrated that the analgesic effect of calcitonin is not necessarily due to its hypocalcemizing effect, nor to an interference in prostaglandin synthesis (9,10). Concerning the hypothesis of a direct analgesic effect on the central nervous system it has been demonstrated that the subarachnoid or epidural injection of calcitonin in man results in analgesia (10-12). This evidence raised the possibility that calcitonin is capable of producing analgesia functioning directly as a neurotransmitter in the central nervous system. Nevertheless, some animal studies do not exclude the possibility that the central analgesic effect of calcitonin may be mediated by monoaminergic systems (13,14).

In animals and man it has been demonstrated that the intravenous infusion of calcitonin determines a sudden increase in circulating beta-endorphin- and ACTH-immunoreactivity (15-17). The parallel increase of beta-endorphin and ACTH indicates that their origin is probably in the pituitary gland. The similar structure of beta-lipotropin and beta-endorphin represents a problem when obtaining specific antisera for radioimmunoassay: this fact implies a cross-reactivity that is elevated for beta-lipotropin vs beta-endorphin. High performance gel permeation chromatography is the technique required to demonstrate in plasma beta-endorphin distinctly separated from beta-lipotropin. The validation of the measurement may be obtained by the employment of labeled human beta-endorphin. With high performance gel chromatography we have clearly documented the increase in circulating beta-endorphin, one hour after the intravenous infusion of salmon calcitonin (10). In order to evaluate a dose-effect relationship between salmon calcitonin and the increase in circulating beta-endorphins, we have recently studied the acute effect of different doses of salmon calcitonin in painful metastatic bone disease, according to a double-blind placebo controlled design. The results clearly demonstrate that the peak of circulating beta-endorphin is dose dependent (10). Controlled studies in man on the analgesic activity of different calcitonins have shown that salmon calcitonin and human calcitonin have different potency in enhancing pain threshold. In these studies salmon calcitonin resulted more effective in reducing pain than human calcitonin and placebo (18). These data support the hypothesis that bone pain relief is associated with the increase in beta-endorphin levels and that salmon calcitonin is more effective than human calcitonin in determining analgesia.

ANALGESIC EFFECT OF CALCITONIN GIVEN BY NASAL SPRAY

To date, calcitonin constitutes one of the major choice for the pharmacologic treatment of involutional osteoporosis. In postmenopausal osteoporosis, calcitonin, analogous to estrogens, determines increase of bone mass. Furthermore, patients treated with calcitonin can also benefit from the analgesic effect of the hormone. Unlike estrogens, these beneficial effects of calcitonin occur with minimal risk and no need for routine gynecological monitoring. The only limitations to the use of calcitonin are linked to the frequent parenteral injections and the occurrence of side effects. These limitations can now be overcome by the availability of the new nasal spray preparation, which has been developed for synthetic salmon calcitonin. The introduction of this new form increases the patients' compliance, and the different pharmacokinetic curtails the side effects, compared to the parenteral administration. At present, one-year controlled studies have been reported, showing a beneficial effect of salmon calcitonin on bone mass not only in patients with established osteoporosis (19), but also in prevention of bone loss of menopause (20).

In osteoporotic patients with a recent vertebral crush fracture the dominant symptom is bone pain, which is felt diffusely in the back, related to movement and reduced by rest. The acute episode may be so painful as to be accompanied by shock, pallor and vomiting. Gentle percussion over the spinous processes may localize precisely the site of the fracture. The radioisotope bone scan is helpful as it will localize fairly precisely the most recent site of fracture. In these cases calcitonin may be effective not only in preventing further deterioration of bone, but also in determining an early and substantial improvement in pain. Although salmon calcitonin, in parenteral form, has been shown to relieve bone pain in acute vertebral crush fracture syndrome (21), daily subcutaneous injection of calcitonin may cause discomfort and inconvenience, resulting in decreased compliance.

Recently, we have conducted a double-blind placebo controlled study in order to evaluate the analgesic activity of salmon calcitonin given by nasal spray (200 IU day for one month) in 21 patients with established osteoporosis presenting an acute episode of vertebral collapse. Bone pain was assessed by measuring spontaneous pain, by a visual analogue scale, and provoked pain, at the site of vertebral crush fracture, by exerting a compression with a digital pain-meter. Salmon calcitonin determined an immediate and consistent relief of pain that was significantly greater than that observed in placebo-treated patients; this response was evident both in the evaluation of spontaneous pain as well as in the measurement of provoked pain (Fig.2).

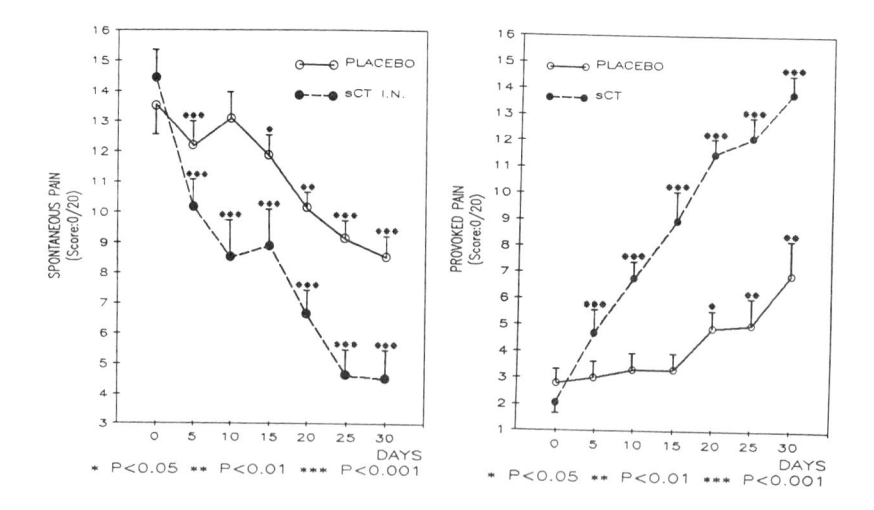

Fig.2. Effect of intranasally administered salmon calcitonin and placebo on the intensity of spontaneous pain (left) and provoked pain (right) in patients with recent osteoporosis spinal fractures. Patient receiving salmon calcitonin had significantly lower pain scores than did patients receiving placebo (p 0.05 for spontaneous pain, p 0.01 for provoked pain).

Some preliminary studies in osteoporotic and pagetic patients have given the impression that the nasal route of administration of calcitonin seems to be more effective in producing analgesia than the parenteral route (22). Recently, a significant beta-endorphin increase after salmon calcitonin nasal spray administration has been demonstrated in healthy adult subjects (23) and patients with metastatic bone disease (24). Given that nasal mucosa is close to the hypotalamic area regulating pain, these findings suggest a central direct effect of calcitonin nasal spray. In three terminal cancer patients with severe pain we have compared the analgesic effect of salmon calcitonin given by nasal spray (200 I.U.) to the analgesia produced by the same dosage of calcitonin given by intramuscular injection. Beta-endorphin-like immunoreactivity was measured before and after 1 hour from the administration of calcitonin in the cerebro-spinal fluid obtained by an intrathecal catheter. The increase in beta-endorphin level resulted more evident after intranasal than after parenteral administration of calcitonin (Fig.3). Furthermore, the improvement in pain was greater with calcitonin nasal spray than with calcitonin parenterally injected.

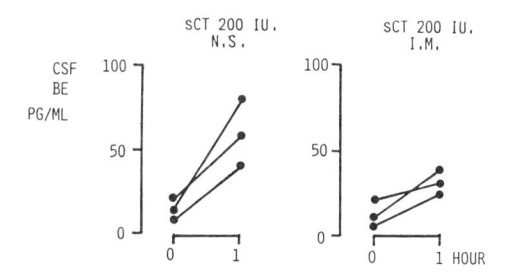

Fig.3. Effect of different route of administration of salmon calcitonin (nasal spray, left; intramuscular, right) on beta-endorphin levels in cerebro-spinal fluid in three terminal cancer patients.

In conclusion, calcitonin shows a precocious and persistent analgesic effect, which appears to be independent of its action on bone. Although the exact biochemical mechanism for this needs further investigation, there is evidence that the analgesic effect of calcitonin may be mediated through the endogenous opioid system. Therefore, calcitonin should be considered therapeutic in diseases characterized by enhanced bone resorption, particularly in patients with bone pain.

REFERENCES

1. C.Gennari, M.S.Chierichetti, S.Gonnelli, C.Vibelli, M.Montagnani, and M.Piolini, Headache 26, 13-16 (1986).
2. D.Welzel in: The effects of Calcitonins in Man, C.Gennari and G.Segre, eds. (Masson, Milano 1983) pp.223-232.
3. C.Gennari, and L.V.Avioli in: The Osteoporotic Syndrome, L.V.Avioli, ed. (Grune and Stratton, Orlando 1987) pp.121-142.

4. M.Satoh, H.Amano, T.Nakazawa, and H.Takagi, Res.Commun.Chem.Pathol. Pharmacol. 26, 213-215 (1979).
5. R.Ceserani, M.Colombo, V.R.Olgiati, and A.Pecile, Life Sci. 25, 1851-1853 (1979).
6. S.Guttman, P.Marbach, and R.Maurer in: The Effects of Calcitonins in Man, C.Gennari and G.Segre, eds. (Masson, Milano 1983) pp.25-31.
7. A.Pecile, S.Ferri, P.C.Braga, and V.R.Olgiati, Experientia 31, 332-333 (1975).
8. C.Gennari in: Calcitonin 1980, A.Pecile, ed. (Excerpta Medica, Amsterdam 1981) pp.277-287.
9. C.Gennari, Triangle 22, 157-163 (1983).
10. C.Gennari, and D.Agnusdei, Curr.Ther.Res. 44, 712-722 (1988).
11. D.Agnusdei, R.Civitelli, S.Gonnelli, G.Francini, A.Camporeale, and C.Gennari in: Pain and Reproduction, A.R.Genazzani, G.Nappi, F. Facchinetti, and E.Martignoni, eds. (Parthenon Publ., Carnforth 1988) pp.23-29.
12. F.Fraioli, A.Fabbri, L.Gnessi, C.Moretti, C.Santoro, and M.Felici, Europ.J.Pharmacol. 78, 381-382 (1982).
13. A.Groppetti, C.Flauto, F.Guidobono, M.Parenti, G.Rotondi, A.Soranzio, and F.Tirone in: Calcitonin 1984, A.Pecile, ed. (Excerpta Medica, Amsterdam 1985) pp.271-278.
14. G.Clementi, F.Drago, M.Amico-Roxas, A.Prato, E.Rapisarda, F.Nicoletti, G.Rodolico, and U.Scapagnini in: Calcitonin 1984, A.Pecile, ed. (Excerpta Medica, Amsterdam 1985) pp.279-286.
15. C.Gennari, G.Francini, S.Gonnelli, and R.Nami in: The Effects of Calcitonins in Man, C.Gennari and G.Segre, eds. (Masson, Milano 1983) pp.213-222.
16. J.Ronher, and D.Planche, Clin.Rheumatol. 4, 218-219 (1985).
17. L.Laurian, Z.Oberman, and E.Graf, Horm.Metab.Res. 18, 268-271 (1986).
18. C.Gennari, S.M.Chierichetti, S.Gonnelli, M.Piolini, G.Francini, R.Civitelli, D.Agnusdei, and M.Montagnani in: Calcitonin 1984, A.Pecile, ed. (Excerpta Medica, Amsterdam 1985) pp.183-188.
19. B.J.Riis, C.Christiansen, and K.Overgaard in: Calcitonin '88, G.F.Mazzuoli, ed. (Esi Stampa Medica, Milano 1988) pp.114-117.
20. J.Y.Reginster, D.Denis, A.Albert, R.Deroisy, M.P.Lecart, M.A.Fontaine, P.Lambelin, and P.Franchimont, Lancet ii, 1481-1483 (1987).
21. G.Attali, J.Levernieux, and F.Caulin in: Osteoporosis 1987, C.Christiansen, J.S.Johansen, and B.J.Riis, eds. (Norhaven, Viborg 1987) pp.930-932.
22. A.E.Pontiroli, G.Pozza, M.Alberetto, A.Calderara, and E.Pajetta in: Calcitonin '88, G.F.Mazzuoli, ed. (Esi Stampa Medica, Milano 1988) pp.34-40.
23. R.Franceschini, A.Cataldi, T.Barreca, and E.Rolandi, Med.Sci.Res. 16, 1279-1280 (1988).
24. M.Montagnani, S.Gonnelli, G.Francini, M.Piolini, and C.Gennari in: Calcitonin '88, G.F.Mazzuoli, ed. (Esi Stampa Medica, Milano 1988) pp.126-133.

EXERCISE AND CALCIUM

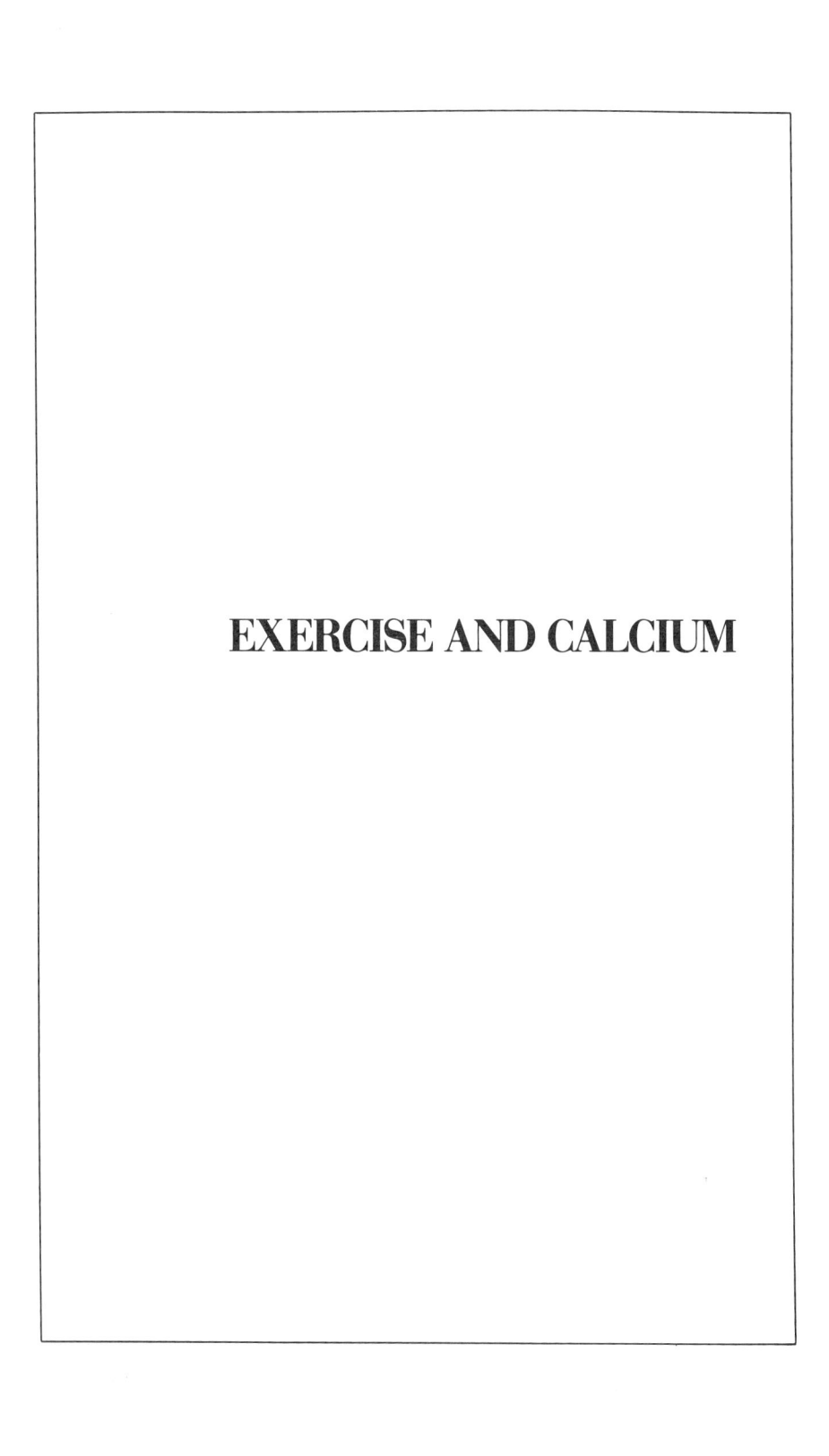

Physical Activity and Bone Mass

John A. Eisman,* P.J. Kelly,* P.N. Sambrook,* N.A. Pocock,†
J.J. Ward,‡ S. Eberl,† and M.G. Yeates†

*Bone and Mineral Research Group, Garvan Institute of Medical Research
†Department of Nuclear Medicine, St. Vincent's Hospital, Sydney, NSW
‡Cumberland College of Health Sciences, Lidcombe, NSW, Australia

ABSTRACT

Osteoporosis is a major and increasing health problem in most Western societies. Part of the increase is due to increasing longevity but part is due to a real increase in incidence per age group. The reasons for such an increase are unclear but changes in life-style and environmental factors may be important. We have examined the effect on bone density of one potentially protective life-style factor, physical activity, which may be declining in Western societies. We have previously shown in cross-sectional studies that physical fitness (estimated as predicted maximal oxygen consumption) and muscle strength (measured on a Cibex II ergometer) are predictors of bone mineral density (BMD) in the spine and hip, independent of age.

A major problem with previous longitudinal studies of interventions on change in bone density is that they have not controlled for the potentially major confounding effect of genetic factors. We have now initiated a longitudinal study of the potential for exercise to modify bone mass and, to control for possible genetic factors, we are performing the study in 20 pairs of identical twins. The long-term defined exercise programme includes strength and fitness building components. Both exercising and non-exercising twin subjects are being monitored for changes in fitness, strength,and BMD (measured by dual photon absorptiometry) at six monthly intervals.

Analysis of the data from 12 month on 12 twin pairs shows significant increases in physical fitness but not muscle strength of the exercising versus the non-exercising twins. Although there were no differences in the changes of BMD at any site between the exercising and non-exercising twins, the changes in BMD in the lumbar spine were significantly correlated with the observed changes in physical fitness ($r = 0.46$, $p < 0.05$) and biceps strength ($r = 0.62$, $p < 0.01$). Interestingly there was no correlation between femoral neck BMD and any parameter of physical fitness or muscle strength consistent with the slower turnover of cortical bone than trabecular bone.

These data support the concept that increased physical activity can result in increased lumbar spine bone mass; however the femoral neck seems less responsive. Clarification of the requirements for an effect on the latter site is most important to public health measures for the prevention and reversal of osteoporosis.

INTRODUCTION

Osteoporosis is a major health care problem around the world, particularly in developed countries where populations are aging at a dramatic rate. Femoral neck fractures are a major part of that problem. In the United States such fractures accounted for most of the estimated $7 billion to $10 billion in health care costs attributed to osteoporosis in 1985 [1-3]. There is growing evidence that excessive trauma associated with falls is an important component of the osteoporotic fracture syndrome [4]. On the other hand, although there is little evidence for femoral neck bone mass being lower in fracture subjects than in age-matched controls, there is no doubt that aged subjects have considerably lower bone mass than young individuals. Thus two factors clearly contribute to the risk of fracture, the strength of the bone and the stress applied to it. Aging is associated with both increased tendency to falls and lowered bone mass, which may explain the exponential increase in fractures with advancing age.

Based on previous studies, it seems that low bone mass in the femoral neck is a necessary if not sufficient requirement for hip fracture. An extension of this premise is that, if the age-related decline in proximal femoral bone mass can be prevented, hip fracture risk (and incidence) could be markedly reduced. This would be the case even if postural instability and falls were not altered. Spinal osteoporosis is reasonably clearly related to post-menopausal bone loss and although a recent study has suggested estrogens may protect against hip fractures [5], bone loss in the proximal femur appears to be related primarily to aging per se in both men and women. It is thus critically important to determine if age-related bone loss in the proximal femur is an inevitable consequence of aging or is consequent upon other age-related phenomena. If the latter is the case then if certain interventions could reverse or prevent such changes, the overall risk of fractures could be significantly altered.

Figure 1. Correlations of femoral neck bone mineral density (gm/cm2) with estimated physical fitness (predicted maximal oxygen consumption, ml/kg/min, left panel) and with quadriceps muscle strength (Newton.metres, right panel).

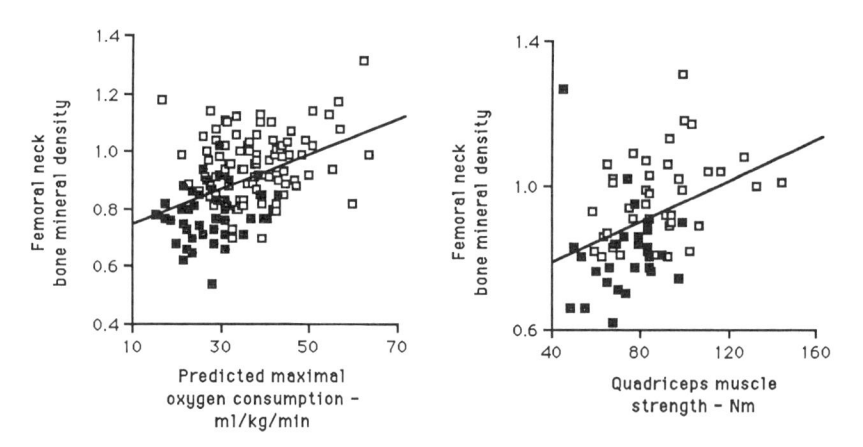

A considerable body of work has shown a biologically relevant relationship between the mechanical force exerted on the skeleton and bone mass, including data on the relationship between muscle strength, physical fitness and bone mass. In both human and animal studies mechanical loading appears to be a major determinant of bone mass. In man immobilization and weightlessness (in zero gravity) have been well documented as leading to an increase in urinary calcium loss and a decrease in bone mineral [6-9]. At the other extreme studies in athletes have shown significant increases in bone mass at various sites consistent with the increased local loading applied [10-14]. However we have shown previously strong genetic determinants on bone density in various skeletal sites [15]. Thus it can not be excluded in the studies in athletes, that genetic factors may contribute to both athletic ability and bone strength.

Although animal studies [16, 17] suggest that the exercise effect is a direct one, it is still important to remember that genetic factors may be operating to modify any bone response to exercise. Several cross-sectional studies have examined correlations between muscle mass and forearm or spine bone mass. Some have found positive correlations [18-21] but others have not done so [22, 23]. Positive correlations have been shown between physical activity or capacity for work (physical fitness) and muscle strength and bone mass in the normal population [18, 24-29]. Our studies in populations unselected for obvious concern about osteoporosis have shown clear correlations between bone density and muscle strength and physical fitness (see figure 1).

Overall the studies outlined above support a protective effect of physical activity on bone mass. However whether there is a direct relationship between muscle strength and bone mass and how aging may affect such a relationship is less clear. Significantly, increased body weight, generally associated with increased strength, has also been reported as having a beneficial effect on bone mass [25,30-32].

Some short term longitudinal studies have found a beneficial effect of exercise programmes on bone density [33-37]. However there are very few data on the possible interaction between physical fitness, muscle strength, weight and aging on the skeleton. In particular the role of these factors in determining bone mass in the proximal femur, the site of osteoporotic fracture with the greatest morbidity, mortality and socio-economic cost, has not been studied. In order to examine these potential interactions we have examined the effect on bone mass in the proximal femur and lumbar spine of a programme to increase muscle strength and physical fitness in a group of normal female twin volunteers.

METHODS

Subjects

The volunteers, who gave informed consent, had a mean age of 51.6 ± 2.2 years (mean ± SEM, range 26 - 71 years). To avoid the potentially important biases inherent in selection of subjects for an exercise programme, we have used identical twins allocated to an exercising programme or normal activities. Twenty pairs of identical twins, who had been recruited through direct mailing and media advertising on the basis of participating in previous studies, were invited to take part in this study. None of the subjects were incapacitated in any way and none were involved in vigorous exercise programmes. Any individuals with a previous history of bone disease, illness, known heart disease or drug use, which could affect bone, muscle strength or fitness were excluded from the study. No subject in the study had a prior history of renal disease and all had normal renal function as assessed by creatinine clearance and/or a serum creatinine. Lumbar spine radiographs were obtained in all subjects older than 40 years to exclude the presence of fractures or severe osteoarthritis, which may falsely elevate calculated lumbar bone mineral density (BMD). Both exercising and non-exercising twin subjects are monitored for changes in muscle strength, physical fitness.and BMD at six monthly intervals. The plan is that the twins will swap over at 18 months and continue for a further 18 months. The data presented here are from the first 12 months of the study on 13 twin pairs; seven of the pairs are postmenopausal.

Exercise Programme

The exercise programme was designed in collaboration with the Department of Occupational Therapy, St Vincent's Hospital to improve physical fitness and muscle strength. It includes a graded series of warm-up exercises progressing to a series of standing and floor exercises and followed by cool-down components. The exercises are graded over time to avoid strains and injuries and to gradually increase the stresses applied. Subjects are encouraged to achieve an elevation of pulse rate to 60-80% of predicted maximum. All participants are encouraged to engage in one-half to one hour of brisk walking three times per week. The pace of walking is also selected to achieve an increase in pulse rate as above.

Muscle Strength

Muscle strength in Newton metres (Nm) was measured using an isokinetic dynamometer (Cybex II, Lumex, Ronkonkoma, New York) as previously described [29]. In the lower limbs strength was measured in the knee extensors of the right leg, primarily the quadriceps, at angular velocities of 30, 60 and 90°/sec. Quadriceps maximum isokinetic strength was taken as the average of these three measures. Maximum isometric torque was measured at a knee angle of 60° from full extension. An overall index of quadriceps strength was determined as the mean of these two measurements. In the upper limb muscle strength was measured in the elbow flexors of the dominant arm, consisting primarily of the biceps, using an upper limb adaptation of the dynamometer. Isokinetic strength was taken as the mean of the values at angular velocities of 30, 60 and 90°/sec. Maximum isometric force was measured at an elbow angle of 60° from full extension and, as in the lower limb, an overall index of biceps strength was determined as the mean of these two measurements. Grip strength was measured in the non-dominant hand to correspond to the side of distal forearm BMC using a grip strength meter (Lafayette Instrument Co. Lafayette, Indiana). Although biceps and quadriceps strength were significantly correlated (r=0.53, p<0.001), grip strength and biceps strength were not correlated [29].

Physical fitness

Physical fitness (VO_2max, ml/kg/min) was estimated as predicted maximal oxygen uptake from measurements during a sub-maximal stress test according to the criteria of Astrand and Ryhming as described previously [27]. Weight (kg) and height (m) were measured in all volunteers and body mass index (BMI) calculated as kg/m^2. Predicted maximal oxygen uptake is a satisfactory estimate of maximal aerobic capacity in our relatively young study population. Problems with this indirect measure of aerobic capacity related to the prediction of maximal heart rate may arise in elderly men and women.

Bone Mineral Density

BMD (g/cm^2) was measured using a Lunar DP-3 dual photon absorptiometer (Lunar Radiation, Madison, Wisconsin, USA) as previously described [38]. The lumbar spine (L2-L4) and three sites in the proximal femur (the femoral neck at a trans-cervical position, the trochanteric region and Ward's triangle) were measured. The coefficient of variation was 2.6% in normal volunteers [38] consistent with published values [39].

Statistical Methods

Bone mineral measurements were correlated at each skeletal site against the measures of muscle strength, fitness, BMI and age. The twin data were examined by paired analysis and individually in relation to observed changes in physical fitness and muscle strength measures. In addition forwards and backwards stepwise multiple regression analyses were performed to determine predictor variables for each skeletal site. Linear regression analysis was used to estimate rates of change of bone density at each site in each individual. Student's t test was used to test the significance of the partial regression coefficients.

RESULTS

The exercising twins improved their physical fitness by comparison with their non-exercising twin co-pairs and both groups of twins increased grip strength (Figure 2). However there were no significant changes in measures of grip strength or biceps or quadriceps muscle strength between the exercising and non-exercising twin pairs (Figure 2). This was due in part to the fact that the "non-exercising" twin pairs had observed the beneficial effects of the exercise programme on the exercising twins and had subtly increased their own levels of physical activity. The exercising twins lost a small amount of weight at six months (approximately 1 kg) but had recovered this weight at 12 months.

Figure 2. Changes in physical fitness and muscle strength in 13 pairs of exercising and non-exercising twins at 12 months (*, $p < 0.05$ compared with baseline studies).

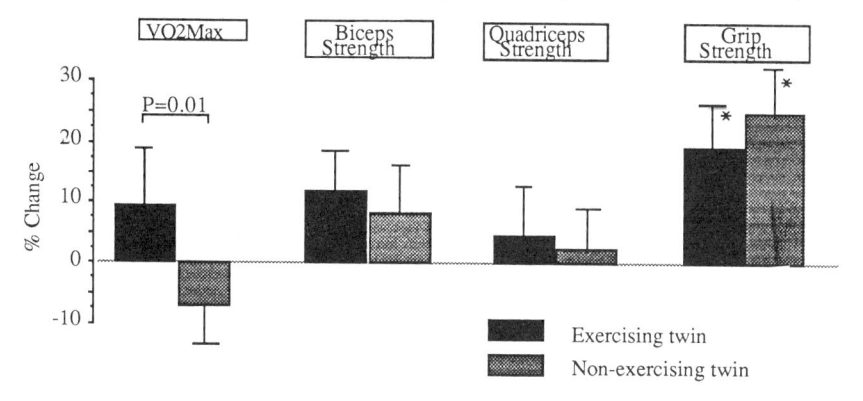

There were no significant differences between the exercising and non-exercising twin pairs in relation to changes in BMD at either the lumbar spine or femoral neck sites. However the changes in BMD in the lumbar spine correlated significantly with changes in physical fitness and biceps strength. Interestingly femoral neck BMD changes did not correlate with changes in these parameters (Figures 3 and 4). Quadriceps strength did not correlate with changes in BMD at either site.

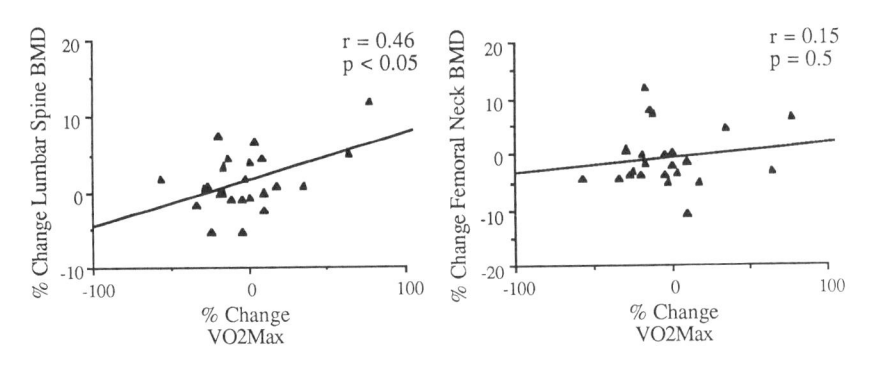

Figure 3. Correlation between changes in physical fitness and changes in lumbar spine and femoral neck BMD.

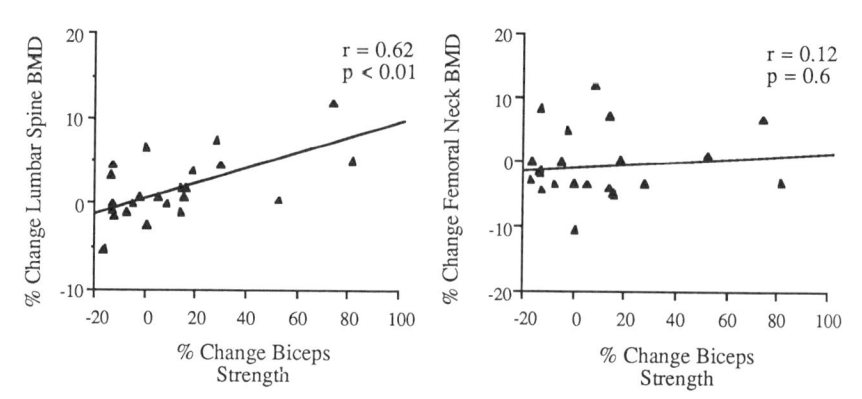

Figure 4. Correlation between changes in biceps strength and changes in lumbar spine and femoral neck BMD.

DISCUSSION

The present studies have shown that an exercise programme can produce significant increases in physical fitness in an exercising group compared with a non-exercising group. The groups were controlled for genetic predisposition by selection of identical twin pairs. However no significant differences were observed in muscle strength parameters. The studies also showed a modest association between both increased physical fitness and biceps strength and bone mass in the lumbar spine but not the femoral neck over the 12 month study period. This effect was observed across the twin pairs from both exercising and non-exercising groups.

It is unclear at this stage why there has been no effect on femoral neck BMD, but this would be consistent with the higher proportion of cortical bone at this site as compared with the predominantly trabecular bone of the lumbar spine. Although it is possible that exercise can not modify femoral neck bone mass, many studies strongly suggest that factors such as muscle strength, physical fitness and weight do exert effects on bone mass at this site [27, 29]. An alternative explanation is that our older subjects were unable to exercise enough to modify bone density. This is not consistent with the effects seen in the lumbar spine or with previous exercise studies in aged groups [33-37]. Moreover our previous studies have shown that the correlation between muscle strength, physical fitness and bone density are independent of age [27, 29]. However one other study, which examined the relationship between quadriceps strength and distal femur BMD in athletes did not find a correlation [10]. As skeletal muscle effects on bone are likely to be regional, it is possible that the exercises were inappropriate in that they may have not increased regional muscle strength.

A number of previous reports have shown an effect of increased body weight or body fat, on bone mass in the spine [30, 31], upper limb [21, 25, 33] and proximal femur [29]. This effect may be related to peripheral oestrogen production in adipose tissue [40] or to the increased mechanical load in weight bearing bones. Although the exercise programme resulted in transient weight loss in the exercising twin, this effect was small and would not seem likely to have offset any beneficial effects of the exercise programme. Another possibility for the modest effect of the exercise programme is that its intensity was gradually increased over the first 6 months and thus that it had not had sufficient time to influence the bone density of the various sites. In this context it is important to stress that none of the subjects was leading a sedentary life style prior to the study. This is in contrast to some studies [33-36] in older subjects who may have been very inactive at the start of the studies and therefore may have been more sensitive to the exercise effects and in which only lumbar spine sites have been studied.

We have shown useful effects of increased physical fitness and muscle strength resulting from an exercise programme on lumbar spine BMD. We are continuing to evaluate the changes in bone density versus changes in muscle strength in local areas as well as in relation to changes in physical fitness over the remainder of the study programme. It is important therefore to continue this study to determine whether this exercise programme, which is achievable by most subjects, can result in useful increases in bone mass in both clinically important sites of lumbar spine and femoral neck.

ACKNOWLEDGEMENTS

This research was supported by the National Health and Medical Research Council of Australia, Sandoz Australia, the Australian and New South Wales Dairy Corporations and by the Garvan Research Foundation.

REFERENCES

1. Riggs BL, Melton LJ III. Involutional osteoporosis. New Engl J Med 1986; 314:1676-1686.
2. National Center for Health Statistics. 1985 Summary: National Hospital Discharge Survey. Advance Data from Vital and Health Statistics. DDHS publication no. 127.
3. Health and Public Policy Committeee, American College of Physicians. Bone Mineral Densitometry. Annals Int Med 1987; 107:932-936.
4. Cooper C, Barker DJP, Morris J, Briggs RSJ. Osteoporosis, falls and age in fracture of the proximal femur. Brit Med J 1987; 295:13-15.
5. Kiel DP, Felson DT, Anderson JJ, Wilson PWF, Moskowitz MA, Hip fracture and the use of estrogens in postmenopausal women, N Eng J Med, 1987; 317, 1169-1174
6. Mack PB, LaChance PA, Vose GP, Vogt FB. Bone demineralization of foot and hand of Gemini-Titan IV, V and VII astronauts during orbital flight. Am J Roentgenol 1967; 100:503-511.
7. Hulley SB, Vogel JM, Donaldson CL, Bayers JH, Friedman RJ, Rosen SN. The effect of supplemental oral phosphate on the bone mineral changes during prolonged bed rest. J Clin Invest 1971; 50:2506-2518.
8. Stewart AF, Adler M, Byers CM, Segre GV, Broadus AE. Calcium homeostasis in immobilization: An example of resorptive hypercalciuria. N Engl J Med 1982; 306:1136-1140.
9. Krolner B, Toft B. Vertebral bone loss: an unheeded side effect of therapeutic bed rest. Clin Sci 1983; 64:537-540.
10. Nilsson BE, Westlin NE. Bone density in athletes. Clin Orthop 1971; 77: 179-182.
11. Brewer V, Meyer BM, Keele MS, Upton SJ, Hagan RD. Role of exercise in prevention of involutional bone loss. Med Sci Sports Exerc 1983; 16:445-449.
12. Dalen N, OlssonKE. Bone mineral content and physical activity. Acta Orthop Scand 1974; 45:170-174.
13. Jones HH, Priest JD, Hayes WC, Tichenor CC, Nagel DA. Humeral hypertrophy in response to exercise. J Bone Joint Surg 1977; 59:204-208.
14. Huddleston AL, Rockwell D, Kulund DN, Harrison RB. Bone mass in lifetime tennis athletes. J Am Med Assn 1980; 244:1107-1109.

15. Pocock NA, Eisman JA, Hopper JH, Yeates MG, Sambrook PN, Eberl S. Genetic determinants of bone mass in adults: A twin study. J Clin Invest 1987; 80:706-710.
16. Saville PD, Whyte MP. Muscle and bone hypertrophy. Clin Orthop 1969; 65: 81-88.
17. Burr DB, Martin RB, Martin PA. Lower extremity loads stimulate bone formation in the vertebral column: implications for osteoporosis. Spine 1983; 8:681-686
18. Black-Sandler R, LaPorte RE, Sashin D et al. Determinants of bone mass in menopause. Prev Med 1982; 11:269-280.
19. Doyle F, Brown J, Lachance C. Relation between bone mass and muscle weight. Lancet 1970; 1:391-393.
20. Sinaki M, McPhee MC, Hodgson SF, Merritt JM, Offord KP. Relationship between bone mineral density of spine and strength of back extensors in healthy postmenopausal women. Mayo Clin Proc 1986; 61:116-122.
21. Meema S, Reid DB, Meema HE. Age trends of bone mineral mass, muscle width and subcutaneous fat in normals and osteoporotics. Calc Tiss Res 1973; 12:101-112.
22. Meema HE. Menopausal and aging changes in muscle mass and bone mineral content. J Bone Joint Surg 1966; 48-A:1138-1144.
23. Sinaki M, Opitz JL, Wahner HW. Bone mineral content: relationship to muscle strength in normal subjects. Arch Phys Med Rehabil 1974; 55:508-512.
24. Krolner B, Tondevold E, Toft B, Berthelssen B, Pors Nielson S. Bone mass of the axial and the appendicular skeleton in women with colles' fracture: its relation to physical activity. Clin Physiol 1982; 2:147-157.
25. Oyster N, Morton M, Linnell S. Physical activity and osteoporosis in post-menopausal women. Med Sci Sport Exercise 1984; 16:44-50.
26. Chow RK, Harrison JE, Brown CF, Hajek V. Physical fitness effect on bone mass in postmenopausal women. Arch Phys Med Rehabil 1986; 67:231-234.
27. Pocock NA, Eisman JA, Yeates MG, Sambrook PN, Eberl S. Physical fitness is a major determinant of femoral neck and lumbar spine bone mineral density. J Clin Invest 1986; 78:618-621.
28. Aloia JF, Vaswani AN, Yeh JK, Cohn SH. Premenopausal bone mass is related to physical activity. Arch Int Med 1988; 148:121-123.
29. Pocock NA, Eisman JA, Guinn T, Sambrook PN, Kelly PJ, Freund J, Yeates MG. Muscle strength, physical fitness and weight but not age predict femoral neck bone mass. J Bone Min Res 1989 ; 4:441-448.
30. Riggs BL, Wahner HW, Dunn WL, Mazess RB, Offord KP, Melton LJ. Differential changes in bone mineral density of the appendicular and axial skeleton with aging. J Clin Invest 1981; 67:328-335.
31. Linquist O, Bengtsson C, Hansson T, Roos B. Bone mineral content in relation to age and menopause in middle-aged women. Scan J Clin Lab Invest 1981; 41:215-223.
32. Hui SL, Wiske PS, Norton JA, Johnston CC. A prospective study of change in bone mass with age in postmenopausal women. J Chron Dis 1982; 35:715-725.
33. Aloia JF, Cohn SH, Ostuni JA, Cane R, Ellis K. Prevention of involutional bone loss by exercise. Ann Intern Med 1978; 89:356-358.
34. Smith EL, Reddan W, Smith PE. Physical activity and calcium modalities for bone mineral increase in aged women. Med Sci Sports Exercise 1981; 13:60-64.
35. Krolner B, Toft B, Pors Nielsen S, Tondevold E. Physical exercise as prophylaxis against involutional vertebral bone loss: a controlled trial. Clin Sci 1983; 64:541-546.
36. Simkin A, Ayalon J, Leichter I. Increased trabecular bone density due to bone loading exercises in postmenopausal women. Calcif Tissue Int 1987; 40:59-63.
37. Margulies JY, Simkin A, Leichter I et al. Effect of intense physical activity on bone-mineral content in the lower limbs of young adults. J Bone Joint Surg 1986; 68-A:1090-1093.
38. Pocock NA, Eberl S, Eisman JA et al. Dual-photon densitometry in normal Australian women: a cross-sectional study. Med J Aust 1987; 146:293-297.
39. Riggs BL, Wahner HW, Seeman E et al. Changes in bone mineral density of the proximal femur and spine with aging. J Clin Invest 1982; 70:716-723.
40. Frumar AM, Meldrum DR, Geola F et al. Relationship of fasting urinary calcium to circulating estrogen and body weight in postmenopausal women. J Clin Endocrinol Metab 1980; 50:70-75.

Exercise and Bone Mass

Everett L. Smith and Catherine Gilligan

Biogerontology Laboratory, Department of Preventive Medicine, University of Wisconsin, Madison, Wisconsin

ABSTRACT

The unique dual function of bone in maintaining serum calcium and providing structural support subjects the tissue to both systemic and local controls.

Like muscle, bone is affected locally by mechanical forces. The response is confined to the area of increased strain. While muscle responds to both dynamic and isometric exercise, however, in bone dynamic strain is necessary for hypertrophy.

Walking, swimming, biking and running, if performed at the same relative intensity, all enhance cardiovascular fitness to the same degree. Their local strain patterns on bone, however, are dissimilar and therefore they have different effects. For example, spine density is less affected by swimming than by running. Various studies of athletes show that the areas and degree of bone hypertrophy are related to the dynamic strains of the activity.

Exercise intervention programs promote bone hypertrophy or reduce bone loss regardless of age or initial bone mass. Research has found benefits of exercise in young men, postmenopausal women, women with Colles', hip or spine fractures, and elderly women. We studied whether exercise was effective in reducing bone loss in healthy premenopausal and postmenopausal women, aged 35-65 [1]. Eighty women participated in an exercise program meeting 45 minutes/session, 3 times/week. Sessions included a wide range of upper and lower body and aerobic activities. Radius and ulna bone loss was significantly lower in the exercise group than in the control group (n = 62). Both premenopausal and postmenopausal subgroups had significantly reduced bone loss. Furthermore, there was no significant difference in the bone response to exercise between premenopausal and postmenopausal women. This supports the concept of a mechanical control system independent of hormonal status.

INTRODUCTION

Bone is homeostatically controlled by both systemic hormones which control serum chemistries and local mechanical loading demands for structural support. These two homeostatic controls are consistent with the three-fold function of bone to provide protection, support, and a repository for calcium. Both systems influence osteoclast and osteoblast function in modelling and remodelling bone. Osteoclasts and osteoblasts are the common pathway for calcium mobilization, bone growth, and geometric change in response to mechanical loading. The function of these cells integrates the competing or coinciding inputs of the systemic and local factors. Local mechanical strain can modulate the response of bone to systemic factors, as seen in athletes in unilateral sports. Bone mass is maintained by maximum strain levels that are "normal", i.e., matching the recent strain history. Rubin [2] reported that peak strain in the limb during locomotion was similar for a wide variety of animals and equivalent to approximately 1/2 to 1/3 of yield strain. Changes in bone with small increases or decreases in physical activity are difficult to detect, and there may be a band of strains around normal for which bone is maintained at the current level. With more pronounced changes in mechanical forces, bone mass changes in a direction that tends to bring peak strain back to normal levels.

When the mechanical load on bone is decreased--such as in bed rest, paralysis, or spaceflight--bone mass correspondingly declines. Kiratli et al. [3] demonstrated that this response was local in her study of spinal cord injured patients. During the first year post-injury, femur bone mineral density (BMD) decreased significantly but spine BMD did not change significantly. Femur BMD declined approximately 2% per month the first five months post-injury and 1% per month from five to eighteen months post-injury [4].

Increasing the mechanical force on bone by physical activity can produce hypertrophy or, rarely, fracture, depending on the strain intensity and number of cycles. On the average, athletes have greater bone mass than their sedentary counterparts. The effect is local, as shown by the normal bone mass in the non-dominant arm and hypertrophy in the dominant arm of tennis players. The extent of hypertrophy is related to the level of strain; for example, subjects who lifted weights had greater spine BMD than subjects who trained aerobically for a similar amount of time per week [5]. Bone response may also be influenced by the subject's age and physical strain history. Various physical activity intervention programs increased bone mass or decreased bone loss in previously sedentary subjects. Very high strain levels and/or number of cycles of peak strain, however, can produce fractures. Stress fractures are not uncommon among runners, and in one intervention study 41% of subjects experienced fractures in the course of training 8 hours/day, six days/week [6].

BONE HYPERTROPHY IN ATHLETES

Runners

Studies of runners have reported bone hypertrophy at various sites. Dalen and Olsson [7] compared bone mineral content (BMC) of 15 male long-term cross-country runners (age 50-59) to that of age- and weight-matched controls. Runners had significantly greater BMC distal radius plus ulna (19%), the head of the humerus (19%), the femur shaft (13%), and the calcaneus (21%). BMC was non-significantly higher in runners at the shaft of the radius plus ulna (6%), third lumbar vertebrae (9%) and femur neck (8%). The greater hypertrophy at some non-weightbearing sites than in weightbearing sites was not explained. Aloia et al. [8] found that total body calcium was 7% above predicted values in male marathon runners (mean age 42) but that radius BMC was nonsignificantly higher by 5%. In a study of women marathon runners (ages 30-49) Brewer et al. [9] found that os calcis bone mineral density was lower in the runners than in the sedentary controls. The authors attributed this to the greater body weight of control subjects. Marathoners had significantly greater radius midshaft BMC (5%) and phalanx V-2 density (12%) but did not differ from controls in distal radius BMC. BMC of the distal and midshaft radius and os calcis increased with age in marathoners while BMC decreased with age in controls. Lane et al. [10] studied spine L-1 bone mineral density (measured by computed tomography) in subjects from the 50+ Runners Association. Eight men and six women runners had spine bone density 40% greater than in matched sedentary controls. This hypertrophy is more than would be expected from other exercise studies, and may be due to the small sample size or the measurement site and method. Further studies are needed to confirm this degree of spinal hypertrophy.

Other Sports Activities

Studies comparing athletes with differing patterns of stress corroborate the importance of strain level and site. Nilsson and Westlin [11] studied distal femur bone density in world class athletes, physically active non-athletes, and sedentary controls. Compared to sedentary controls, weightlifters had 47% hypertrophy, throwers 42%, runners 40%, soccer players 39%, and swimmers 34% (nonsignificant). Physically active non-athletes had significantly greater bone density than their sedentary counterparts. Nilsson and colleagues [12] studied BMC of the proximal tibia and fibula in weightlifters, and confirmed that bone was hypertrophied at these weightbearing sites as well as the femur. In another cross-sectional study comparing forms of activity, Block et al. [5] evaluated spine bone density by computed tomography. Young men who reported participating in vigorous physical activity for at least one year were categorized into three groups: aerobic, weight training, and aerobic plus weight-training (combined). Compared to controls, the combined training group had the greatest hypertrophy in trabecular bone density (22%), followed by the weight training group (14%) and the aerobic group (7%). Jacobson et al. [13] compared bone mineral of the lumbar spine, distal radius, and metatarsal in women inter-collegiate tennis players (n = 11) and swimmers (n = 23) and sedentary controls (n = 46). Distal and midshaft radius BMC and W were higher in both swimmers (7-16%) and tennis players (12-17%) than in controls. Metatarsal density was 10% higher in swimmers and 23% greater in tennis players than in controls. Lumbar bone mineral density, however, while 11% higher in tennis players, was non-significantly lower in swimmers than in controls.

Unilateral Sports

Athletes in unilateral sports such as baseball and tennis have bone hypertrophy of the dominant arm relative both to control subjects and to the non-dominant arm. Watson [14] studied 200 male baseball pitchers ages 8-19. Bone mass in the dominant humerus was 17% greater in the dominant than in the non-dominant humerus. Studying professional tennis players, Jones and his colleagues [15-16] reported that combined cortical thickness of the playing arm compared to the non-playing arm was 35% greater in males and 28% greater in females. The increase in cortical thickness was due to both smaller medullary cavity and larger periosteal diameter. Hypertrophy of the proximal radius and ulna was less pronounced but significant. Bone hypertrophy in unilateral sports is not confined to young subjects. Montoye et al. [17] studied 61 senior male tennis players (mean age 64). The dominant arm had 8% greater BMC and 4% greater width at the 1/3 distal radius, and 10% greater BMC and 4% greater width in the humerus midshaft than in the nondominant arm. Cortical area of the dominant hand was 15% greater in the second metacarpal and 7% greater in the third metacarpal. This increase occurred primarily due to periosteal widening, since medullary area was greater. Huddleston et al. [18] observed similar differences in senior male tennis players (ages 70-84). BMC of the 1/3 distal radius was 13% greater in the playing arm than in the non-playing arm.

EXERCISE INTERVENTION IN HUMANS

Arm

Studies of arm bone (primarily radius) response to increased physical activity have produced conflicting results. Several studies reported that physical activity intervention did not significantly affect BMC in the arm, while others indicated a reduction in bone loss or an increase in BMC. The major difference between the two types of studies appears to be the level of local loading on the site measured.

Lack of Response. Aloia et al. [19] measured total body calcium by neutron activation analysis and distal (8 cm) radius BMC by single photon absorptiometry in postmenopausal women. Nine women (mean age 53) participated in exercise sessions 3 times/week for one year, and nine women (mean age 52) served as controls. The supervised exercise program consisted of warm-up, conditioning and aerobic exercises recommended by the President's Council on Physical Fitness. Subjects progressed in number of repetitions (5 levels) according to tolerance. Total body calcium increased in the exercise group and decreased in the control group. The change in total body calcium differed significantly between groups. Radius BMC and BMC/W, however, were not significantly affected by this exercise protocol.

Krolner et al. [20] studied thirty-one women (ages 50-73) with previous Colles' fractures. Sixteen subjects were assigned to an exercise group (3 dropouts) and 15 to a control group (1 dropout) based on distance from the research site. Spine and distal forearm bone mineral were assessed by dual photon absorptiometry. Exercise sessions were held for one hour, twice a week, for eight months. The exercise regime included walking, running, exercises while standing, sitting, lying or on all fours, and ball games. The program did not focus on training of the forearms. Spine bone mineral increased 3.5% in the exercise group and decreased 2.7% in the control group. In contrast, forearm bone mineral was essentially unchanged in the exercise group and decreased 3.7% in the controls, but this difference was not significant.

Sandler et al. [21] performed a three-year randomized clinical trial on the effects of walking on bone tissue density (BTD) of the radius measured by computed tomography. The measurement site was 70% of the distance from the elbow to the wrist. The purpose of the study was to determine whether exercise had generalized skeletal effects. Two hundred fifty-five postmenopausal women were randomized into increased physical activity and control groups. Exercise subjects were instructed to increase physical activity by approximately seven miles of walking per week (about 672 kilocalories). Exercise subjects increased physical activity levels by 330 kcal per week and control subjects by 160 kcal per week. Since the physical activity group had a higher activity level at the start of the study, the difference between groups at the end of the study was about 330 kcal/week (3.5 miles). Changes in BTD or cross-sectional area of the area did not differ significantly between groups. The authors subdivided the control and exercise groups based on grip strength above or below the median at the beginning of the study. Walkers with high grip strength had significantly greater increases in cross-sectional area than controls with high grip strength. This difference did not occur in BTD or between low grip strength walkers and controls.

Reduction in Bone Loss. Simkin et al. [22-23] studied bone loss of the 3 cm distal radius by two methods -- single photon absorptiometry (SPA) and Compton scattering. Subjects (mean age 63) were women diagnosed as osteoporotic based on morphology of the spine, divided into control (n=26) and exercise intervention (n=14) groups. Exercise sessions met 3 times per week, 50 minutes per session, for five months. Each session included 15-20 minutes of forearm loading exercises, 10-15 repetitions each. Exercises for tension, compression, bending and torsion were utilized each session. The remainder of the session consisted of warm-up, stretching, strength exercises and relaxation. Trabecular bone mineral density (BMD), measured by Compton scattering, increased 3.8% in the exercise group and decreased 1.9% in the control group over the five month period. In contrast, bone mineral content (BMC), measured by SPA, tended to decrease in the exercise group (-3.3%) and to increase in the control group (+3.1%). These results raise questions regarding trabecular vs. cortical bone response and measurement techniques. The authors noted that SPA at the 3 cm distal radius was imprecise and measured both cortical and trabecular bone, while Compton scattering was more precise and measured only trabecular bone.

White et al. [24] studied postmenopausal women, ages 50-63, divided into a control group (n=21, mean age 55), and two exercise intervention groups--walkers (n=27, mean age 56) and dancers (n=25, mean age 57). Exercise subjects were assigned semi-randomly to the two intervention groups, and the control group was matched for age, height and weight. Bone mineral content of the 1/3 distal radius was measured by single photon absorptiometry. Subjects exercised 2-4 days/week for 6 months. The investigators supervised one session per week. During the first 11 weeks, walkers progressed from walking 1 mile on 2 days per week to walking 2 miles on 4 days per week. Over the same period, dancers progressed from 2 dances on 2 days per week to 5 dances on 4 days per week. Investigators supervised one session per week. BMC declined significantly by 1.6% in the control group and 1.7% in the exercise group, and nonsignificantly by 0.8% in the dance group. Width increased significantly by 1.6% in the walkers and 1.3% in the dancers, and nonsignificantly by 0.9% in the controls. The groups did not differ significantly at the end of the study. The authors hypothesized that the aerobic dance routines provided stress to the arms, and reported a significant increase in arm strength (elbow flexion) in the dance group. However, no strength measurements were performed on the controls.

Smith et al. [25] studied elderly women (mean age 82) in a nursing home over a period of three years. Single photon absorptiometry was used to assess BMC and BMC/W of the 1/3 distal radius. Subjects were assigned to one of four groups: control, calcium supplementation (with vitamin D), exercise, and exercise plus calcium. Exercise subjects (n=12) participated in three sessions per week of mild chair exercises. Control subjects (n=18) lost 3.3% in BMC and 2.6% in BMC/W over the three year period. Exercise subjects gained 2.3% in BMC and 1.7% in BMC/W. Calcium supplementation (750 mg elemental calcium and 400 IU vitamin D; double blinded) had an effect similar to the exercise effect. Calcium supplemented subjects (n=10) gained 1.6% in BMC and 3.5% in BMC/W. The exercise plus calcium group (n=11), however, was less affected by the intervention, losing 0.3% in BMC and having no change in BMC/W. The authors hypothesized that the lower response in the exercise plus calcium group was due to declining health and mobility in these subjects.

Smith et al. [1] studied the effects of exercise in women ages 35-65. BMC and W were measured by single photon absorptiometry at the 1/3 distal radius and ulna and at the humerus midshaft, bilaterally. Exercise sessions, held three days/week for four years, included 10-15 minutes warmup, 5-10 minutes cooldown, and 25-30 minutes of aerobic exercise progressing from 70% of maximum heart-rate reserve the first year to 85% the fourth year. The aerobic portion of the class incorporated exercise routines designed to improve upper body strength by the use of light weights (0.5-2 kg) on the wrists. In addition, the non-aerobic portions of class included upper body strength exercises such as pushups and activities using elastic tubing. Subjects were instructed not to take calcium supplements. Bone loss in the radius and ulna was significantly reduced by exercise in both premenopausal and postmenopausal women. Humerus bone loss was not as strongly affected. Premenopausal control subjects lost 0.4-1.4% per year in radius and ulna BMC and BMC/W, while premenopausal exercise subjects changed by -0.2% to +0.1% per year. For postmenopausal subjects, the control group lost 1.3-2.3% per year, and the exercise group 0.0-1.4% per year.

Weightbearing Bones

Os Calcis.
Rundgren et al. [26] analyzed os calcis BMC in elderly subjects by a modified dual photon absorptiometry system. Fifteen women from 63 to 84 years old (mean age 72) participated in a training program. Twenty-one women from 65 to 81 years old (mean age 73) agreed to serve as

controls. The training sessions took place twice a week for 40 minutes for nine months, excluding a 10 week summer break. The emphasis of the program was on muscular strength. For 25 minutes per session, subjects performed 'light' periods of dynamic exercises emphasizing the lower extremities. Some exercises were performed seated or using elastic bands. Four 'heavy' periods of high speed walking or jogging lasting 2.5 to 4 minutes alternated with the light periods. Average attendance was 75%. BMC increased about 5% in the exercise group and decreased about 2% in the control group. The exercise group tended to have greater BMC at the beginning of the study, and had significantly higher BMC than the control group at the end of the study.

Williams et al. [27] measured os calcis BMC by single photon absorptiometry in 20 men (ages 36-68, mean age 49) before and after a nine-month marathon training program. Ten men (ages 41-58, mean age 47) served as controls. Consistent runners (n=7) were defined as those running more than 16 km in each of the 9 months of training. Inconsistent runners (n=13) ran less than 16 km during at least one month. Mean training was 141 km/month for consistent runners and 65.3 km/month for inconsistent runners. (Competitive marathoners train approximately 320-448 km/month.) While final BMC did not differ significantly between groups, the group of consistent runners increased significantly in os calcis bone mineral by 3%. Inconsistent runners and controls increased nonsignificantly by about 1% and controls by about 0.5%.

Dalen & Olsson [7] trained 19 men (ages 25-52) for three months. Bone mineral content was measured at seven skeletal sites (distal and shaft radius plus ulna, humerus, L3, femur neck and shaft, calcaneus) by x-ray spectrophotometry. Subjects walked three km five times/week (n=10) or ran five km three times/week (n=9). BMC was not significantly affected by this short-term training protocol.

Tibia. Margulies et al. [6] studied BMC of the tibia (measured by single photon absorptiometry) in young male military trainees. Two hundred and six infantry recruits trained for fourteen weeks in a rigorous program including walking, jogging with and without weights, and calisthenics for at least eight hours a day, six days a week. One hundred and ten subjects were unable to complete the training course, primarily due to stress fractures of the lower limbs. Sixty-three percent of fractures occurred during the first four weeks of training. BMC of the tibia increased 8.3% in the right leg and 12.4% in the left leg in subjects who completed training. In subjects who did not complete training, BMC increased 1.0% in the right leg and 9.4% in the left. Tibia width (measured on an anteroposterior radiograph) did not change significantly. The authors had no explanation for the lateral difference in response.

Trunk. Chow et al. [28] studied the effects of exercise on the calcium bone index (CaBI, bone mass of the trunk measured by neutron activation analysis and adjusted for age and body size) in osteoporotic women. Women (mean age 66) who entered the program were concurrently receiving fluoride therapy and calcium supplementation of 1 gram per day. Subjects were divided into home exercise and hospital exercise groups by self-selection. Seven subjects of the original 26 home exercisers and 3 of the original 22 hospital exercisers dropped out of the study. Exercise sessions, held 3 days/week for 12.5 months, included 20 minutes of low-load strength exercises and 30 minutes of aerobic exercise. Subjects performed 10 repetitions for each major muscle group of the upper and lower extremities at 50-75% repetition maximum using free weights. Target heart rates for the aerobic portion of the class were set at 80% of the maximum heart rate on a progressive treadmill test. Most subjects in the home exercise group did not exercise. Subjects who exercised (n=20) improved CaBI from 0.69 to 0.81 over the course of the study. Non-exercising subjects had a smaller increase from 0.65 to 0.69. CaBI was significantly higher in the exercise group than the non-exercise group at the end of the study.

Chow et al. [29] compared the effects of an aerobic exercise program with an aerobic plus strengthening exercise program. Forty-eight of fifty-eight postmenopausal women (ages 50-62, mean age 56) who were invited to join the program elected to participate. Subjects were randomly assigned into control (n = 19, 4 dropouts), aerobic exercise (n = 19, 2 dropouts) and aerobic plus strength (n = 20, four dropouts) groups. One of the subjects in the aerobic group and 3 subjects in the aerobic plus strength group dropped out because of pain resulting from exercise. Exercise sessions were held for one year, three times per week. The aerobic exercise consisted of 5-10 minutes of warmup and 30 minutes of aerobic activities at 80% of maximum heart rate. Subjects in the aerobic plus strength group had an additional 10-15 minute session. Subjects performed 10 repetitions for each muscle group at 10 repetition maximum using free weights attached to the wrists and ankles. Control subjects declined by 0.011 in CaBI. The aerobic exercise group increased by 0.039 and the aerobic plus strength group by 0.066. The tendency for greater increase in CaBI in the aerobic plus strength group was not significant.

Spine. Two studies which were unable to detect an exercise effect on forearm bone mineral reported that total body calcium or spine BMC were affected. Aloia et al. [19] reported that postmenopausal exercise subjects increased significantly in total body calcium compared to controls. In the study of women with previous Colles' fracture, Krolner et al. [20] reported that spine bone mineral increased 3.5% in the exercise group and decreased 2.7% in the control group.

Dalsky et al. [30] studied spine (L2-L4) BMC change, measured by dual photon absorptiometry, in 35 postmenopausal women ages 55-70 (mean age 62). Nineteen subjects joined an exercise group and 16 a control group. Two subjects in the exercise group dropped out of the exercise program and were included in the analysis as control subjects. Exercise sessions were held 3 days/week, 50-60 minutes, for nine months. Weightbearing exercise consisted of walking, jogging and treadmill walking at 60-70% maximum work capacity during the first three months. After 3 months, stair-climbing (30-40 minutes) was added. Each session also included 15-20 minutes of non-weightbearing activities such as cycling, rowing and weight training. Twelve women exercised on the treadmill an additional 20-25 minutes at 70-90% maximum. All subjects received calcium supplementation sufficient to raise calcium intake to 1500 mg/day. In nine months, spine bone mineral content increased 5.2% in the exercise group and declined 1.4% in the control group. Eleven exercise subjects who continued in an exercise program for a total of 22 months increased spine BMD by 6.1% and fourteen control subjects lost 1.1% in 27 months. Fifteen exercise subjects who were followed for an average of 13 months of detraining lost 4.8% of the final exercise spine bone mass.

OPTIMAL PHYSICAL ACTIVITY STRATEGIES

The studies described above indicate that the effect of physical activity on bone is primarily local, and related to the intensity of mechanical loading. Similar results have been obtained in animal studies [31]. No research has yet, however, compared the effects of differing physical activity interventions on bone in humans. Lanyon [32], performing animal studies, has provided insight into some of the parameters governing bone response to mechanical loading. In his isolated wing preparations, transverse osteotomies are made across the proximal and distal submetaphyseal region of a turkey or rooster ulna. Each end of the ulna shaft is covered with a stainless steel cap and pierced with a Steinmann pin. The pin protrudes from the skin on both dorsal and ventral surfaces of the wing, and is fixed dorsally and ventrally with an external fixator to prevent accidental loading. The external fixators are removed and the pins engaged in the forks of an Instron loading machine for planned mechanical loading. Lanyon determined that static loading at 0.002 strain was ineffective in deterring the 15-20% reduction in cross-sectional area due to disuse. Dynamic loading at the same strain level, however, produced bone hypertrophy of 24% [33]. With dynamic loading (100 cycles at 1.0 Hz daily), strain level was directly related to the amount of hypertrophy. Bone atrophied at strains less than 0.001 and hypertrophied at strains greater than 0.001. The change in bone mass was linearly related to the strain magnitude (r = 0.82) [34]. Number of load cycles appeared to be less important than strain magnitude. When strain was held constant at 0.002, as few as 4 loading cycles at 0.5 Hz per day prevented bone atrophy. Thirty-six cycles per day increased cross-sectional are by 30-40%. Hypertrophy was similar at 36, 300, 1800 and 3600 loading cycles per day [35]. In a study of competing systemic and local influences, artificial loading reduced bone loss due to disuse in calcium-deficient turkeys. Bone loss in the isolated, artificially loaded ulna, however, was greater than in the intact ulna [36]. Even a single cycle of mechanical loading produced mitogenic activity [32]. Pead and Lanyon [37] suggested that the mediator of strain to chemical stimuli may be prostaglandin. To test this concept, they assessed osteoblastic activity in isolated wing preparations under four conditions: with and without mechanical loading; with and without indomethacin (a prostaglandin inhibitor). Osteoblastic activity (evaluated by tetracycline labeling) was minimal in unloaded preparations. Periosteal osteoblastic activity was greater in mechanically loaded bones than in unloaded bones, under both the presence and absence of indomethacin. Indomethacin injections, however, significantly reduced the bone response to mechanical loading.

Based on these data, an optimal bone loading program should utilize activities that provide relatively high strain levels and relatively few loading cycles. Further research is needed to determine which activities meet these suggestions, and their effect on bone in humans, particularly postmenopausal women at risk of fracture.

REFERENCES

1. E.L. Smith, C. Gilligan, M. McAdam, C.P. Ensign, and P.E. Smith, Calcif. Tissue Int. 44, 312-321 (1989).
2. C.T. Rubin, Calcif. Tissue Int. 36, S11-S18 (1984).
3. B.J. Kiratli, J.C. Agre, M.A. Wilson, and E.L. Smith, J. Bone Min. Res. 3, S121 (1988).
4. B.J. Kiratli, J.C. Agre, M.A. Wilson, and E.L. Smith, Arch. Phys. Med. Rehab. 69, 711 (1988).
5. J.E. Block, H.K. Genant, and D. Black, West. J. Med. 145, 39-42 (1986).
6. J.Y. Margulies, A. Simkin, I. Leichter, A. Bivas, R. Steinberg, M.Giladi, M. Stein, H. Kashtan and C. Milgrom, J. Bone Joint Surg. 68A, 1090-1093 (1986).
7. N. Dalen and K.E. Olsson, Acta Orthop. Scand. 45, 170-174 (1974).
8. J.F. Aloia, S.H. Cohn, T. Babu, C. Abesamis, N. Kalici, and K. Ellis, Metabolism 27, 1793 (1978).
9. V. Brewer, B.M. Meyer, M.S. Keele, S.J. Upton, and R.D. Hagan, Med. Sci. Sports Exer. 15, 445-449 (1983).
10. N.E. Lane, D.A. Bloch, H.H. Jones, W.H. Marshall, P.D. Wood, and J.F. Fries, J. Am. Med. Assoc. 255, 1147-1151 (1986).
11. B.E. Nilsson and N.E. Westlin, Clin. Orthop. Rel. Res. 77, 177-182 (1971).
12. B.E. Nilsson, S.M. Andersson, T. Havdrup, and N.E. Westlin, Am. J. Roentgen. 13, 541-542 (1978).
13. P.C. Jacobson, W. Beaver, S.A. Grubb, T.N. Taft, and R.V. Talmage, J. Orthop. Res. 2, 328-332 (1984).
14. R.C. Watson, in: International Conference on Bone Mineral Measurements,ed. (DHEW #NIH 75-683, Washington, DC 1974) 380-385.
15. H.H. Jones, J.D. Priest, and W.C. Hayes, J. Bone Joint Surg. 59A, 204-208 (1977).
16. J.D. Priest, H.H. Jones, C.J.C. Tichnor, and D.A. Nagel, Minnesota Med. 60, 399-404 (1977).

17. H.J. Montoye, E.L. Smith, D.F. Fardon, and E.T. Howley, Scand. J.Sports Sci. 2, 26-32 (1980).
18. A.L. Huddleston, D. Rockwell, D.N. Kulund, and R.B. Harrison, J. Am. Med. Assoc. 244, 1107-1109 (1980).
19. J.F. Aloia, S.H. Cohn, J. Ostuni, R. Cane, and K. Ellis, Ann. Int. Med. 89, 356-358 (1978).
20. B. Krolner, B. Toft, S.P. Nielson, and E. Tondevold, Clin. Sci. 64, 541-546 (1983).
21. R.B. Sandler, J.A. Cauley, D.L. Hom, D. Sashin, and A.M. Kriska, Calcif. Tissue Int. 41, 65-69 (1987).
22. A. Simkin, J. Ayalon, and I. Leichter, Calcif. Tissue Int. 40, 59-63 (1986).
23. J. Ayalon, A. Simkin, I. Leichter, and S. Raifmann, Arch. Phys. Med. Rehabil. 68, 280-283 (1987).
24. M.K. White, R.B. Martin, R.A. Yeater, R.L. Butcher, and F.I. Radin, Intl. Orthop. 7, 209-214 (1984).
25. E.L. Smith, W. Reddan, and P.E. Smith, Med. Sci. Sports Exer. 13, 60-64 (1981).
26. A. Rundgren, A. Aniansson, P. Ljungberg, and H. Wetterqvist, Arch. Gerontol. Geriat. 3, 243-248 (1984).
27. J.A. Williams, J. Wagner, R. Wasnich, and L. Heilbrun, Med. Sci. Sports Exer. 16, 223-227 (1984).
28. R.K. Chow, J.E. Harrison, W. Sturtbridge, R. Josse, T.M. Murray, A. Bayley, J. Dornan, and T. Hammond, Clin. Invest. Med. 10, 59-63 (1987).
29. R.K. Chow, J.E. Harrison, and C. Notarius, Br. Med. J. 292, 607-610 (1987).
30. G.P. Dalsky, K.S. Stocke, A.A. Ehsani, E. Slatopolsky, W.C. Lee, and S.J. Birge, Ann. Intern. Med. 108, 824-828 (1988).
31. E.L. Smith and C. Gilligan, in: Bone and Mineral Research/6, W.A. Peck ed. (Elsevier, Amsterdam 1989) 139-173.
32. L.E. Lanyon, Topics Geriat. Rehab. 4, 13-24 (1989).
33. L.E. Lanyon and C.T. Rubin, J. Biomechanics 17, 897-905 (1984).
34. C.T. Rubin and L.E. Lanyon, Calcif. Tissue Int. 37, 411-417 (1985).
35. C.T. Rubin and L.E. Lanyon, J. Bone Joint. Surg. 66A, 397-402 (1984).
36. L.E. Lanyon, C.T. Rubin, and G. Baust, Calcif. Tissue Int. 38, 209-216 (1986).
37. M.J. Pead and L.E. Lanyon, Calcif. Tissue Int. (in press).

Calcium and Bone Loss in Postmenopausal Women

Bess Dawson-Hughes, Elizabeth A. Krall, and Gerard E. Dallal

Calcium and Bone Metabolism Laboratory, USDA Human Nutrition Research Center on Aging at Tufts University, Boston, Massachusetts

ABSTRACT

Despite increased research focus, there is currently no concensus on the relationship between calcium intake and the rate of age- or menopause-related loss of bone mass. In a pilot study, we noted that bone loss from the lumbar spine in 76 healthy postmenopausal women was greatest in those with low usual dietary intakes of calcium. We therefore recruited 360 healthy postmenopausal women with self-selected daily intakes generally under 650 mg into a longitudinal, placebo-controlled calcium intervention trial. The women were randomly assigned to either a placebo or one of two calcium treatment groups, each receiving 500 mg of elemental calcium as either calcium carbonate or calcium citrate malate. Baseline bone mineral density (BMD) of the spine (L2-4), hip, and radius, measured by single (SPA)- and dual-photon absorptiometry (DPA), was significantly influenced by years since last menses and by % reference weight. There was no association between calcium intake and BMD at these sites at the time of enrollment. The effect of increased calcium intake on the rate of bone loss from the spine, hip and radius is currently under investigation in this cohort.

INTRODUCTION

Calcium intake and its relationship to bone mineral status has been a popular subject over the last 5 years. With the population over the age of 65 years in the United States expected to double between the years of 1980 and 2030, loss of bone mass will become an increasingly common medical, social, and economic problem. Determination of safe and cost-effective means to retard bone loss and reduce the number of spontaneous fractures is appropriate. A number of factors contribute to loss of bone mineral. Of these, estrogen loss at menopause is the most important. Others include aging, weight, physical activity level, heredity, smoking, and use of alcohol and caffeine. Because of the large number and varying importance of factors known to influence bone mass, it is difficult to isolate the specific role of calcium.

There is general agreement that calcium alone is not an effective agent in building bone in osteoporotic patients who are fracturing. However, calcium is an important concommitant therapy. For example, calcium given along with fluoride prevents the osteomalacia which results from treatment with fluoride alone [1]. In addition, calcium along with estrogen may allow use of a lower dose of estrogen to achieve bone sparing.

There is little agreement at this time about the effectiveness of increased calcium intake in mitigating age- or menopause-related loss of bone mineral. This lack of concensus has been presented eloquently in two recent position papers, one concluding that the calcium deficiency model of bone loss is viable [2] and the other that calcium intake is not relevant to the development of osteoporosis [3,4]. The task of defining any role for calcium is made more difficult because of the slow and varied lifetime patterns of bone loss and because of variable self-selected calcium intakes within the populations of interest.

PATTERNS OF BONE LOSS

The effects of aging and menopause on bone loss have been reexamined in recent cross-sectional studies [5-7]. Gallagher et al observed that total bone mineral in women declined by 20% over a lifetime. Of this, 4.0% was lost prior to menopause, 10% was lost in the first 10 years after menopause and the remaining 6% thereafter [5]. A similar pattern of loss was observed for spine mineral [5]. Earlier estimates of lifetime bone loss of women were greater, around 40% [8]. Given the slow, chronic nature of bone loss in adult women and the state of current technology, large sample sizes are required to detect positive effects of any intervention in mitigating bone loss, particularly when those being studied are not in the perimenopausal period of more rapid bone loss. Although identification of an intervention which reduces the rate of bone loss from 0.7 to 0.4% per year, for example, is very difficult, such a modest reduction over many years should substantially postpone the time when a subject reaches the fracture threshhold. SPA- and DPA- determined bone mineral content (BMC) and fracture incidence have been inversely related in large population studies [9].

VARIABILITY IN EFFECT OF CALCIUM ON BONE LOSS

Calcium supplementation has been reported to retard loss of mineral from cortical sites in the appendicular skeleton in several controlled studies [10-12]. In one of these studies [10] the women were an average of 5 years since menopause and received 800 mg of calcium daily; however, their usual calcium intake was not reported. In another, women were 9 years since menopause, had mean self-selected calcium intake of 600 mg, and received 1 g of elemental calcium as a supplement [11]. In the third of these reports, [12], the women studied were perimenopausal (within 3 years of last menses), had a usual dietary calcium intake estimated at 1,000 mg [13], and received 2,000 mg of calcium as supplements daily. These data indicate that added calcium does not prevent but does mitigate bone mineral loss from the appendicular skeleton in both peri- and postmenopausal women. Furthermore, the benefit is not dependent upon a low usual calcium intake.

There are fewer published controlled studies of the effect of increased calcium intake on rate of bone loss from the central skeleton because the technology required to make the measurement is newer. Of the available methods, CT scanning of the lower thoracic and upper lumbar vertebrae measures the trabecular bone mineral content, and DPA and the newer dual-energy absorptiometry measure cortical and trabecular BMC of lumbar vertebrae. Riis et al reported the first controlled study of calcium supplementation and rate of lumbar spine mineral loss determined by DPA [12]. The study population was healthy women within 3 years since last menses and the treatment was 2 g of calcium daily. As indicated above, the usual calcium intake of the study population was approximately 1,000 mg daily [13]. During the 2 yr treatment period, rates of bone loss from the lumbar spine were similar in the calcium treated and placebo groups. Thus, in perimenopausal women, increasing calcium intake from 1,000 to 3,000 mg daily was of some benefit in curbing cortical bone loss (cited above) but of no benefit to the spine.

TABLE I. Pilot study - bone loss by quartile of calcium intake.

	1	2	3	4
Ca intake, mg	303±14.2[a]	488±11.8	652±14.6	1,032±47.7
Ca intake range, mg	198-405	409-565	572-761	777-1416
Years after menopause	12±1.9	13±2.2	13±1.8	13±1.9
% Reference wt	126±4.9	114±2.8	117±3.1	108±2.7
Tot vit D intake IU/d.	102±21[b]	118±13	135±18.5	262±20.7
Basal L2-4 BMD, g/cm^2	1.065±0.037	1.014±0.035	1.025±0.030	0.958±0.036
Change in L2-4 BMD, %	-3.4±1.5[c]	0.7±1.6	-1.1±1.6	1.2±1.4

[a] Mean ± SEM.   [b] Differs from quartile 4, p<0.001.
[c] Significant measured loss within quartile 1, p=0.02.

Table II. Longitudinal trial - correlations of physical characteristics with bone mineral density.

	Radius	L2-4	Femoral neck
n	324	308[a]	326
Years since last menses			
r	-0.378	-0.272	-0.187
p	<0.001	<0.001	0.001
1-5 years			
n	84	78	83
r	-0.216	-0.108	-0.142
p	0.048	ns	ns
slope[b]	-9.7±4.8	-9.1±9.6	-10.5±8.2
5-30 years			
n	240	230	243
r	-0.262	-0.196	-0.156
p	<0.001	0.003	0.015
slope[b]	-3.6±0.8	-5.1±1.7	-2.9±1.2
% Reference wt			
r	0.249	0.402	0.414
p	<0.001	<0.001	<0.001

[a] Sample size is smaller because truncal thickness measurements needed to correct for drift were not available in all women.

[b] Slope ± SE in 10^{-3} gm/cm^2/year. Differences between slopes at each bone measurement site are not significant.

Currently no randomized, controlled, calcium-treatment studies of populations with low usual intakes of calcium have been reported. Given the obligatory urinary and endogenous fecal losses of calcium, there must be an intake below which more calcium in the diet is beneficial. This critical intake would be expected to vary greatly among individuals and to be affected by their absorption capacity (which is known to vary with aging), adequacy of vitamin D intake, diet composition, gastric acidity, renal function, and other variables.

CALCIUM SUPPLEMENT FIELD TRIAL

Pilot Study

In preparation for a prospective calcium-intervention trial, we first performed a pilot study which was designed to determine the variability in the rate of bone mineral loss from the spine [14]. This information was needed to estimate the sample size required for a trial. Seventy-six healthy postmenopausal women completed the pilot study. None had diseases associated with altered bone loss or evidence of vertebral fracture on spine radiographs. None used calcium supplements, estrogen,

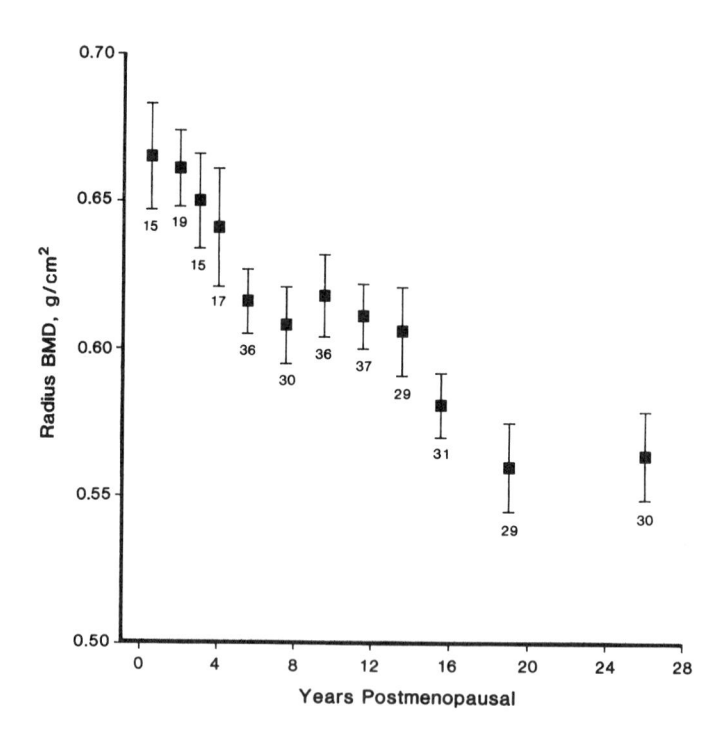

Figure 1. Radius (1/3 distal) density (mean $\pm$ 1 SE) for postmenopausal women in the following groups: 1, 2, 3, 4, 5-6, 7-8, 9-10, 11-12, 13-14, 15-16, 17-21 and 22-30 years since last menses. Subject number is given for each group.

or steroids prior to or during the study. Their usual dietary calcium intake at enrollment ranged from 198 to 1,416 mg daily. Loss of BMD from the spine in the 76 women stratified by quartile of calcium intake is shown in Table I [14]. Women with an intake below 400 mg daily incurred significant bone loss over a 7-month period and lost at a greater rate than did women with an intake of over 777 mg. The women with low calcium intake also had lower vitamin D intake. Any contribution of the latter to their accelerated bone loss can not be determined in this study. Bone loss of the women in relation to time since menopause was not evaluated in this study. Barden et al found that low calcium intake (<595 mg daily) was associated with slightly decreased BMD in the spine, radius and femur in normal premenopausal women [15]. In a study of a mixed group of pre-, peri- and postmenopausal women, rates of loss of BMD were similar in women in the lowest (mean, 501 mg) and highest (mean, 1,397 mg) quartiles of calcium intake [16]. In these 3 studies correlations between calcium intake and both bone mass [14-16] and bone loss [16] were not significant.

Longitudinal Trial-Baseline Measurements

To identify whether more calcium is beneficial in retarding loss of bone mineral from the spine in peri- and postmenopausal women with low

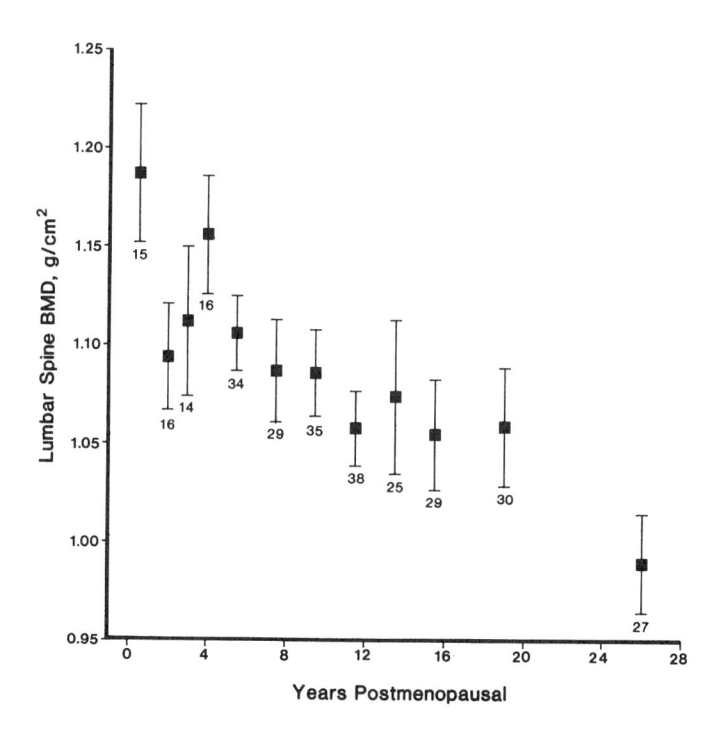

Figure 2. Lumbar spine (L2-4) density (mean ± 1 SE) for postmenopausal women grouped as described in Figure 1.

usual calcium intakes, a double-blind, 2-year, calcium-intervention trial is being conducted. Each woman had normal screening laboratory tests and no history of disorders associated with altered bone metabolism. None had a history of estrogen or glucocorticoid use and no evidence of a compression fracture on spine roentenogram. Of the 360 postmenopausal women participating, approximately one quarter were within 5 years since last menses at enrollment. Women with low usual calcium intakes (<650 mg except for 9 subjects who ingested between 651 and 900 mg) were recruited and randomly assigned to a placebo or to 1 of 2 calcium treatment groups (each receiving 500 mg of calcium, as either calcium citrate malate or calcium carbonate). Calcium with the naturally occurring fruit acids, citrate and malate, was selected because absorption of calcium from this form is excellent in the populations tested [17,18]; the carbonate was selected because it is widely used. Bone mass measurements are being made at enrollment and after 1 and 2 years of treatment.

Bone mineral density of the nondominant radius (1/3 distal site), lumbar spine, and femoral neck in relation to years since menopause at the time of enrollment are shown in Figures 1-3. Values are given for those women with good scans and in whom years since menopause could be determined. Women treated for hypothyroidism who had abnormal thyroid stimulating hormone levels were also excluded. Radius measurements were

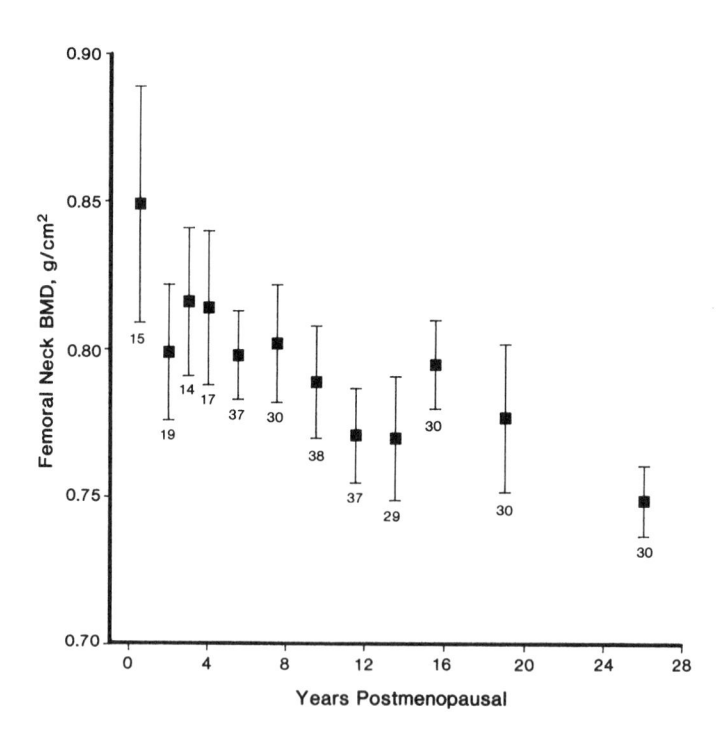

Figure 3. Femoral neck density (mean ± 1SE) for postmenopausal women grouped as described in Figure 1.

Table III. Longitudinal trial - calcium intake and baseline bone mineral density.

	Quartile of calcium intake			
	1	2	3	4
N	85	82	83	83
Ca intake, mg	210±65[a]	361±33	462±34	599±64
Ca intake range, mg	58-296	299-408	409-523	524-926
Years since last menses	11.0±6.9	10.8±6.6	10.5±6.9	11.1±6.8
% Reference wt	119±22	119±19	117±17	118±19
Caloric intake, kcal/day	1,555±440	1,660±426	1,664±366	1,643±405
BMD, g/cm^2				
Spine (L2-4)	1.086±0.152 (78)[b]	1.078±0.144 (76)	1.067±0.133 (78)	1.089±0.146 (76)
Femoral neck	0.793±0.106 (83)	0.784±0.105 (82)	0.772±0.102 (79)	0.808±0.110 (82)
Radius	0.620±0.080 (85)	0.600±0.083 (80)	0.604±0.071 (79)	0.609±0.077 (80)

[a] Mean ± S.D.
[b] Values in parentheses indicate study number if different from above.

made with an SP-2 model SPA (Lunar Radiation Corp, Madison, WI) by the method of Cameron and Sorenson [19]. Spine measurements were made on a DP-3 model DPA from Lunar Radiation Corp and analyzed with software version 08B. All spine BMD values were corrected for inter- and intra-gadolinium variation and for truncal thickness-related drift with the use of an external standard, as described previously [20]. Femoral neck measurements were also made on the DPA scanner. Correlations between BMD and years since menopause and % reference weight in these subjects are given in Table II. As expected, years since menopause is a significant predictor of bone mass. To estimate whether the rate of loss varied in the early menopausal period, we performed separate regression analyses in those within 5 and those over 5 years since menopause. Although the slopes of the decrease in bone mass at all three measurement sites tended to be greater in the 0-5 than in the over 5 year group, the differences in the slopes were not significant for any site. A more accurate estimate of the effect of menopause on rate of bone loss can be made with the longitudinal data.

Percent reference weight is a strong predictor of radius, spine and hip BMD in these women (Table II). The importance of weight in this population has been reported previously [21] and recently emphasized by Stevenson [22]. The relative contributions of fat and lean body mass in predicting BMD in the elderly are not yet established. There is reason to believe that both are important. For example, muscle and bone mass are closely linked in women and decline at similar rates with aging [23]. On the other hand, adipocytes convert androstenedione to estrone, the major postmenopausal estrogen and one expected to enhance bone sparing.

Finally, baseline BMD and other clinical and laboratory parameters are examined in relation to quartile of dietary calcium intake at enrollment (Table III). Calcium and intake was assessed by food frequency questionnaire and calorie intake by 3-day diet records. There were no significant differences among the quartiles in a number of parameters known to affect bone mass, including years since last menses, % reference weight, and calorie intake. The similarities in caloric intake and % reference weight suggest that physical activity levels among the quartiles did not differ. There were no differences in baseline BMD of the spine, hip or radius among the quartiles. This lack of association emphasizes the point that any effect of calcium in this population is likely to be subtle.

Although their baseline BMD is not related to recent dietary calcium intake, it remains to be learned whether rates of loss of bone mineral in these peri- and postmenopausal women are influenced by increased calcium intake.

ACKNOWLEDGEMENTS

This work was supported by the USDA (Contract No. 53-3K06-5-10) and by the Procter and Gamble Company.

REFERENCES

1. J.E. Compston, S. Chadha and A.L. Merrett, Brit Med J 281 910-911 (1980).
2. B.E.C. Nordin and H.A. Morris, Nutrition Reviews 47 65-72 (1989).
3. J.A. Kanis and R. Passmore, Br Med J 298 137-140 (1989).
4. J.A. Kanis and R. Passmore, Br Med J 298 205-208 (1989).
5. J.C. Gallagher, D. Goldgar, and A. Moy, J Bone Min Res 2, 491-96 (1987).
6. A. Gotfredsen, A. Hadberg, L. Nilas and C. Christiansen, J Lab Clin Chem 110 362-368 (1987).
7. P.J.M. Elders, J.C. Netelenbos, P. Lips, F.C. van Ginkel and P.F. van der Stelt, Bone and Min 5 11-19 (1988).
8. B.L. Riggs, H.W. Wahner, W.L. Dunn, R. B. Mazess, and K.P. Offord, J Clin Invest 67 328-335 (1981).
9. P.D. Ross, R.D. Wasnich and J.M. Vogel, J Bone Min Res 3 1-11 (1988).
10. A. Horsman, J.C. Gallagher, M. Simpson and B.E.C. Nordin, Br Med J 2 789-792 (1977).
11. R.R. Recker, P.D. Saville and R.P. Heaney, Ann Int Med 87 649-655 (1977).
12. B. Riis, K. Thomsen and C. Christiansen, N Engl J Med 316 173-177 (1987).
13. R. Pacifici and L.V. Avioli, New Engl J Med 317 1025 (1987).
14. B. Dawson-Hughes, P. Jacques and C. Shipp, Am J Clin Nutr 46 685-687 (1987).
15. H.S. Barden, G.M. Green and R.B. Mazess, J Bone Min Res 1 (Suppl 1) abstr 64 (1988).
16. B.L. Riggs, H.W. Wahner, L.J. Melton III, L.S. Richelson, H.L. Judd and W. M. O'Fallon, J Clin Invest 80 979-82 (1987).
17. K.T. Smith, R.P. Heaney, L. Flora and S.M. Hinders, Calcif Tissue Int 41 351-352 (1987).
18. J.Z. Miller, D.L. Smith, L. Flora, C. Slamenda, X. Jiang and C.C. Johnston, Jr., Am J Clin Nutr 48 1291-1294 (1988).
19. J.R. Cameron and J. Sorenson, Science 142 230-232 (1963).
20. B. Dawson-Hughes, M.S. Deehr, P.S. Berger, G.E. Dallal and L.J, Sadowski, Calcif Tissue Int 44 251-257 (1989).
21. B. Dawson-Hughes, C. Shipp, L. Sadowski and G. Dallsl, Calcif Tissue Int 40 310-314, 1987.
22. J.C. Stevenson, B. Lees, M. Davenport, M.P. Cust and K.F. Ganger, Br Med J 298 924-928 (1989).
23. S.H. Cohn, A. Vaswani, I. Zanzi, J.F. Aloia, M.S. Roginsky, and K.J. Ellis. Metabolism 25 85-96 (1976).

Calcium Requirements

Robert P. Heaney

Creighton University, Omaha, Nebraska

ABSTRACT

Calcium intake is required for skeletal growth up to about age 30, and to offset excretory losses at all ages. New data on calcium absorption efficiency and obligatory excretion at different life stages, and on continued bone mass accumulation in the 10–12 years after completion of growth, permit re-evaluation of current estimates for intake requirements.

Growth up to age 12 adds 100 mg Ca/day to bone. Absorption and excretory loss during childhood are such that this need can be met with an intake of 500–600 mg Ca/day. While the RDA would be somewhat higher, the current US value for children (800 mg) seems adequate.

During adolescence, growth consumes an average of 230–250 mg Ca/day, and at the peak of the growth spurt, 360–400 mg. At prevailing rates of obligatory loss and absorption, these demands require an average intake across adolescence of 1000–1200 mg Ca/day, or at the growth spurt, about 1500 mg/day. Thus, by either criterion, the RDA should be substantially higher than the current US value (1200 mg). From age 18 to 30, the RDA needs to be about 1000 mg to accommodate the slow bone accumulation that is still occurring then.

In the absence of pregnancy or lactation, it is likely that a lower RDA will suffice from age 30 to 50. Since estrogen enhances calcium absorption and decreases excretory losses, a woman is probably most tolerant of low intakes at this period of life. At menopause, bone mass falls as a result of estrogen loss; the calcium transiently released thereby meets homeostatic needs independently of intake. Thus, most women exhibit calcium resistance in the early postmenopause. However later, without ERT, intestinal absorption falls and obligatory loss rises. As a result, the mean requirement rises to about 1100 mg/day. Adolescence and senescence are, thus, the times of highest calcium requirement in a woman's life.

INTRODUCTION

Under steady state conditions of health, the requirement for a nutrient is that quantity which must be ingested both to provide for tissue growth (when applicable) and to offset metabolic degradation and/or excretion. For calcium, of course, there is no metabolic degradation, so only growth and excretion need to be provided for.

The need of calcium for growth is conceptually straightforward and is reflected in the generally higher values of the recommended dietary allowances (RDAs) that most nations have adopted for adolescents and for pregnant or lactating women [1]. In the United States these values are 1200 mg Ca/day for both groups [2] (and higher still when both conditions occur in the same woman). However, the standards are surprisingly different for different nations. For example they range from a low of 500 mg for adolescents in Hungary to 1400 mg in the USSR [1]. National differences in requirements for calcium during growth can be explained only in part by genetic differences in growth potential of the respective populations or by growth limitations imposed by availability of other nutrients.

While the need for calcium during growth is generally accepted – at whatever level the RDA may be set – the need for a maintenance intake to offset excretory and other losses has been less universally acknowledged. These losses are of three sorts: dermal, urinary, and intestinal. Whatever the route, such loss must be offset by absorption of ingested calcium if an individual is to maintain calcium balance.

DETERMINATION OF THE REQUIREMENT FOR CALCIUM

Intake and Retention. The relation between intake, excretory loss, and retention of calcium is complicated, inasmuch as both absorption and excretion are themselves related to intake, to some extent in a non-linear manner. In brief, as intake rises, absorption fraction falls and both urinary and endogenous fecal losses rise. As a result, an increase in intake of 1000 mg in an individual with a 30 percent absorption efficiency would not increase net absorption by 300 mg, but by a substantially smaller amount, and retention by a smaller amount still. Enough is now known about these relationships to permit theoretical calculation of the intake required for any specified level of retention. Still, such a calculation would not be likely to attract scientific acceptance were it not for the fact that its conclusions are supported by recent observational data. In what follows I shall review first the empirical relation between intake and absorption, and then between absorption and excretion.

Wilkinson gathered published data concerning net absorption from 212 balances in normal individuals [3], and found, for intakes above 500 mg/day, a slope of net absorption on intake close to +0.110. In over 500 studies of our own in healthy perimenopausal women, we found a value of +0.096. These very similar values mean that net absorption rises by only about 10 percent of an increment in intake. While a fraction this low may seem an inefficient arrangement, it can help to put this relationship in perspective if we note that current estimates of the natural calcium intake for the human species, according to Eaton and Konner [4], are in excess of 1500 mg/day. Thus the system may well have been designed (or have evolved) to deal with relative surplus rather than with relative deficiency.

The relation of intake to retention is even less efficient. Both in the extensive studies of Nordin [5] and in our own work [6,7], the slope of urinary calcium on intake in mature women is approximately +0.06. Thus, with roughly 10 percent of an intake increment absorbed, and 6 percent excreted in the urine, it follows that only about 4 percent will be retained (exclusive of dermal losses). In fact, this is almost exactly the value we have found empirically in our own studies for the slope of measured balance on intake [6,7].

Obligatory Loss. Obligatory loss consists of calcium secretion and excretion that is either not controlled by any known component of the calcium regulatory apparatus or would continue even in the face of calcium deficiency. Non-excretory losses are a particularly important component of obligatory loss, because they are so often ignored in computations concerning the calcium economy. Dermal losses in the form of sweat and desquamated epithelium are a good example. They amount to 15–25 mg/day under sedentary conditions, and are known to be higher under exercising conditions. This figure needs to be augmented by hair, nail, and various non-excretory, secretory losses, and may total up to 60 mg/day [8]. At prevailing adult levels of absorption efficiency, this non-excretory loss adds perhaps as much as 420–550 mg/day to the intake requirement.

Quantitatively somewhat larger are the excretory losses, and particularly that component which may properly be considered obligatory. "Obligatory" for these losses, as for the dermal route, means losses that occur even under conditions of calcium conservation, such as urinary calcium excretion after an overnight fast or on a low calcium intake. While some women can reduce fasting urinary loss to extremely low levels, not all can do so. Sodium and protein intakes are major determinants of obligatory calcium loss through the kidney, and caffeine a minor one. There are probably many others as well. Inter-population differences in apparent requirement may reflect differences in intake of these other nutrients, with their associated effect on obligatory loss in the urine.

Also obligatory is the calcium contained in the digestive juices and in desquamated intestinal epithelium, neither of which is related to ECF [Ca^{++}] nor to circulating PTH. Together they may be thought of as the calcium cost of digestion [9]. This digestive juice calcium averages about 140 mg/day in adult women [10]. While some of this amount is reabsorbed along with food calcium, at absorption fractions typical of the adult US female, most is lost in the feces. For this reason digestive juice calcium can be a substantial route of loss, particularly when absorption efficiency is low. This is also the reason why net absorption can even be negative at low intakes or low absorption efficiencies.

Table 1 summarizes these relationships and expresses them in concrete form, namely, as the ingested calcium intakes required to produce equilibrium for four arbitrarily selected (but typical) levels of obligatory loss, and for various levels of absorption efficiency. The equation used in these calculations, derived from the studies previously cited, is as follows:

$$\text{Required Intake} = \frac{\text{TIC} + \text{Net Abs} - \text{Absfx}*(\text{Prox})}{\text{Absfx}},$$

where TIC = total intestinal calcium secretion (in mg/day), Net Abs = the difference between ingested intake and fecal output (in mg/day), Absfx = fractional absorption, and Prox = that portion of the TIC – generally 80–85 percent – secreted sufficiently orad to be absorbed at the efficiency of food calcium [10]. In all these calculations, typical adult levels of digestive juice calcium secretion are presumed (140 mg/day TIC; 115 mg/day Prox).

Table 1. Intakes Required for Calcium Equilibrium (mg/day)

Absorption Fraction	Extraintestinal Obligatory Loss (mg Ca/day)			
	100	150	200	250
0.20	1085	1335	1585	1835
0.25	845	1045	1245	1445
0.30	685	852	1018	1185
0.35	571	714	856	999
0.40	485	610	735	860

The values in Table 1 show dramatically the importance not just of absorption efficiency, but of obligatory loss. What the Table cannot directly show, however, is the adjustments that must be made when obligatory loss changes (for example, an increase from 150 to 200 mg/day). Thus, at an absorption efficiency of 0.25, the table shows that the intake required to offset such an increased loss would rise by 200 mg (from 1045 to 1245 mg). But this obtains only if absorption fraction remains constant, which, unfortunately does not occur. Instead, as intake rises, absorption efficiency falls, and while more calcium is absorbed, the absorption fraction is lower. If, for the sake of illustration, we assume that fractional absorption drops only 10 percent (i.e., to 0.225), then, applying the foregoing equation, the required intake is no longer 1245 mg/day, but 1396, or an overall increment in required intake of c. 350 mg just to offset an increase in obligatory loss of 50 mg/day. This is a ratio of 7:1. Empirical data, previously cited, suggest that the ratio may be even higher (i.e., as much as 9:1 or 10:1).

Application. Recent studies of factors influencing obligatory losses, as well as of absorptive performance itself, have added significantly to the understanding of the maintenance requirement and have shown, as well, that this requirement changes at different life stages. Further, new epidemiological data show that low life-long calcium intakes increase hip fracture risk two- to threefold [11,12], underscoring the practical importance of assuring an adequate calcium intake throughout life, and putting to rest – one would hope – the dangerous notion that, practically speaking, there is no calcium deficiency state in humans [13].

In what follows I review current evidence in regard to calcium requirement during three life stages: skeletal accumulation, maturity, and involution. My focus is exclusively on women – because they have been studied far more extensively than men, because they carry a much greater osteoporosis burden than do men, and because, in the US at least, their calcium intakes average 40 percent lower than those of men [14].

CALCIUM REQUIREMENT AT VARIOUS LIFE-STAGES

Skeletal Accumulation

Skeletal mass accumulation extends from birth, past the completion of linear growth at roughly 16–18 years, to approximately age 30.

Childhood. From birth to age 10–12 bone mass increases from an average of 25 g to about 390–450 g. The increase is approximately linear and thus daily retention averages about 100 mg. Recent isotope-based studies in children indicate that absorption efficiency averages 40–45 percent [18]. Endogenous fecal losses in children have not been measured, but may be estimated from body size, since body size is known to be one of their determinants in adults. Taking a conservative estimate for excretory and dermal losses of 100–150 mg/day, it follows that an intake of 550–650 mg/day should suffice to meet the needs of bone growth during childhood. Allowing for interindividual variation leads to an estimated RDA value close to the present US figure (800 mg for children up to age 12), which must thus be judged to be adequate.

Adolescence. During adolescence, skeletal growth accelerates, and at the peak of the adolescent growth spurt requires daily retention of 360–400 mg [19]. Even averaged over the years from 12–18, daily retention must be 230–250 mg, or better than twice the rate during childhood. Oddly, the calcium economy changes for the worse at this time of greatest need: absorption efficiency falls from the childhood high, and at the same time excretory losses rise. Newly available, isotope-based studies of absorption fraction in adolescents in their mid-teens yield values in the 30–35 percent range [20], and no estimates in contemporary adolescents from any source are higher than 40–45 percent [18,21]. Further, obligatory losses, principally through the urine, are relatively high (180–220 mg/day [21]). It seems paradoxical that utilization efficiency for calcium should fall at the time of greatest need, and it may be that the explanation for this change in US adolescent women needs to be sought in concomitant changes in other dietary or lifestyle factors.

Whatever the explanation, this performance has obvious implications for calcium requirement. To retain enough calcium to mineralize the growing skeleton and to offset known excretory losses as well requires, at prevailing absorption efficiencies, a *mean* intake close to 1200 mg/day throughout adolescence. This is the value for the present RDA. Thus, allowing for population variances, the adolescent RDA should be higher still – perhaps 1400–1500 mg. This conclusion is supported by the balance studies of Matkovic *et al.* [21] in which increasing dietary calcium from 250 to 1600 mg/day in adolescent females produced a *non*significant increase in urine calcium. This finding strongly suggests that, even at an intake of 1600 mg/day, the capacity of the growing skeleton to utilize dietary calcium has not been saturated.

Young Adulthood. Skeletal accumulation continues from age 20 to about age 30, though at a slower rate. There had been some thought in recent years that bone mass, rather than continuing to increase, actually started to decline as early as age 20. This suggestion was based mainly on cross-sectional studies of spine bone mass at that age that seemed to show a decline after age 20 [15], but a recent longitudinal study by Davies *et al.* has shown a clear *increase* in bone mass, even at the spine, between ages 20 and 30 [16]. In this study spine BMC increased at a rate of about 7 percent per decade, and if this value is extrapolated to the whole skeleton, it computes to a retention of about 20 mg/day. Garn's cortical data [17] would suggest a slightly higher daily retention rate. So a 20 mg figure is a conservative one. At the same time it should be noted that the mean calcium intake of the young women in the Davies study was 760 mg/day, which is less than the foregoing calculations indicate is optimal, and hence it is possible that an even higher accumulation rate might have been found had the intake been higher.

Absorption efficiency has been extensively studied in this age group, and is known to average about 32 percent. Obligatory losses average 200 mg/day, and hence, taking a conservative estimate for skeletal retention of 20 mg/day, a mean intake of 900–1000 mg should suffice. Again, making allowance for population variation in absorption and excretion, the RDA should probably be 1200 mg through age 30.

Maturity

In the absence of pregnancy and lactation, a woman's requirement from age 30 to time of menopause is probably the lowest since childhood. Absorption averages 30–35 percent and extraintestinal excretory losses, 150–200 mg/day, values that translate to a *mean* requirement of 600–700 mg/day. Nordin's balance data [5] point to an only slightly lower figure, 500–600 mg/day. Hence the two estimates are essentially congruent. Both lead to a calculated RDA for this age of 800–1000 mg.

Involution

Involutional bone loss in women has two major components. The first is related to estrogen withdrawal (either at time of menopause, or after termination of estrogen replacement therapy), and is self-limited. The same kind of rapid bone loss occurs in young women who become estrogen deficient for any reason, and has been reported as well for castrated males. It is as if the skeleton has different mass set-points for the hormone-replete and hormone-deprived states, and the bone loss that occurs immediately following gonadal hormone withdrawal represents a transition from one steady state to another. This transition can be approximated by an exponential function, with very rapid loss occurring in the first 1–3 years [23]. To the extent that such a model is accurate, this bone loss can be said to be intrinsic, and thus to have essentially no extrinsic (i.e., nutritional) cause.

Estrogen-withdrawal bone loss is at best only partially offset by such modalities as high calcium intake, and exercise.* In the case of calcium, this is because, for a short period of time, a great deal of calcium is made available from the downward revision of skeletal mass. Since a calcium ion loses its identity once it enters the extracellular fluid, the homeostatic system cannot tell whether the calcium it sees has come from bone or from diet. Hence, practically speaking, there may be only a very low requirement for calcium ingestion during this brief period of life. That realization helps to explain why it has been so difficult to see a calcium effect in immediately postmenopausal women [7].

The second component of involutional loss is a slower, but continuing process that is probably due in part to such factors as decreased mechanical loading, decreased muscle mass, accumulation of structural errors, and, in some women, nutritional deficiency. Within probably five years after menopause, when bone approaches its new equilibrium mass, the calcium economy gradually becomes more dependent upon external factors once again. At this life-stage an estrogen-deprived woman is put at two additional disadvantages. Estrogen lack results in a fall in absorption efficiency, amounting to about a 7 percent reduction from immediate premenopausal levels [24]. At the same time urinary calcium loss increases [5,6].** Since calcium requirement is a function of the balance between absorbed intake and obligatory losses, it follows inexorably that a

---

* Curiously such loss is minimal or non-existent in obese women [22] and may be less in blacks as well [Garn, SM, personal communication].

** These steady state effects need to be understood as quite distinct from the transient effect of estrogen loss on bone mass. They not only persist but dominate the scene after the new, hormone-deficient skeletal steady state is achieved.

simultaneous deterioration in both absorption and excretion will lead to an increased requirement. In a very large group of studies from my laboratory [6,7], in which both calcium balances and double-isotope absorption methods were employed, the estrogen-deprivation effect appears to increase the calcium requirement by about 500 mg/day [7]. This observation is part of the reason for the recommended intakes of both by the NIH Consensus Development Conference on Osteoporosis [25], and the National Osteoporosis Foundation [26].

Table 2 summarizes the foregoing requirement estimates for the various life stages.

Table 2. Estimated Calcium Requirements in US Women

Life stage	Mean Requirements (mg/day)	Estimated RDA (mg/day)
Skeletal Accumulation:		
1–12	500–600	800
12–18	1200	1500
18–30	800–1000	1200
Maturity:*		
30–mpse	600–800	800–1000
Involution:		
Mpse + 5 y	?	?
Senescence	1000–1200	1500+

*non-pregnant, non-lactating women

COMMENT

Requirement varies with stage of growth, with physiological drains (e.g., pregnancy and lactation), and with factors that influence absorption and excretory loss (e.g., gonadal hormone status and sodium and protein intakes). While for certain life-stages the cited requirement values are higher than currently recommended, they are below the intakes of both contemporary hunter-gatherers [4] and our closest primate relatives (adjusted for body size). Hence, they can be considered high only in comparison with current US practices. However, it also needs to be emphasized that bone health is a multifactorial affair and that meeting calcium requirements alone will neither guarantee optimal bone growth nor protect against bone loss if other critical factors are missing. For example, calcium affords only minimal protection against either immobilization or estrogen-withdrawal bone loss. Thus, while assuring an adequate calcium intake remains a sound strategy, it cannot be considered a panacea.

REFERENCES

1. Recommended Dietary Intakes Around the World. Nutr. Abstracts and Reviews in Clinical Nutrition 53 (11), 939-1015 (1983).
2. Recommended Dietary Allowances, Committee on Dietary Allowances, Food and Nutrition Board, Commission of Life Sciences, National Research Council. 9th ed. Washington DC: National Academy Press (1980).
3. R. Wilkinson, in: Calcium, Phosphate and Magnesium Metabolism, B.E.C. Nordin, ed. (Churchill Livingstone, London 1976) pp. 36-112.
4. S.B. Eaton and M. Konner, N. Engl. J. Med. 312, 283-289 (1985).
5. B.E.C. Nordin, K.J. Polley, A.G. Need, H.A. Morris, and D. Marshall, Am. J. Clin. Nutr. 45, 1295-1304 (1987).
6. R.P. Heaney, R.R. Recker, and P.D. Saville, J. Lab. Clin. Med. 92, 953-963 (1978).
7. R.P. Heaney, Public Health Reports S104, (1989).
8. F.T. Jensen, P. Charles, L. Mosekilde, and H.H. Hansen, Clin. Physiol. 3, 187-204 (1983).
9. R.P. Heaney and R.R. Recker, Am. J. Clin. Nutr. 43, 299-305 (1986).
10. R.P. Heaney and T.G. Skillman, J. Lab. Clin. Med. 64, 21-28 (1964).
11. V. Matkovic, K. Kostial, I. Simonovic, R. Buzina, A. Brodarec, and B.E.C. Nordin, Am. J. Clin. Nutr. 32, 540-549 (1979).
12. T.L. Holbrook, E. Barrett-Connor, and D.L. Wingard, Lancet 2, 1046-1049 (1988).
13. J.A. Kanis and M. Passmore, Br. Med. J. 298, 137-140, 205-208 (1989).
14. National Center for Health Statistics, M.D. Carroll, S. Abraham, and C.M. Dresser: Dietary intake source data: United States, 1976-80. Vital and Health Statistics. Series 11-No. 231. DHHS Pub. No. (PHS) 83-1681. Public Health Service. Washington. U.S. Government Printing Office, March 1983.
15. B.L. Riggs, H.W. Wahner, E. Seeman, K.P. Offord, W.L. Dunn, R.B. Mazess, K.A. Johnson, and L.J. Melton, III, J. Clin. Invest. 70, 716-723 (1982).
16. K.M. Davies, R.R. Recker, M.R. Stegman, R.P. Heaney, D.B. Kimmel, and J. Leist. J. Bone Min. Res. (in press) (1989).
17. S.M. Garn, The earlier gain and the later loss of cortical bone. (Charles C Thomas, Springfield, Illinois 1970).
18. J.Z. Miller, D.L. Smith, L. Flora, M. Peacock, and C.C. Johnston, Jr., Clinica Chimica Acta (in press) (1989).
19. I. Leitch and F.C. Aitken. Nutr. Abstracts and Reviews 29, 393-407 (1959).
20. J.Z. Miller, D.L. Smith, L. Flora, C. Slemenda, X. Jiang, and C.C. Johnston, Jr., Am. J. Clin. Nutr. 48, 1291-1294 (1988).
21. V. Matkovic, D. Fontana, C. Tominac, P. Goel, and C.C. Chesnut, III, Am. J. Clin. Nutr. (submitted) (1989).
22. C. Ribot, F. Tremollieres, J-M. Pouilles, M. Bonneu, F. Germain, and J-P. Louvet, Bone 8, 327-331 (1987).
23. R.P. Heaney, Bone and Mineral (submitted) (1989).

24. R.P. Heaney, R.R. Recker, M.R. Stegman, and A.J. Moy, J. Bone Min. Res. (in press) Aug. (1989).
25. National Institutes of Health Osteoporosis Consensus Development Conference Statement. JAMA 252, 799-802 (1984).
26. National objectives for disease prevention and health promotion for the year 2000. National Osteoporosis Foundation (1988).

ADFR

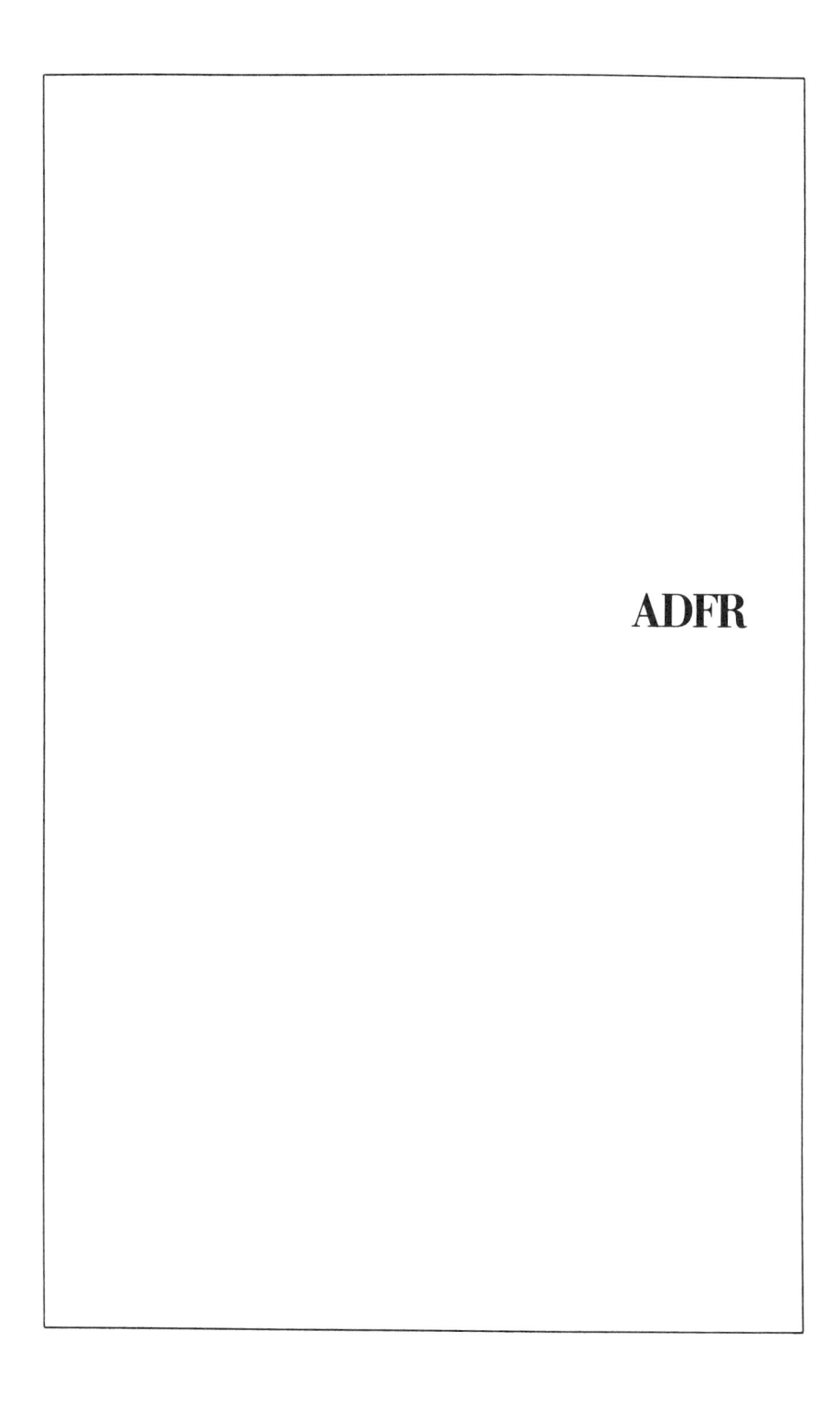

ADFR, or Coherence Therapy, for Osteoporosis

A.M. Parfitt,

Bone and Mineral Research Laboratory, Henry Ford Hospital, Detroit, Michigan

ABSTRACT

Bone remodeling cycles in different locations are normally out of step or incoherent. Frost proposed giving an activator of remodeling as a brief pulse followed by a depressor of osteoclast function, in the hope that many cycles would be initiated simultaneously and evolve coherently, and the new osteoclast teams constrained to resorb shallower cavities. If the subsequent new osteoblast teams made the same amount of bone as normal, a net gain in bone volume would result. Activation can be increased in several ways, but validation of the other steps is lacking. Patients with the osteoblast defect of osteoporosis in its most severe form could lose more bone following the activation than could be recovered during the remainder of the cycle, particularly if a trabecular plate is perforated. Published clinical trials using phosphate as an activator and sodium etidronate as a depressor have disregarded Frost's recommendation by using calcium with or without estrogen in the free period; not surprisingly the results have been conflicting. Many regimens called ADFR or coherence therapy bear even less resemblance to Frost's conception. The beneficial results of cyclical etidronate administration depend on sustained reduction in remodeling activation; they have no bearing on the validity of Frost's concept, but highlight a potential hazard. Because crucial experiments have been omitted and clinical trials begun prematurely, 10 years after its first description we still do not know if ADFR will work.

INTRODUCTION AND BACKGROUND

In all branches of medicine most treatment regimens consist of continuous administration of one or more agents. Many continuous regimens have been applied to osteoporosis, but few have proved useful. Several features of the skeleton may have limited the effectiveness of this approach, including the long time scale of bone remodeling, the intrinsic life-long negative balance on the endosteal envelope and the sequential nature of bone remodeling and its regulation by changing the size of cell populations rather than the activity of differentiated cells [1,2]. Most pharmacologic interventions in osteoporosis depress remodeling activation and retard bone loss, but do not add bone except for the small and non-sustained effect of reducing the reversible mineral deficit associated with remodeling [3]. But if fracture risk is already high, reducing it to a worthwhile extent requires a substantial increase in bone strength.

Pending greater understanding of the qualitative aspects of bone fragility, a substantial increase in amount of bone is necessary, which might be more successfully achieved with intermittent or sequential than with continuous treatment [4,5].

Normally, bone formation occurs only at locations where bone resorption has recently been completed, and after age 30 each remodeling episode puts back less bone than was removed (by about 10%) on the endosteal envelope. Reversing the normal endosteal negative balance requires some combination of diminishing the depth of resorption cavities and increasing the thickness of new packets of bone deposited within them. It is both a necessary and a sufficient condition for bone gain that wall thickness exceeds resorption depth. This has been accomplished on the cancellous surface by sodium fluoride, human parathyroid hormone, and several types of cyclical regimen; in each case it is likely that some of the added bone is formed at the expense of accelerated loss from the endocortical and intracortical surfaces [2].

OTHER INTERMITTENT AND SEQUENTIAL REGIMENS

It is important to distinguish between intermittent administration of a single agent alone, the same in combination with another agent given continuously, sequential administration of two agents, and coherence therapy as originally conceived and defined by Frost [5]. An example of the first method is giving sodium etidronate for two weeks followed by a rest period of 13 weeks and continuing the cycles as often as needed to obtain a satisfactory response. In a controlled trial, this treatment led to a significant increase in spinal bone mineral measured by dual energy photon absorptiometry (DPA) [6]. The response was similar in timing and magnitude to that observed with continuous administration of calcitonin [7], and presumably was mainly the result of a sustained fall in remodeling activation, possibly due to prolonged binding of bisphosphonates to bone surfaces. However, cyclical etidronate reduces the rate of vertebral deformation [6], an effect not yet demonstrated with calcitonin.

An example of the second method is daily supplemental phosphate combined with intermittent calcitonin [8,9]. The theory was that phosphate would both stimulate osteoblasts and increase endogenous parathyroid hormone (PTH) secretion, which in turn would increase the rate of remodeling activation and bone turnover, while intermittent calcitonin would depress the activity of osteoclasts but not the activation of remodeling, so that cell recruitment would continue. This treatment has been shown in a controlled trial to increase cancellous bone mass measured in iliac bone biopsies, and to retard appendicular cortical bone loss measured by single photon absorptiometry [8]. No data on axial bone density, or on vertebral or long bone fracture rates have been reported. The histologic effects of this regimen [9] will subsequently be examined in more detail.

An example of sequential administration is sodium fluoride and calcium given alternately for six month periods instead of continuously in combination [10]. The basis was the observation that the increase in osteoblast number in response to fluoride peaked at 6-9 months [11], together with suggestive evidence of osteoblast toxicity after several years of continuous therapy [12]. Short-term results of uncontrolled trials appeared promising [10], but long-term results have been equivocal [13]. A more complex example is giving sustained released sodium fluoride, calcidiol and calcium for three months, followed by calcidiol and calcium alone for six weeks, with or without a preceding two week period of calcitriol [14]. In an uncontrolled trial this regimen increased spinal bone mineral content measured by DPA, but no fluoride based regimen has been shown in a controlled trial to reduce fracture rate. An example of intermittent and sequential treatment combined is growth hormone given for 2 months, followed by calcitonin for 3 months with a 3 month rest period, which increased total body calcium measured by neutron activation [15].

THE COHERENCE CONCEPT-VALIDATION AND POTENTIAL PITFALLS

None of the regimens just described should be referred to as coherence therapy, but this assertion is intended, not to criticize or to denigrate, but to clarify. Coherence therapy is a specific combination of intermittent and sequential administration in which the timing and duration are based on the characteristics of the bone remodeling system [5,16]. Cycles of remodeling in different skeletal locations are normally out of step, or incoherent, so that at any instant all stages of the cycle are represented. An activator of remodeling is given as a brief pulse in high dose, to initiate many new cycles simultaneously, so that their evolution will be coherent. This is followed by a depressor of resorption, to constrain the recently recruited teams of osteoclasts into eroding shallower cavities than usual. The depressor is then withdrawn, in the hope that the subsequently appearing teams of osteoblasts will make amounts of bone appropriate to cavities of normal depth. The net result would be to form more bone at each location than was resorbed, to move the bone surfaces outward towards the marrow, and to increase the thickness of the bone structures. The concept is known by the acronym ADFR, for Activate-Depress-Free-Repeat.

Activation of remodeling is the conversion of a small region of bone surface from remodeling quiescence to activity [2]. Activation in this sense is frequently confused with activation of osteoclasts, a process not yet shown to be relevant to human bone physiology and which could not occur on a quiescent surface where there are no osteoclasts [3]. Activation of remodeling is increased by endogenous thyroid and parathyroid hormones [17], and probably by short term high dose calcitriol administration [18], but it is not known if a large number of new remodeling episodes can be started within a short enough time to be coherent. Most depressors of bone resorption act mainly as anti-activators; whether the dose and time relationships of an activator followed by a depressor can be adjusted to separate the effects on osteoclast recruitment from those on osteoclast activity is not known. Only for intermittent calcitonin is there evidence that resorption depth can be reduced, a cumulative effect inferred from an increase in cancellous interstitial bone thickness [9]. The evidence is suggestive rather than conclusive, because the change reported was improbably large in relation to the time interval between the biopsies.

Whether osteoblasts can be deceived into laying down more bone than is needed to refill the cavity, which is the limit of their normal task [2], has also not been demonstrated. If osteoblast recruitment is governed by the release of a mitogen from resorbed bone [19], the number of osteoblasts in the new team would be expected to fall in proportion to the size of the resorbed cavity, and no experimental evidence to the contrary has been reported. The increase in wall thickness observed with continuous phosphate administration [9] is important, but not relevant to the ADFR concept. In osteoporotic patients with impaired recruitment and activity of osteoblasts, manifested as a reduction in wall thickness [2], the combination of increased remodeling activation with only a modest reduction in resorption depth could promote bone loss rather than bone gain [Figure 1; 20]. The risk of trabecular perforation and its structural consequences [21] increases with more frequent activation [22]. Furthermore, thin vertical trabeculae that have lost their lateral bracing [23] will be more likely to undergo Euler buckling if activation is increased, even if not perforated. [Figure 2].

THE COHERENCE CONCEPT - IMPLEMENTATION

The concept has been applied using high dose sodium and/or potassium phosphate for three days to stimulate endogenous PTH secretion as an activator of remodeling, followed by sodium etidronate for two weeks as a depressor of resorption, with the cycle repeated every three months. In the first uncontrolled trial fully reported, there was a significant increase in spinal bone density, measured by DPA during the first two years of treatment [24]. Both in timing and magnitude, the response was very similar to those

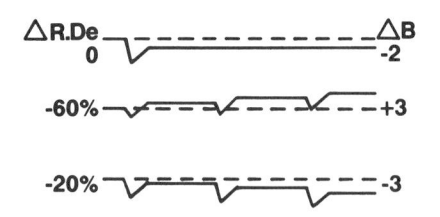

Figure 1: Possible outcomes of coherence therapy. In each panel is depicted the movement of a small element of bone surface as a function of time in a patient with low bone turnover and reduced wall thickness. If resorption depth [R.De] is reduced by 60% [middle panel], each remodeling cycle will add a small amount of bone, and the sign of bone balance [ΔB] will be reversed. If R.De is reduced only by 20% [lower panel], each cycle will remove less bone than before, but because the number of cycles is increased, the net effect is that more bone is lost.

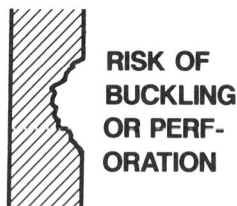

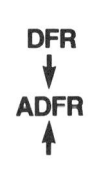

Figure 2: Biomechanical effects of different regimens. A vertical trabecular plate is depicted in diagrammatic form. Because horizontal trabeculae are lost preferentially, the unsupported length and the liability to buckling are increased [23]. If the width of the trabecula is slightly less than normal [100 μm], a resorption cavity of normal depth [50μm] represents a significant focal weakness. Consequently, the risk of both buckling and perforation will be in proportion to the rate of remodeling activation, and will change with the regimen as shown.

obtained by cyclical etidronate alone (sometimes known as DFR), and by continuous calcitonin, consistent with a sustained depression of remodeling activation as the major consequence of the intervention. There was equivocal evidence for parathyroid stimulation, but no evidence that remodeling activation was increased, even transiently. Using each patient as her own historical control, vertebral deformation rate appeared to fall after the first year of treatment, a common finding in trials without concurrent controls [25], probably due to the clustering of fracture episodes in time, analogous to the behavior of urinary tract stones [26]. In a second uncontrolled trial, giving phosphate for seven days and etidronate for only five days, and repeating the cycle every 60 days, the results were very similar [27].

In the only randomized controlled trial so far reported in detail, a regimen similar to the first trial prevented bone loss only in the radius; in the spine it was less effective than calcium and much less effective than estrogen [28], possibly because concurrent calcium depressed absorption. There was a small increase in PTH secretion during one three day period of phosphate administration; the response was greater with longer administration [27], but there was no demonstration in either study that the same effect could be obtained repetitively. In patients with post-menopausal osteoporosis, the increase in serum immunoreactive PTH in response to oral phosphate is substantially less than in healthy subjects of the same age [29,30]. Consequently, how increased remodeling activation contributed to the effect of the regimen, and whether the contribution was favorable or unfavorable, cannot be reliably inferred from any of the three studies. Better methods are needed, not only for activation of remodeling, but for verifying its continued occurrence, before adequate tests of its therapeutic importance can be conducted.

An important issue in applying the coherence concept is the treatment given during the free period. Frost stipulated that all medication be withheld, to ensure the unencumbered evolution of the new cycles of remodeling that had been initiated [5,16]. In all three studies just mentioned this requirement was disregarded by giving supplemental calcium continuously [24,27,28], and in one study, varying amounts of estrogen and calcitriol were given as well [24]. Frost did not explain how more bone could be made without supplying its constituents, and reliance on adaptive mechanisms known to be inefficient in osteoporosis [31] could be hazardous. Only one investigator has adhered to Frost's recommendations [32,33]; the histologic response has been more convincing, with increases both in wall thickness and trabecular thickness not found when calcium was given during the free period (Shih, M.S. personal communication), but no densitometric data, either appendicular or axial, and no fracture rates have been reported. It is important to determine if calcium does indeed have an adverse effect in this particular situation, and if so, by what means it is exerted.

A major practical difficulty with the coherence concept is the large number of possible regimens [34]. Allowing only two choices each for type of agent, dose and duration of administration for both activator and depressor, and in duration of free period and amount of calcium provided, would give rise to $256[2^8]$ plausible and distinct combinations. A reasonable choice among this large number, together with adequate validation of each component of the regimen, is clearly impossible without extensive animal and human experimentation. Until such studies are completed, further long term clinical trials will represent a gamble with the health of patients that is without scientific or ethical justification. It is deplorable, and a collective discredit to pharmaceutical companies, scientific funding agencies, and biomedical investigators that this novel and important idea still has not received the experimental attention it needs and deserves before it can be translated into a safe and effective form of treatment.

CONCLUSIONS

1. Coherence therapy (ADFR) is soundly based on bone remodeling theory, but none of its components has been validated; it is not known whether coherent remodeling activation, reduced resorption depth, and net bone gain can be sequentially and repetitively achieved.

2. The regimen could promote bone loss rather than bone gain in patients with too few or inactive osteoblasts, and increase the risk of buckling and perforation in patients with thin trabeculae.

3. Most cyclical and/or intermittent regimens are not coherence therapy, and should not be so described.

4. Phosphate is an unreliable activator of remodeling because the PTH response is blunted in patients with osteoporosis; Etidronate is a poor choice for a depressor of resorption in an ADFR regimen, because its skeletal half life is too long to achieve the intermittent effect essential for testing the concept.

5. Published clinical trials have been premature and inconclusive; ten years after its first description, we still don't know if ADFR will work.

6. Further long term trials of coherence therapy should be suspended until crucial gaps in knowledge have been filled by appropriate animal and human experiments.

REFERENCES

1. H.M. Frost in: The Skeletal Intermediary Organization. A Synthesis, W. Peck, ed. (Elsevier, Amsterdam 1985) pp. 49-107.
2. A.M. Parfitt in: Osteoporosis, Etiology, Diagnosis and Management, B.L. Riggs, L.J. Melton, eds. (Raven Press 1988) pp. 45-93.
3. A.M. Parfitt in: Clinical Pharmacology of Calcium Metabolism, J.A. Kanis, ed. (S. Karger, Basel) (in press).

4. P.J. Meunier, G.G. S-Bianchi, C.M. Edouard, et al., Orthop. Clin. North Am. 3,745-776 (1972).
5. H.M. Frost, Clin. Orthop. 143,227-244 (1979).
6. T. Storm, G. Thamsborg, H. Genant, et al. J. Bone. Min. Res. 4, Supp 1, (1989).
7. C. Gennari, S.M. Chierichetti, S. Bigazzi, et al., Current Therapeutic Research 38,3,155-161 (1985).
8. P.J. Marie, C. Alexandre, D. Chappard, et al., in: Calcium Regulation and Bone Metabolism: Basic and Clinical Aspects 9, D.V. Cohn, T.J. Martin, P.J. Meunier, eds. (Elsevier Science Publishers B.V. 1987) pp 943-947.
9. P.J. Marie, F. Caulin, Bone 7,17-22 (1986).
10. M. Kleerekoper, B. Frame, A.R. Villanueva, et al., in: Osteoporosis: Recent Advances in Pathogenesis and Treatment, H.F. DeLuca, H. Frost, W. Jee, C. Johnston, A.M. Parfitt, eds. (University Park Press, Baltimore 1981) pp. 441-448.
11. R.K. Schenk, W.A. Merz, F.W. Reutter, in: Fluoride in Medicine, T.L. Vischer, ed. (Hans Huber Publishers, Bern 1970) pp. 153-168.
12. D. Baylink, D.S. Bernstein, Clin. Orthop. 55,51 (1967).
13. M. Kleerekoper, R. Balena, E. Peterson, et al., Abstract, Steenbock Symp. on Osteoporosis, June 4-7 (1989).
14. C.Y.C. Pak, D. Sakhaee, J.E. Zerwekh, et al., J. Clin. Endocrinol. Metab. 68,1,150-159 (1989).
15. J.F. Aloia, A. Vaswani, P.J. Meunier, Calcif. Tissue Int. 40,253-259 (1987).
16. H.M. Frost, Calcif. Tissue Int. 36,349-353 (1984).
17. F. Melsen, L. Mosekilde, E.F. Eriksen, et al., in: Clinical Disorders of Bone and Mineral Metabolism, M. Kleerekoper, S. Krane, eds. (Mary Ann Liebert Publishers, Inc., New York 1989) (in press).
18. J.C. Gallagher, R.R. Recker in: Vitamin D: A Chemical, Biochemical and Clinical Update, Norman et al, ed. (Walter de Gruyter & Co., Berlin 1985) pp. 971-975.
19. J.R. Farley, N. Tarbaux, L.A. Murphy, et al., Metabolism 36,314-321 (1987).
20. A.M. Parfitt in: Second International Conference on Osteoporosis: Social and Clinical Aspects, A. Vagenakis, P. Soucacos, A. Avramides, G. Segre, L. Deftos, eds. (Masson Italia Editori SIA, Milano 1986) pp. 197-209.
21. A.M. Parfitt, Am. J. Med. 82, Suppl. 1B,68-72 (1987).
22. P.J. Meunier in: Calcium Regulation and Bone Metabolism: Basic and Clinical Aspects, 9, D.V. Cohn, T.J. Martin, P.J. Meunier, eds. (Elsevier Science Publishers B.V. 1987) pp. 941-942.
23. M. Kleerekoper, D. Dickie, L.A. Feldkamp, et al., in: Osteoporosis 1987, C. Christiansen, C. Johansen, B.J. Riis, eds. (Osteopress Aps, Copenhagen 1987) pp. 301-308.
24. A.B. Hodsman, Bone and Min. 5,201-212 (1989).
25. J.A. Kanis, Lancet 1,27-33 (1984).
26. B. Ettinger, Amer. J. Med. 61,200-206 (1976).
27. L.E. Mallette, A.D. LeBlanc, J.L. Pool, et al., J. Bone Min. Res. 4,2,143-148 (1989).
28. R. Pacifici, C. McMurtry, I. Vered, et al., J. Clin. Endocrinol. Metab. 66,747-753 (1988).
29. J. Ittner, M.A. Dambacher, R. Muff, et al., Min. Electrolyte Metab. 12,199-203 (1986).
30. S.J. Silverberg, E. Shane, L. DeLa Cruz, et al., New Eng. J. Med. 320,5,277-281 (1989).
31. A.M. Parfitt, Drugs 36,513-520 (1988).
32. C. Anderson, R.D.T. Cape, R.G. Crilly, et al., Calcif. Tissue Int. 36,341-343 (1984).
33. C.A. Anderson in: Calcium Regulation and Bone Metabolism: Basic and Clinical Aspects, 9, D.V. Cohn, T.J. Martin, P.J. Meunier, eds. (Elsevier Science Publishers B.V. 1987) pp. 948-951.
34. S.T. Harris in: Osteoporosis Update 1987, H.K. Genant, ed. (Radiology Research and Education Foundation, California 1987) pp. 287-291.

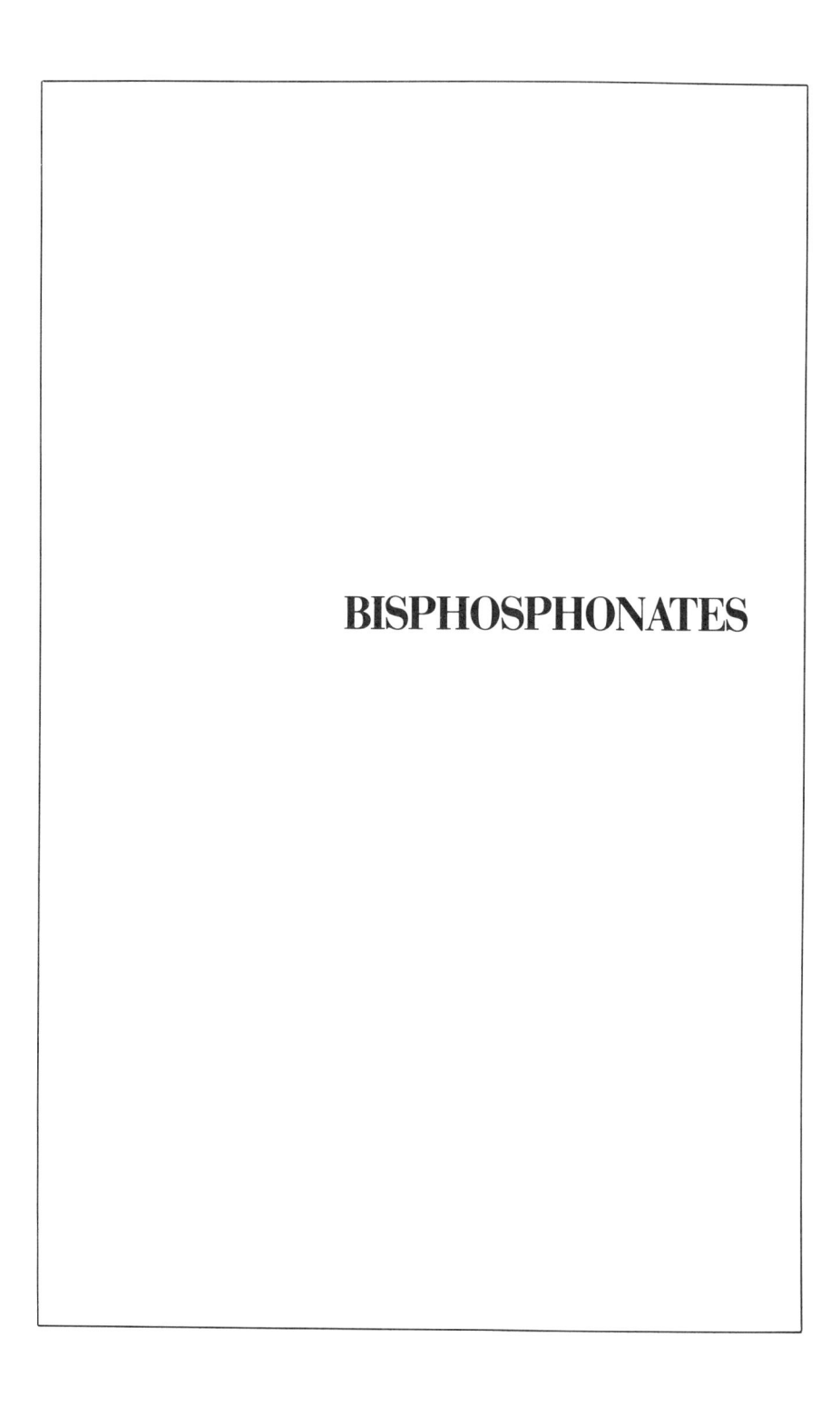

BISPHOSPHONATES

The Possible Use of Bisphosphonates in Osteoporosis

H. Fleisch

Department of Pathophysiology, University of Berne, Berne, Switzerland

ABSTRACT

Bisphosphonates are analogues of pyrophosphate and are marked by their strong affinity to mineralized tissues. Some of them have the property to inhibit bone resorption even when administered in low amounts and for this reason are currently used in the treatment of bone diseases with high bone destruction.

Bisphosphonates can lead to an increase of bone mass in the animal and prevent various types of experimental osteoporosis. First results in humans suggest that they also prevent bone loss and in some cases even induce an increase of bone mass in high turnover osteoporosis.

Based on preliminary results it appears worthwhile, although it promises to be arduous, to elucidate the most suitable bisphosphonate as well as its dosage, its mode of administration and its possible association with other drugs for a potential use in some types of osteoporosis.

CHEMISTRY

The bisphosphonates, previously incorrectly called diphosphonates, are compounds characterized by two C-P bonds. If the two bonds are linked to the same carbon atom, the compounds are named geminal bisphosphonates. Thus they are analogues of pyrophosphate, but contain a carbon instead of an oxygen atom. Commonly, the geminal bisphosphonates are simply referred to as bisphosphonates, a term used not quite correctly.

The basic P-C-P structure allows to synthesize bisphosponates in many different forms, either by changing the two lateral chains on the carbon atom or by esterifying the phosphate groups. A large number of various bisphosphonates has been and are still synthesized. Based on numerous studies, it has emerged that small changes in the structure can lead to extensive alterations in the physicochemical and biological characteristics. This means that it is not possible to extrapolate from the results of one compound to others, and hence it would be incorrect to talk generally of "effects of bisphosphonates". Each compound has to be considered separately and statements should be restricted to specific compounds.

To date the following bisphosphonates have been investigated to be used as therapeutic agents in human bone disease, whereof the first two listed are commercially available in some countries.

1-hydroxyethylidene-1,1-bisphosphonic acid (HEBP or etidronate), previously called 1-hydroxyethane-1,1-diphosphonic acid (EHDP); dichloromethylenebisphosphonic acid (Cl_2MBP or clodronate) previously called dichloromethylenediphosphonic acid (Cl_2MDP); 3-amino-1-hydroxypropylidene-1,1-bisphosphonic acid (AHPrBP or pamidronate), previously called 3-amino-1-hydroxypropane-1,1-diphosphonic acid (APD); 4-amino-1-hydroxybutylidene-1,1-bisphosphonic acid (AHBuBP); 6-amino-1-hydroxyhexylidene-1,1-bisphosphonic acid (AHHexBP); 4-chlorophenylthiomethylenebisphosphonic acid. Very recently two new compounds have been synthesized, which appear to be of

Copyright 1990 by Elsevier Science Publishing Co., Inc.
Osteoporosis: Physiological Basis, Assessment, and Treatment
Hector F. DeLuca and Richard Mazess, Editors

great potential clinical interest, namely 1-hydroxy-3-(methylpentylamino)-propylidenebisphosphonic acid [1] and 2-(3-pyridinyl)-1-hydroxyethylidene-bisphosphonic acid [2].

Bisphosphonates cause physical-chemical effects very similar to those of pyrophosphate. Thus many of them inhibit the precipitation of calcium phosphate from clear solution [3], block the transformation of amorphous calcium into hydroxyapatite [4], and delay the aggregation of apatite crystals into larger clusters [5]. They also slow down the dissolution of these crystals [6,7]. All these effects are related to their affinity for the calcium phosphate solid phase [8].

ANIMAL WORK

Effects on calcification

The physical-chemical properties suggest that the bisphosphonates might be also active in vivo by inhibiting both calcification and bone dissolution. This hypothesis proved to be correct. Indeed, some of these compounds were found to prevent experimentally induced calcification produced e.g. in arteries, kidneys, skin and heart [3,9]. The bisphosphonates are active both when given parenterally and orally. The inhibitory action was not confined to only ectopic calcification but in certain cases also ectopic ossification is effectively inhibited [10]. If administered in sufficient doses, certain bisphosphonates, such as HEBP, also retard the mineralisation of normal calcified tissues such as bone and cartilage [11,12,13] and dentin. The doses required for this to occur vary according to the bisphosphonate used, the animal species, the length of the treatment and the route of administration. The inhibition of ectopic mineralisation is most probably due to the physical-chemical inhibition of crystal growth. Indeed, there is a close relationship between the ability of individual bisphosphonates to inhibit calcium phosphate formation in vitro and their effectiveness to act on ectopic calcification in vivo [3,14]. This effect on mineralisation has been made use of in the treatment of patients with ectopic calcification and ectopic ossification [for review see 15].

Effects on bone resorption

Many of the bisphosphonates also proved to be very powerful inhibitors of bone resorption when tested in a variety of conditions both in vitro [16] and in vivo. In growing rats they block the destruction of both bone and cartilage so that the metaphysis becomes radiologically more dense than normal [13]. The inhibition of bone resorption has also been documented by ^{45}Ca kinetic studies and by hydroxyproline excretion [17]. Bisphosphonates also reduce bone resorption induced experimentally by various means. Thus they blunt the effect of parathyroid hormone [7], and of a retinoid [18], inhibit tumour invasion of bone [19] as well as various types of tumoral hypercalcemia [20].

The degree of activity of the individual bisphosphonates varies greatly from compound to compound. Thus for example an increase of the aliphatic carbon backbone increases the activity [14]. Amino derivatives with an amino group at the end of the side chain are extremely active, whereby the highest activity was found with a backbone of four carbons (AHBuBP) [21]. If the amino group of AHPrBP is dimethylated, the potency is likewise increased [22]. The activity is even more increased if the amino group is methylated and pentylated; 1-hydroxy-3-(methylpentilamino)propylidenebisphosphonate has been found in our laboratory to be the most active compound, doses as low as 0.1 µg P/kg per day administered s.c. in the rat showing an effect already (unpublished results). Cyclic geminal bisphosphonates are also active, especially those containing a N atom in the cycle, such as 2-(3-pyridinyl)-1-hydroxyethylidenebisphosphonate [2]. Of the six bisphosphonates tested clinically AHBuBP appears to be the most potent in the rat, followed by AHPrBP, AHHexBP and Cl$_2$MBP while HEBP and 4-chlorophenylthiomethylenebisphosphonate are less effective [13].

The mechanism of the inhibition on bone resorption is still not clear. No correlation has been found between the inhibition of bone resorption in vivo and that of crystal dissolution in vitro [14]. Furthermore, the fact that extremely small amounts of some of the bisphosphonates are active in vivo also makes the initially postulated physical-chemical mechanism unlikely. It appears now that the effect is cellular in nature, osteoclasts serving as target cells. This is supported by the fact that bisphosphonates can alter the morphology of osteoclasts both in vitro and in vivo [13] and when added to osteoclasts in vitro inhibit their bone resorbing activity [23]. Besides their effect on osteoclast activity, bisphosphonates also induce a decrease in the number of osteoclasts, either because already formed cells are destroyed or recruitement of new cells is inhibited. Studies in vitro have shown that bisphosphonates can inhibit the recruitement of osteoclasts in culture [24] and the formation of multinuclear cells in long-term bone marrow culture [25].

The mechanism by which the bisphosphonates act on the osteoclasts is still unknown. These compounds have been found to induce a variety of different biochemical effects in cultured bone cells, among others reduction of lactic acid production [26], inhibition of lysosomal enzymes [27] and innibition of prostaglandin synthesis [28]. Since the bisphosphonates have a strong affinity for calcium phosphate, they are efficiently taken up by calcified tissues, especially bone. When the latter is resorbed they are released into the surrounding environment from which they can be taken up by the resorbing cells where they may exert any one of the above mentioned or other effects.

Bisphosphonates have been used in various diseases characterized by increased bone destruction such as Paget's disease, tumoral bone destruction and hypercalcemia of malignancy (for review see 15).

Effect on bone mass in normal animals

The fact that bisphosphonates inhibit bone resorption raises the question whether this inhibition could lead to an increase in bone mass. This was found to be the case, especially in the metaphysis of the growing rat [13], and the density of the metaphysis is used as a scanning system to assay new bisphosphonates [21]. Increased density was also obtained following bisphosphonate treatment over longer time periods [29]. Balance and ^{45}Ca kinetic studies in the growing rat have shown that Cl$_2$BP caused an increase in Ca balance [17], due to a drastic decline of bone resorption. Bone formation was found to be decreased as well, but to a lesser degree. Intestinal Ca absorption was increased as the result of an increase in plasma 1,25(OH)$_2$D$_3$ [30]. Similar results occur with APD [31] and as recently shown with 1-hydroxy-3-(methylpentilamino)propylidenebisphosphonate (unpublished results), while HEBP is less effective.

Besides inhibiting bone resorption the bisphosphonates also provoke a decrease in bone formation. This can be visualised at the level of longitudinal growth [13], midshaft expansion [32] and by Ca incorporation measured with ^{45}Ca [17,31]. It is possible that this effect is not due primarily to the bisphosphonate but may be secondary to bone resorption and due to the so called "coupling" between resorption and formation. Whatever the mechanism may be, the extent of the observed decrease in bone formation will determine whether bisphosponate can be used in osteoporosis.

Effect on experimental osteoporosis

A series of bisphosphonates have been tested on a number of experimental osteoporosis models. All compounds tested prevent bone loss induced by sciatic nerve section [33-39] or by spinal cord section [40] in the rat. Cl$_2$ MBP was found to be more effective than HEBP. Bisphosphonates not only inhibit bone loss induced by immobilization, but in certain cases the treatment leads to a bone mass higher than in controls [34]. Bone loss elicited by hypokinesis is also prevented [41,42]. Cl$_2$MBP and HEBP counteract bone loss induced by ovariectomy in the rat [39,43,44], and HEBP prevents the loss induced by heparin [45]. The results on bone loss induced by low Ca diet are ambiguous; while one study failed to show an effect [46], in an other report an inhibition was demonstrated [39]. Finally bone loss induced by cortisol in rabbits was prevented by Cl$_2$MBP [47].

HUMAN STUDIES

Effect on osteoporosis

Recently some bisphosphonates have been investigated on their possible effects in human osteoporosis. The first controlled detailed study was performed with HEBP at a dose of 20 mg/kg per day for 6 months. The results were not very encouraging because both bone resorption and accretion decreased approximately to the same extent, meaning that the effect on Ca balance was only small [48]. Intestinal Ca absorption as well as urinary Ca was increased. However, at the above dose an inhibition of mineralisation was induced which resulted in an increase in osteoid tissue [49]; therefore a positive effect on bone balance, if present, would have been obscured by the induced osteomalacia. Later studies confirmed the increase in intestinal Ca absorption [50], probably induced by the increase of serum PTH [49,50]. HEBP administered at 5 mg P/kg per day produced no effect on Ca balance during bed rest, but seemingly diminished the negative balance when given at 20 mg P/kg. However, calcaneal loss assessed by gamma ray absorptiometry was not altered (51, 52). On the other hand a daily dose of 400 mg of HEBP for 3 months did reverse the increase of whole body retention of ^{99m}Tc-bisphosphonate, as well as the increase in calcemia and urinary calcium occurring after surgical menopause [53].

Recently a series of so called coherence therapies have been performed using multiple cycles of short periods of an activator of bone resorption before or together with HEBP [54-57]. The first results of such studies [54] on 5 osteoporotic patients and no controls, using P as an activator, suggested that an increase in the mean trabecular diameter and volume can be found in biopsy samples of the iliac crest. Unfortunately, these results could not be substantiated after more patients were investigated, but a 6 % increase in lumbar bone mineral density and a decrease in fracture rate was observed [55]. Another non controlled study also suggested that an increase in vertebral bone might occur [56]. The results on axial bone mineral density are strengthened by more recent controlled studies where the same dose of HEBP given discontinuously, but without activator were used. In these studies HEBP was given for 2 weeks followed by a 13 weeks interruption. The cycles were repeated for 100 to 150 weeks [58-60]. The results showed an increase between 4 and 12 % of lumbar bone mineral content, as assessed by DPA or by QCT, while the controls decreased or increased only slightly. The difference between the two groups ranged between 4 and 11 % . No effect was however observed on the radius. Contrary to the above results, another study using a similar protocol showed some effect on the bone loss in the forearm but none in the spine [61].

Fewer studies have been carried out with Cl_2MBP. Indeed this compound was withdrawn for a certain time from investigational trials because of a possible relation with the development of leukemia, an effect that has not been substantiated in later studies. The first results were encouraging, since after 18 months the discontinuous administration led to an increase of about 6 % in total body Ca measured by neutron activation as compared to a decrease of 2 % in patients given placebo [62]. Daily doses of 400 and 1600 mg given continuously prevented the bone loss occurring in paraplegia [63,64].

More information is available for APD. A short term treatment with this bisphosponate resulted in an increase of the Ca balance of about 220 mg per day. The increase, although less, was still present after 1 year of treatment [65]. This finding was supported by bone mineral measurements in patients treated with ADP between 1.4 and 6.2 years. These data showed a steady yearly increase of about 3 % as compared to a non-significant change of 0.4 % in the controls. In yet another study APD was found to prevent not only the metacarpal cortical loss in steroid induced osteoporosis [66, 67] but appeared to increase lumbar mineral density [66]. When given in a patient with juvenile osteoporosis, APD normalized the increased bone resorption within a week and changed the negative Ca balance into a positive one, while urinary Ca was decreased and intestinal Ca absorption increaed [68]. $1,25(OH)_2D_3$ and PTH were increased as described by others for APD [69] and Cl_2MBP [70]. In summary it appears that APD not only reverses a negative Ca balance but transforms it into a positive one, leading to an increase in bone mass.

CONCLUSION

Based on data currently available it appears that bisphosphonates not only inhibit bone resorption but induce in some cases an increase in Ca balance and in bone mass. This suggests that these compounds may possibly be used in the future to prevent bone loss or perhaps even to reverse it in osteoporosis. The cases most likely to respond are those with high rates of bone resorption. In low turnover osteoporosis the success is less likely unless the compounds are given together with a substance which stimulates the turnover. Presently it is not possible to predict which of the compounds will be most suitable. It should be active at a dose where no inhibition of mineralisation occurs, which is the case with the more recent compounds. Furthermore since the bisphosphonates are "bone seekers" they remain for a long period in the skeleton, and since they are not degraded in the body, special care must be taken with respect to chronic toxicity. The dose, the mode of administration, continuous or discontinuous, and the association with other drugs will have to be worked out.The elucidation of these various parameters, although a long and arduous undertaking, appears a more than worthwhile endeavour in view of the aim of a new treatment in osteoporosis.

REFERENCES

1. A. Stutzer, R.C. Mühlbauer, M. Janner, and H. Fleisch, Calcif. Tissue Int. 44 (Suppl. 1), S-107 (1989).
2. J.A. Bevan, A.F. Franks, J.E. McOsker, R.W. Boyce, and K.W. Buckingham, J. Bone Min. Res. 3 (Suppl. 1, S193 (1988).
3. H. Fleisch, R.G.G. Russell, S. Bisaz, R.C. Mühlbauer, and D.A. Williams, Eur. J. Clin. Invest. 1, 12-18 (1970).
4. M.D. Francis, Calcif. Tissue Res. 3, 151-162 (1969).
5. N.M. Hansen Jr., R. Felix, S. Bisaz, and H. Fleisch, Biochim. Biophys. Acta 451, 549-559 (1976).
6. H. Fleisch, R.G.G. Russell, and M.D. Francis, Science 165, 1262-1264 (1969).
7. R.G.G. Russell, R.C. Mühlbauer, S. Biasz, D.A. Williams, and H. Fleisch, Calcif. Tissue Res. 6, 183-196 (1970).
8. A. Jung, S. Bisaz, and H. Fleisch, Calcif. Tissue Res. 11, 269-280 (1973).
9. I.Y. Rosenblum, H.E. Black, and J.F. Ferrell, Calcif. Tissue Res. 27, 151-159 (1977).
10. C.M.T. Plasmans, W. Kuypers, and T.J.J.H. Slooff, Clin. Orthop. Rel. Res. 132, 233-243 (1978).
11. J. Jowsey, K.E. Holley, and J.W. Linman, J. Lab. Clin. Med. 76, 126-133 (1970).
12. W.R. King, M.D. Francis, and W.R. Michael, Clin. Orthop. 78, 251-270 (1971).
13. R. Schenk, W.A. Merz, R. Mühlbauer, R.G.G. Russell, and H. Fleisch, Calcif. Tissue Res. 11, 196-214 (1973)
14. H. Shinoda, G. Adamek, R. Felix, H. Fleisch, R. Schenk, and P. Hagan, Calcif. Tissue Int. 35, 87-99 (1983).
15. H. Fleisch in: Handbook of Experimental Pharmacology, Vol. 83, P.F. Baker, ed. (Springer-Verlag, Berlin, Heidelberg 1988) pp. 441-466.
16. J.J. Reynolds, C. Minkin, D.B. Morgan, D. Spycher, and H. Fleisch, Calcif. Tissue Res. 10, 302-313 (1972).
17. A.B. Gasser, D.B. Morgan, H.A. Fleisch, and L.J. Richelle, Clin. Sci. 43, 31-45.
18. U. Trechsel, A. Stutzer, and H. Fleisch, J. Clin. Invest. 80, 1679-1686 (1987).
19. A. Jung, J. Bornand, B. Mermillod, C. Edouard, and P.J. Meunier, Cancer Res. 44, 3007-3011 (1984).
20. K.Y. Johnson, M.A. Wesseler, H.M. Olson, R.R. Martodam, and J.W. Poser in: Diphosphonates and Bone, A. Donath, and B. Courvoisier, eds. (Editions Médecine et Hygiène, Genève 1982) pp. 386-394.
21. R. Schenk, P. Eggli, R. Felix, H. Fleisch, and S. Rosini, Calcif. Tissue Int. 38, 342-349 (1986).
22. P.M. Boonekamp, C.W.G.M. Löwik, L.J.A. van der Wee-Pals, M.L.L. van Wijk-van Lennep, and O.L.M. Bijvoet, Bone and Mineral 2, 29-42 (1987).
23. A.M. Flanagan, T.J. Chambers in: Osteoporosis 2, C. Christiansen, J.S. Johansen, and B.J. Riis, eds. (Osteopress ApS, Nørhaven A/S, Vinborg, Denmark 1987) pp. 776-777
24. P.M. Boonekamp, L.J.A. van der Wee-Pals, M.M.L. van Wijk-van Lennep, C.W. Thesing, O.L.M. Bijvoet, Bone and Mineral 1, 27-39 (1986).
25. D.E. Hughes, B.R. MacDonald, R.G.G. Russell, and M. Gowen, J. Bone Min. Res. 2 (Suppl. 1), abstract 265.
26. D.K. Fast, R. Felix, C. Dowse, W.F. Neuman, and H. Fleisch, Biochem. J. 172, 97-107 (1978).
27. R. Felix, R.G.G. Russell, and H. Fleisch, Biochim. Biophys. Acta 429, 429-438.
28. R. Felix, J.D. Bettex, and H. Fleisch, Calcif. Tissue Int. 33, 549-552 (1981).

29. O.L.M. Bijvoet, W.B. Frijlink, K. Jie, H. van der Linden, C.J.L.M. Meijer, H. Mulder, H.C. van Paassen, P.H. Reitsma, J. te Velde, E. de Vries, and J.P. van der Wey, Arthr. Rheum. 23, 1193-1204 (1980).
30. D. Guilland, U. Trechsel, J.-P. Bonjour, and H. Fleisch, Clin. Sci. Mol. Med. 48, 157-160 (1975).
31. P.H. Reitsma, O.L.M. Bijvoet, H. Verlinden-Ooms, and L.J.A. van der Wee-Pals, Calcif. Tissue Int. 32, 145-147 (1980).
32. C.S. Wink, and E.M. Hill, Acta anat. 132, 321-323 (1988).
33. H. Fleisch, R.G.G. Russell, B. Simpson, and R.C. Mühlbauer, Nature 223, 211-212 (1969).
34. R.C. Mühlbauer, R.G.G. Russell, D.A. Williams, and H. Fleisch, Europ. J. Clin. Invest. 1, 336-344 (1971).
35. W.R. Michael, W.R. King, and M.D. Francis, Clin. Orthop. Rel. Res. 78, 271-276 (1971).
36. M.E. Cabanela and J. Jowsey, Calc. Riss. Res. 8, 114-120 (1971).
37. J.M. Lane and M.E. Steinberg, J. Trauma 13, 863-869 (1973).
38. K. Lindenhayn, H. Hähnel, U.J. Schmidt, and I. Kalbe, Z. Alternsforsch. 34, 173-176 (1979).
39. E. Shiota, Fukuoka Acta Med. 76, 317-342 (1985).
40. A. Schoutens, M. Verhas, N. Dourov, P. Bergmann, F. Caulin, A. Verschaeren, M. Mone, and A. Heilporn, Calcif. Tissue Int. 42, 136-143 (1988).
41. V.N. Shvets, A.S. Pankova, O.E. Kabitskaya, Z.E. Vnukova, and B.V. Morukov, Kosm. Biol. Aviakosm. Med. 20, 45-49 (1986).
42. V.N. Shvets, A.S. Pankova, and O.E. Kabitskaia, Kosm. Biol. Aviakosm. 22, 49-53 (1988).
43. C.S. Wink, M.St. Onge, and B. Parker, Acta anat. 124, 117-121 (1985).
44. C.S. Wink, Acta anat. 126, 57-62 (1986).
45. H. Hähnel, R. Mühlbach, K. Lindenhayn, P. Schaetz, and U.J. Schmidt, Z. Alternsforscn. 27, 289-292 (1973).
46. J. Jowsey and K.E. Holley, J. Lab. Clin. Med. 82, 567-575 (1973).
47. W.S.S. Jee and J.E. Gotscner, Clin. Ortnop. Rel. Res. 156, 39-51 (1981).
48. R.P. Heaney and P.D. Saville, Clin. Pharmacol. Ther. 20, 593-604 (1976).
49. J. Jowsey, B. L. Riggs, P.J. Kelly, D.L. Hoffman, and P. Bordier, J. Lab. Clin. Invest. 78, 574-584 (1971).
50. R. Nuti, G. Righi, V. Turchetti, and A. Vattimo, Cl. Therap. 99, 33-42 (1981).
51. D.R. Lockwood, J.M. Vogel, V.S. Schneider, and S.B. Hulley, J. Endocrinol. Metab. 41, 533-541 (1975).
52. V.S. Schneider and J. McDonald, Calcif. Tissue Int. 36, 151-154 (1984).
53. M.L. Smith, I. Fogelman, D.M. Hart, E. Scott, J. Bevan, and I.Leggate, Calcif. Tissue Int. 44, 74-79 (1989).
54. C. Anderson, R.D.T. Cape, R.G. Crilly, A.B. Hodsman, and B.M.J. Wolfe, Calcif. Tissue Int. 36, 341-343 (1984).
55. A.B. Hodsman, Bone and Mineral 5, 201-212 (1989).
56. P.D. Miller, B.J. Neal, D.O. McIntyre, M.J. Yanover, and L. Kowalski in: Osteoporosis 1987, C. Christiansen, ed. (Osteopress Aps, Nørhaven A/S, Viborg, Denmark 1987) pp. 41-42
57. R.D. Hesch, J. Heck, G. Delling, E. Keck, J. Reeve, H. Canzler, O. Schober, and H. Harms, Klin. Wochenschr 66, 976-984 (1988).
58. T. Storm, G. Thamsborg, O.H. Sørensen, and B. Lund in: Osteoporosis 1987, C. Christiansen, ed. (Osteopress ApS, Nørhaven A/S, Viborg, Denmark 1987) pp. 20-24
59. H.K. Genant, S.T. Harris, P. Steiger, P.F. Davey, and J.E. Block in: Osteoporosis 1987, C. Christiansen, ed. (Osteopress ApS, Nørhaven A/S, Viborg, Denmark 1987) pp. 25-29

60. T. Steiniche, C. Hasling, G. Thamsborg, T. Storm, O.H. Sørensen, L. Mosekilde, and F. Melsen in: Osteoporosis 1987, C. Christiansen, ed. (Osteopress ApS, Nørhaven A/S, Viborg, Denmark 1987) pp. 30-35
61. R. Pacifici, C. McMurtry, I. Vered, R. Rupich, and L.V. Avioli, J. Endocrinol. Metab. 66, 747-753 (1988).
62. C.H. Chesnut III in: Osteoporosis, Etiology, Diagnosis and Management, B. L. Riggs and L.J. Melton III, eds. (Raven Press, New York 1988) pp. 403-414.
63. P. Minaire, E. Berard, P.J. Meunier, C. Edouard, G. Goedert, and G. Pilonchery, J. Clin. Invest. 68, 1086-1092 (1981).
64. P. Minaire, J. Depassio, E. Berard, P.J. Meunier, C. Edouard, G. Pilonchery, and G. Goedert, Bone 8 (Suppl. 1), S63-S68 (1987).
65. R. Valkema, F.-J.F.E. Vismans, S.E. Papapoulos, E.K.J. Pauwels, and O.L.M. Bijvoet, Bone and Mineral 5, 183-192 (1989).
66. I.R. Reid, C.J. Alexander, A.R. King, and H.K. Ibbertson, Lancet i, 143-146 (1988).
67. I.R. Reid, S.W. Heap, A.S. King, H.K. Ibbertson, Lancet ii, 1144 (1988).
68. K. Hoekman, S.E. Papapoulos, A.C.B. Peters, and O.L.M. Bijvoet, J. Clin. Endocrinol. Metab. 61, 952-957 (1985).
69. S. Adami, W.B. Frijlink, O.L.M. Bijvoet, J.L.H. O'Riordan, T.L. Clemens, and S.E. Papapoulos, Calcif. Tissue Int. 34, 317-320 (1982).
70. P.J. Meunier, C. Alexandre, C. Edouard, L. Mathieu, M.C. Chapuy, C. Bressot, E. Vignon, and U. Trechsel, Lancet ii, 489-492 (1979).

The Use of Bisphosphonate in Osteoporosis

Olav L.M. Bijvoet,* Roelf Valkema,† Clemens W.G.M. Löwik,* and Socrates E. Papapoulos*

*Clinical Investigation Unit of the Department of Clinical Endocrinology, University Hospital Leiden, Leiden, The Netherlands
†Divison of Nuclear Medicine of the Department of Diagnostic Radiology, University Hospital Leiden, Leiden, The Netherlands

INTRODUCTION

Forthcoming reports suggest that bisphosphonates may increase bone mass in osteoporosis [1-12]. These reports further attribute the efficacy of the treatments to the specific regimes that have been applied. Many use cyclic regimes, in accordance with special bone biodynamic considerations [5-12]. Bone remodelling is considered to be achieved through cycles of non synchronized bone-resorption and -formation sequences, taking place at sundry sites of the bone surface. In 1979 Frost proposed that an increase in trabecular bone volume could be achieved by activating a synchronized or "coherent" population of such sequences with a pulse of a stimulatory drug, and then suppressing the resorptive phase by giving, at the proper time, a short course of an inhibitory drug, allowing bone formation to proceed normally after the resorptive phase had been curtailed [13]. The resulting positive transients in calcium balance would be exploited time and again by repeating these treatment cycles at appropriate intervals. Such a regime is dubbed ADFR (Activation of the cycle, Resorption inhibition, Free of treatment, Repeat) A different approach considers formation- and resorption-cycles as mutually dependent elements of a cybernetic equilibrium. If permanent pressure is exerted on one of the phases of such a cycle, compensation will occur but will never be complete, since the driving force for the compensatory event is the presence of a disequilibrium [4]. Since bone formation should be allowed occur at a reasonable rate in order for the slight positive balance to remain effective, the suppressive force should remain small. The treatment should use long-term administration of low dose bisphosphonate[1-4].

A discussion of the results of trials with bisphosphonate in osteoporosis needs to consider the physiologic mechanisms by which effects are achieved. This requires a pharmacokinetic, pharmacodynamic and biodynamic background.

EFFECTS OF BISPHOSPHONATE ON BONE REMODELLING ARE OF LONG DURATION

Bisphosphonate compounds enable to modulate bone metabolism in disease. They offer effective and safe treatment for Paget's disease and hypercalcemia of malignancy [14-21]. In the latter, the serum calcium is normalized through suppression of an excessive, and unopposed bone resorption. In Paget's disease in which the primary elevation of bone resorption rate is associated with a secondary increase in bone formation rate, the bisphosphonates normalize bone remodelling [15,16]. Although here too, the primary action of the drugs is on resorption, bone formation is secondarily affected through adaptive regulation mechanisms proper to the organ. The ultimate effect of this is that all the elements of the excessive bone turnover are normalized. The difference in nature between these two results: suppression of resorption, and suppression of turnover, is not related to the mode of treatment: short in hypercalcemia, and prolonged in Paget's disease. Actually, a short 10 day course of a potent bisphosphonate in Paget's disease, sufficient to achieve suppression of resorption, has within that period no visible effect on the bone formation rate. Yet, after that, and in the absence of further treatment, there is a slow and steady decline in bone formation rate until, after three to six months this has normalized as well[16,18]. The kinetics are in accordance with the hypothesis that they reflect the natural survival of the osteoblast populations that were already operating before suppression of resorption [22]. It is not certain wether the delay in adaptation of formation merely reflects the survival of preexisting osteoblasts, or if, according to the cyclic concept, previously mentioned, it includes a period of osteoblastic "repair" of the lacunae formed by "inhibited osteoclasts". The answer to this question, of obvious importance in relation to the cyclic treatment concept, depends on the mechanism of action of the bisphosphonates and will be discussed later. In any case, the kinetics of bone remodelling subsequent to administration of bisphosphonate imply that a single resorption-suppressing course of high dose bisphosphonate will have protracted effects and will, after some delay, end with suppression of bone turnover. The transient is of course associated with a transient positive bone balance.

Experiments in dogs with rigorous long-term suppression of bone turnover have resulted in an impressive increase in the rate of pathological fractures [23]. One should therefore not only know how long it takes to recover from a suppressive bisphosphonate course, but also if continuous administration of low doses will not result in cumulation. In rats, dog and man, 20 to 50% of the systemic load of bisphosphonate is distributed in the bone with the remaining drug being excreted in the urine within 24 hours. The half life of bisphosphonate in bone is not known but may be long and exceed many months [24]. But even if bisphosphonates have a long residence in bone, akin to that of bone seekers in general [25], like strontium or the tetracyclins, this does not necessarily imply that their biologic action is equally prolonged. This depends on wether the biologic effects is related to the total-bone-bisphosphonate or only to the amount of bisphosphonate within a relevant, special bone compartment.

Biodynamic as well as pharmacokinetic arguments suggest therefore that the action of bisphosphonate on bone remodelling could be prolonged. Interpretation of the available data is impossible without considering the mode of action of bisphosphonate.

THE MODE OF ACTION OF BISPHOSPHONATE

Bisphosphonates contain a carbon atom with two non-hydrolyzable phosphates. This bisphosphonate group conveys the ability to strongly bind to crystals of calcium salts precipitated from a solution. Even small amounts of adsorbed bisphosphonate alter the distribution of surface energy in such a way that the interaction of the crystal surface with the solution is altered.[24]. One consequence is a reduction in the rates of crystal growth and dissolution. The impressive consequence for crystal growth kinetics of these changes of the crystal surface properties were the reason for investigating the action of bisphosphonates on bone metabolism [26]. With hindsight it is perhaps their ability to alter crystal-surface properties in general, rather than the specific consequences of this for crystal growth or dissolution, that is responsible for the biological efficacy of the bisphosphonates.

The affinity to calcium containing crystals causes circulating bisphosphonates to adsorb to the calcified skeleton. This underlies their usefulness as carrier for scanning agents [27,28]. Most bisphosphonates that are used in clinical medicine, but not all, are without effect on the mineralization process proper. The notable exception is Etidronate, that can cause a particular form of osteomalacia, when not used with proper restrictions[29] Surprisingly, some bisphosphonates appear to be potent inhibitors of osteoclastic bone resorption. This effect is not merely a purely physicochemical one, inhibition of the dissolution of hydroxyl apatite, since it is associated with large changes in cellular kinetics in the direct environment of bone. Views on the mechanism through which this inhibitory effect is achieved, vary widely.

These views can be classified in three groups. One possibility is that ingested bisphosphonate is toxic for the resorbing osteoclast [30-32]. The phenomenon has been seen in-vitro, in particular with Clodronate. For two reasons this may not be the explanation for the in-vivo activity. One is that the relative molar potency of bisphosphonates with respect to this property does not reflect their relative potencies as resorption inhibitors in-vivo; the second that whole animal, and clinical studies have not shown similar toxic changes in osteoclasts. The studies do however show that some bisphosphonates may be more toxic than others, a phenomenon that could be considered in relation to clinical acceptability.

A second view postulates that surface bound bisphosphonate may maintain a concentration gradient of bisphosphonate near the bone surface, sufficiently large to let bisphosphonates have a direct influence on osteoclast progenitor cells or on other cell systems that are operative in initiating bone resorption [33-35]. Isolated cells will alter a variety of metabolic properties and even the ability to proliferate in the presence of quite low doses of bisphosphonate. Some of these effects vary widely and are sometimes opposite, between bisphosphonates, but other effects, like those on proliferation of osteoclast-precursors, do vary according to the in-vivo potency of the bisphosphonate. We still consider it to be unlikely that this is represents the mechanism of action. In-vivo, inhibition of resorption is not associated with a reduction in osteoclasts or osteoclast precursors, but even, depending on the circumstance, with an increase in osteoclast like cells. Furthermore, subsequent exposure of a bisphosphonate-pretreated bone explant to resorbing cells results in less resorption, without bisphosphonate in the medium [30,36,37]. The molar potency of the bisphosphonate is the same wether used for pre-treatment, or only added during exposure to osteoclasts. Although bisphosphonates do desorb from bone it is unlikely that they can maintain a sufficiently high bisphosphonate concentration in the bone environment, for this mechanism to be relevant. But again, the studies show that circulating bisphosphonates can have surprisingly large effects on cell metabolism. It would be wise to avoid high circulating concentrations during treatment.

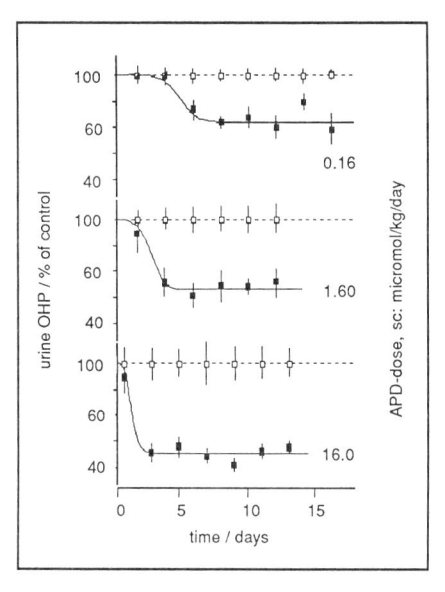

Fig. 1 Rate and Degree of bone resorption suppression in groups of 6 rats, treated with daily injections of APD. Closed symbols are treated animals, open symbols are controls.

The third explanation considers that osteoclastic bone resorption requires a signal from matrix bound cytokines to osteoclast precursors in order to activate their resorptive potential [30,36,37,38]. Osteoclast precursors accede to the bone surface through chemo-attraction and subsequent, after having come into contact with osteoblast derived cytokines, bound to the calcified matrix, their potency to resorb is activated [22,39,40]. In-vitro model systems, consisting of bone explants that have been prepared in such a way that their resorption depends on prior activation by the bone matrix of osteoclast precursors, have been used to show that pre-treatment of those explants with bisphosphonate does inhibit the ability of the explant to induce differentiation of the osteoclast precursor into a mature resorbing osteoclast. Subsequent resorption is prevented to a degree that depends on the bisphosphonate concentration to which the explants had been exposed. The relative molar potencies of bisphosphonates in these systems do closely reflect their inhibitory potential in-vivo [30,36,37]. In those systems, inhibition depends solely on matrix bound bisphophonate and does not require the presence of bisphosphonate in the medium. Within the identical experiment, tissue that has calcified after the exposure to the drug, and that is therefore not not covered with bisphosphonate, retains the potential to be resorbed. It is therefore likely that surface bound and not the circulating bisphosphonate is responsible for the inhibitory action. For the various reasons that have been mentioned, this third mechanism is the more likely one to be responsible for the inhibitory effect of the bisphosphonates in-vivo. Bisphosphonates prevent resorption, rather than inhibit it. If bisphosphonates do preclude, rather than inhibit osteoclastic resorption, their great clinical efficacy has to reflect a large dependency of normal resorption on continuous generation of new osteoclasts. Data on osteoclast turnover are not incompatible with the possibility that these cells depend on continued fusion with new precursors to replace loss of nuclear material, the replacement rate of the latter being quite rapid, in the order of 5 days [22,41]. It is now accepted that the maintenance of the viability of bone as a tissue, depends on close cyclic interaction of the various cell systems present within this organ, an interaction mediated through local messenger molecules, the cytokines. Activation of new osteoclast precursors, their accession to bone under chemotactic influence, their differentiation upon contact with the bone acting as a solid cytokine -the bisphosphonate sensitive process-, are all modulated or mediated by cytokines originating from osteoblasts [40]. Even the stimulation of bone resorption by Parathyroid hormone is mediated through the osteoblast.

The inhibitory action has a certain analogy with the way bisphosphonate act in pure crystal systems: altering surface properties. The presence of a basic group, as in the nitrogen containing drugs, has significance for their potency [36,37]. The importance of surface binding has consequences for the interpretation of pharmacokinetic studies. Bone-surface bound bisphosphonate should be considered as a compartment distinct from the remainder of the bisphosphonate taken up into bone. Surface bound bisphosphonate could theoretically disappear by three mechanisms, physicochemical desorption, removal by resorbing osteoclasts, and incorporation into the bone mass during osteoblastic bone formation. Since the last two may contribute considerably to the turnover of surface bound bisphosphonate, the biological activity in low bone-turnover states may be more prolonged than in high remodelling states. Moreover, inhibition of the rate of bone remodelling would lead to a reduction in the rate of disappearance of surface bound bisphosphonate. Whatever, the disappearance of the pharmacological effect of a given bisphosphonate dose may be much faster than the overall disappearance of bisphosphonate from bone.

PHARMACODYNAMICS

With this information one can resume the discussion of pharmacokinetics and biodynamics relevant to the treatment of osteoporosis. In the absence of proper pharmacokinetic data, one should use pharmacodynamic information. Figure 1 shows that both rate and degree of bone resorption suppression by bisphosphonate are dose dependent [42,43]. The differences in rate, according to dose applied correspond with a similar finding in Paget's disease. The result relevant to the present discussion is, that the pharmacologic effect on bone resorption, measured as decrease of hydroxyproline excretion reaches a plateau, and remains constant thereafter, the level of the plateau too being different according to the dose applied. We have made a similar observation in patients with osteoporosis treated with low dose oral Pamidronate (APD) for more than three years continuously, at a level of 150 mg per day. At 12 months from the start of treatment there was a significant reduction of urine hydroxyproline and serum alkaline phosphatase, with 15 to 20%. The reduction remained stable thereafter, with 6 monthly measurements, for at least two years [4]. This accords with the hypothesis, developed in the previous section, that it is possible to reach a steady state of suppression of bone resorption, at a level dependent upon the dose, and that an equilibrium is obtained between decreasing pharmacologic activity due to disappearance of bisphophonate from a pharmacologic relevant compartment and increasing pharmacologic activity, due to daily dosing.

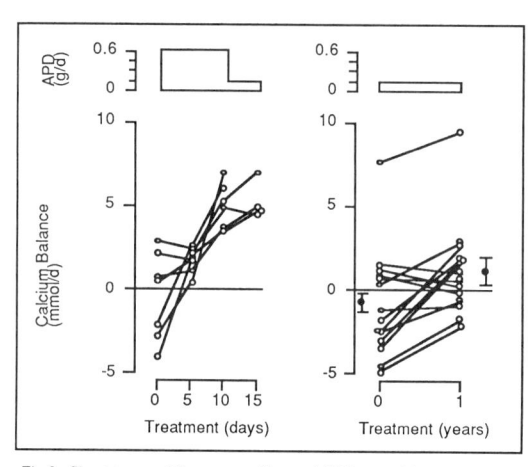

Fig.2 Short-term and long-term effects of APD on calcium balance in patients with osteoporosis. Open circles are results in individuals. Closed circles depict means with sem. APD-dosage on top.
Valkema et al 1989

This provides a setting for discussion of biodynamic changes during continued bisphosphonate. Heaney [1] treated ten patients with postmenopausal osteoporosis for 6 to 12 months with oral disodium Etidronate (EHDP) at 20 mg/Kg/day. Absorption of EHDP averaged 10%, and the effective retained dose was approximately 1.6 mg/kg/day. EHDP reduced bone resorption by about 50% and depressed bone mineralization by almost as much. At 12 months, when a steady state was presumed to have been reached, the calcium balance had shifted slightly but significantly in the positive direction by 57 mg per day. At this dose, however, EHDP reduced bone mass in the iliac crest by interfering with mineralization; this makes further interpretation of the data difficult.

Frijlinck [15], and later Harinck [16], have studied the relative kinetics of bone formation and resorption in APD treated patients with Paget's disease together with their external calcium balance. As expected this treatment was followed by an impressively positive calcium balance, in the order of 8-10 mmol (320-400 mg) per day on the average at around the second treatment week. Thereafter there was a steady decline, but even when around 200 days a new steady state had developed, with a stable reduced remodelling rate, calcium balances still were slightly more positive, though not significantly so, than before. This data encouraged two types of study. The first concerned the acute short-term effects of APD on calcium balance in osteoporosis to obtain an idea of the order of change one can expect at all. The second study was based on the insight obtained in calcium kinetics in Paget's disease which implied that the study of long-term effects of bisphosphonate on calcium balance requires repeat studies at least one year apart [4]. The initial investigations employed a medium dosage of 600 mg APD daily. The absorption of APD is in the order of 1%. The molar potency of APD being about tenfold that of EHDP, this dose could be equivalent to around 10 mg/kg/day EHDP. The results, depicted in fig 2 showed a mean increase in calcium balance of 6 mmol (240 mg) per day within 3 weeks. This is surprisingly high since bone remodelling in these patients is presumably much slower than in Paget's disease. The limit to the degree to which a calcium balance becomes positive may well be set by a maximum limit of calcium absorption by the gut. The dose for long-term studies was much lower, in order to prevent excessive suppression of bone remodelling. This employed 150 mg daily (equivalent to around 2.5 mg/kg/day of EHDP) The

TABLE I. Effects of different cyclic treatment combinations on bone mineral density of postmenopausal women (After Genant [6])

Treatment	Duration (Weeks)	BMD (QCT)	BMD (DPA)	BMC (SPA)	(n)
Placebo/Placebo	60	4.0 ± 2.8	2.5 ± 2.2	-2.4 ± 0.6*	7
Phosphate/Placebo	60	-2.0 ± 2.3	0.1 ± 1.5	-2.4 ± 0.7*	20
Placebo/Etidronate	60	12.2 ± 4.8*	5.8 ± 1.2*	-2.8 ± 0.8*	20
,,	105	9.1 ± 3.2*	5.5 ±1.1*	-3.3 ± 0.9*	17
Phosphate/Etidronate	60	6.5 ± 2.6*	6.8 ±1.3*	-1.2 ± 1.1	14
,,	105	5.1 ± 2.7	6.3 ±1.8*	-1.2 ± 1.2	13

* Significant change from baseline, $p < 0.034$

average pre-treatment calcium balance was -0.72 ± 0.59 and rose with 2 mmol/d (80 mg) to a value of 1.33 ± 0.87 mmol/day ($p < 0.005$) after one year. This amount may seem small, but translated into bone mass, the absolute positive bone balance of 1.3 mmol/day translates into a rate of 3% of the total skeletal calcium mass per year. The data, both from Heaney's [1], and from Valkema's study, suggest therefore that continued low dose bisphosphonate generates a positive skeletal balance which after one year is of a sufficiently large degree to be of interest in terms of bone mass. This result would support the hypothesis that, if continued minor inhibitory pressure is exerted on the resorptive phase of the bone remodelling cycle, compensatory decrease of bone formation will remain incomplete, since the driving force for the compensatory event is the presence of a disequilibrium.

THE USE OF BISPHOSPHONATE IN OSTEOPOROSIS

Valkema and co-workers [4] continued the previous open studies in 24 patients with osteoporosis, who were treated with 150 mg/day oral APD, 30 minutes before meals for a mean period of 3,7 years and compared with 19 concurrent not APD treated patients [4]. Comparison of first with last available bone mineral measurements (L2-L4, NOVO BMC dual photon) showed a mean increase in bone mass of 6.8 ± 1.7% over 2.2 ± 0.2 years ($p < 0.0005$) for the osteoporotic patients, while no significant changes occurred in the patients who did not use bisphosphonate. In character and degree these results are in accordance with the previous kinetic results. The mean rate of increase in bone mass measured over more than 3 years was 3.3% per year and remained unchanged throughout, together with a stable mean decrease of 20% in hydroxyproline excretion and serum alkaline phosphatase. Results of similar nature have been obtained by Reid [2,3], using the same dose and mode of administration in a controlled study on the prevention of steroid osteoporosis. These results permit the conclusion that addition of daily low dose oral bisphosphonate to conventional treatments of osteoporosis is feasible, may not only prevent the loss of bone, but even induce continued gain of bone mass. They warrant undertaking of long-term prospective studies on uninterrupted treatment schemes.

"Cyclic Intermittent" or "Coherence therapy" schedules have been, or are being used in open, as well as in double blind, controlled prospective studies [5-12]. The basis schedule for the prospective, double blind trials [6,7,11,12] consisted of activation with 3 grams of phosphate during 3 days, followed by 400 mg etidronate daily for two weeks, and 88 days without treatment (allowing 500 mg calcium).The bisphosphonate was given outside meals, with particular care for eliminating the possibility that it would complex with calcium in the gut. This makes bisphophonate unabsorbable. One of the open studies (Pacifici [10]) in a population of 30 women used slightly less phosphate and a somewhat shorter free interval, used 500 mg calcium carbonate twice daily, also in the bisphosphonate period, and does not mention specific measures to avoid contamination of oral Etidronate with calcium. This study has completely negative results: After 2 years the women in the ADFR group had a mean reduction of 8% in spinal QCT ($p < 0.05$), more than the 3.8% reduction found with calcium alone, while hormone treatment appeared to protect against bone loss. The results become however un-interpretable, because the mode of administration leaves doubts about the bioavailability of the given etidronate. This doubt is strengthened by the fact that no change at all was seen in the serum alkaline phosphatase levels.

Preliminary, uncontrolled open studies of Mallette et al [9] used 1 to 2 gm of phosphate for 7 days, followed by a quite high dose of 600 mg Etidronate thrice daily for 5 days, followed by 47 days 500 mg calcium twice daily. Lumbar bone density (BMD Lunar) had increased with 7.2 ± 5.3% after 6 months. In 8 women in whom treatment was continued thereafter, no visible further change occurred. The study has too short a duration to offer relevant information. Hodsman [8], with a similar setup on 20 patients obtained the same results, a significant increase in lumbar BMD by around 7% over the first 6 to 12 months, with no further gain thereafter.

The most interesting results are perhaps those, revealed in preliminary communications from the prospective studies given by Genant and by Storm. Their preliminary results have been detailed in the proceedings of the 1987 Aalborg symposium and need not be repeated here [6,11]. Table I summarizes more complete and recently reported data from the Genant study and revealing two interesting phenomena [7]. It appears that there is no difference in results between treatments with phosphate and without phosphate in the schedule, and that Etidronate is equally effective, wether given with or without the so called "activating" treatment. This suggests that the "activation" or "coherence" aspect of the treatment is a doubtful element. A second point that needs conformation is, that the increase in bone mass is not continued beyond the first 14 months. This will have to be confirmed as well as the observation that continuous low dose administration does achieve a continued bone mass gain. In relation to the duration of the compensation cycle observed during bisphosphonate treatment in Paget's disease, the duration of the cycles used by Genant and by Storm seems short. It may also be that the cycles are short in relation to the disappearance of pharmacologically active substance from the bone surface. If that is the case the term cyclic should not be used relative to this treatment, and all that has happened is that continuous treatment has been replaced with intermittent administration. From a pharmacokinetic and toxicologic point of view continuous administration would be preferable above intermittent, since the same bone coverage would be achieved at the cost of lower potentially toxic, circulating as well as peak bone surface concentrations. One could even ask the question, if the suggestion that cyclic treatment seems to produce a transient, and continuous a continued gain in bone mass, is not related to differences in pharmacokinetics. The intermittent schedule would be apt to induce series of ever smaller transients of bone gain, fluctuating around a mean. It would so fail to lead to a cybernetic equilibrium, characterized by a permanent small positive shift in bone balance.

An exiting finding has been that Storms study included patients with more severe osteoporosis, than that of Genant. His study was the only one that demonstrated progressive vertebral deformity for the control group, whereas the Etidronate treated patients remained stable and started to differ from controls with respect to the development of new fractures from one year after that start of treatment onwards [12].

We should conclude that available data suggest a surprising degree of efficacy for bisphosphonate in osteoporosis and merit further study on a wider scale. They seem to alter the vulnerability of bone in the steady state, a phenomenon that has also been observed in relation to the development of partial resistance against metastatic bone disease in breast cancer. The approach in both chronic conditions should probably be different from that used in the exploitation of bisphosphonate for the acute suppression of a pathological, and excessive bone resorption. There is no reason to believe that so called cyclic or ADFR schedules offer an advantage, and what is known or can be surmized about the pharmacokinetics of bisphosphonates makes it unlikely that such schedules will prove to be realistic.

REFERENCES

1. Heaney RP, Saville PD. Etidronate disodium in potmenopausal osteoporosis. Clin Pharm Ther 1976; 20: 593-604
2. Reid IR, Heap SW, King AR, Ibbertson HK. Two-year follow-up of bisphosphonate (APD) treatment in steroid osteoporosis. (Letter). Lancet 1988; 2: 1144
3. Reid IR, King AR, Alexander CJ, Ibbertson HK. Prevention of steroid-induced osteoporosis with (3-amino-1-hydroxypropylidene)-1,1-bisphosphonate (APD). Lancet 1988; 1: 143-46
4. Valkema R, Vismans F-JFE, Papapoulos SE, Pauwels EKJ, Bijvoet OLM. Maintained improvement in calcium balance and bone mineral content in patients with osteoporosis treated with the bisphosphonate APD. Bone and Mineral. 1989; 5: 183-192
5. Anderson C, Cape RDT, Vrilly RG et al. Preliminary observations of a form of coherence therapy for osteoporosis. Calcif Tissue Int. 1984; 36: 342-343
6. Genant HK, Harris ST, Steiger P, Davey PF, Block JE. The effect of etodronate therapy in postmenopausal osrteoporotic women: Preliminary results. In: Osteoporosis 2. 1987, C Christiansen, JS Johansen and BJ Riis, Ed. Osteopress ApS, København, 1989 pp. 177-1181
7. Genant HK, Harris S, Daveys PF, Steiger P. The effect of cyclic etidronate therapy woith or without phosphate in postmenppausal osteoporotic women: Three year study results. In: Cyclical Etidronate. A new dimension in therapy for osteoporosis. Le Grand Hôtel, Paris, April 1989 (in press)
8. Hodsman AB. Effects of cyclical therapy for osteoporosis using an oral regime of inorganic phosphate and sodium etidronate: a clinical and bone histomorphometric study. Bone and Mineral 1989; 5: 201-212

9. Mallette LE, LeBlanc AD, Pool JL, Mechanick JI. Cyclic therapy of osteoporosis with neutral phophate and brief, high-dose pulses of etidronate. J Bone and Miner Res 1989; 4: 143-148
10. Pacifici R, McMurtry C, Vered I, Rupich R, Avioli AV. Coherence therapy does not prevent axial bone loss in osteoporotic women: A preliminary comparatieve study. J clin Endocrin Metab 1988; 66: 747-753
11. Storm TL, Thamsborg G, Sørenseb OH, Lund B. The effects of etidronate therapy in postmenopausal osteoporotic women: Preliminary results. In: Osteoporosis 2. 1987, C Christiansen, JS Johansen and BJ Riis, Ed. Osteopress ApS, København, 1989 pp. 1172-1176
12. Storm TL, Thamsborg GM, Sørensen OH. The effect of etidronate cyclical therapy in postmenopausal osteoporosis. In: Cyclical Etidronate. A new dimension in therapy for osteoporosis. Le Grand Hôtel, Paris, April 1989 (in press).
13. Frost HM. 1979 Treatment of osteoporosis by manipulation of coherent cell population. Clin Orthop Rel Res 1979; 143: 227-244
14. Body JJ, Borkowski A, Cleeren A et al. treatment of malignancy associated hypercalcaemia with intravenous aminohydroxypropylidene diphosphonate. J clin Oncol 1986; 4: 1177-1183
15. Frijlink WB, TeVelde J, Bijvoet OLM, Heynen G. Treatment of Paget's disease of bone with (3-amino-1-hydroxypropylidene)-1,1- bisphosphonate (APD). Lancet 1979; 1: 799-803.
16. Harinck HIJ, Bijvoet OLM, Blanksma HJ, Dahlinghaus-Nienhuis PJ. Efficaceous management with aminobisphosphonate (APD) in Paget's disease of bone. Clin Orthop 1987; 217: 79-98.
17. Harinck HIJ, Bijvoet OLM, Plantingh AST, Body J, Elte JWF, Sleeboom HP, Wildring J, Neyt JP. The role of bone and kidney in tumour hypercalcaemia and its treatment with bisphosphonate and sodium chloride. Am J Med 1987; 82:1133-1142.
18. Harinck HIJ, Papapoulos SE, Blanksma HJ, Moolenaar BAJ, Vermey P, Bijvoet OLM.. Paget's disease of bone: early and late responses to three different modes of treatment with aminohydroxypropylidene bisphosphonate (APD). Brit Med J 1987; 295: 1301-1305.
19. Papapoulos SE, Hoekman K, Löwik CWGM, Vermeij P, Bijvoet OLM. Application of an in vitro model and a clinical protocol in the assessment of the potency of a new bisphosphonate. J Bone Miner Res 1989; (in press)
20. Sleeboom HP, Bijvoet OLM, van Oosterom AT et al. Comperison of intravenous (3-amino-1-hydroxy propylidene)-1,1-bisphosphonate and volume repletion in tumour induced hypercalcaemia. Lancet 1983; ii: 239-243
21. Thiébaud D, Jaeger P, Burkhardt P. A single day treatment of tumour induced hypercalcaemia by intravenous aminohydroxypropylidene diphosphonate. J Bone Miner Res 1986; 1: 555-562
22. Baron R, Vignery A, Horowitz M. Lymphocytes, macrophages and the regulation of bone remodeling. In: Bone and Mineral Research, WA Peck Ed, Elsevier, Amsterdam 1984 pp. 175-243
23. Flora L, Hassing GS, Cloyd GG, Bevan JA, Parfitt AM, Villanueva AR. The long-term skeletal effects of EHDP in dogs. Metab. Bone Dis. Rel. Res. 1981; 4: 289-300.).
24. Francis MD, Martodam RR. Chemical, biochemical and medicinal properties of the diphosphonates. In: The role of phosphonates in living Systems. RL Hildebrand, Editor. CRC Press Inc, Boca Raton, Florida, 1983, pp 55-96)
25. Marshall JH. Measurements and models of skeletal metabolism. In: Mineral Metabolism II, CL Comer and F Bronner Eds. Academic Prees, New York, 1969 pp. 2-122
26. Fleisch H. Bisphosphonates: Mechanism of action and clinical application. In: Bone and mineral research. Annual 1. WA Peck ed. Amsterdam. Excerpta Medica 1983; pp. 319-357.
27. Pauwels EKJ, Blom J, Camps JAJ, Hermans J, Rijke AM. A comparison between the diagnostic efficacy of 99mTc-MDP, 99mTc-DPD and 99mTc-HDP for the detection of bone metastases. Eur J Nucl Med 1983; 25: 166-9
28. Subramanian G, McAfee JG, Blair RJ, Kallfelz FA, Thomas FD. Technetium-99m-methylene diphosphonate – a superior agent for skeletal imaging: comparison with other technetium complexes. J Nucl Med 1975; 16: 744-55
29. Boyce BF, Fogelman I, Ralston S. Focal osteomalacia due to low dose bisphosphonate therapy in Paget's disease. Lancet 1984; i: 821-824
30. Boonekamp PM, van der Wee-Pals LJA, van Wijk-van Lennep M, Thesingh CW, Bijvoet OLM. Two modes of action of bisphosphonates on osteoclastic resorption of mineralized matrix. Bone Mineral 1986; 1: 27-40.
31. Flanagan AM, Chambers TJ. Dichloromethylenebisphosphonate (Cl2MBP) inhibits bone resorption through injury to osteoclasts that resorb Cl2MBP-coated bone. Bone Mineral 1989; 6: 33-43
32. Reitsma PH, Teitelbaum ST, Bijvoet OLM, Kahn AJ. Differential action of the bisphosphonates (3-amino-1-hydroxypropylidene)-1,1-bisphosphonate (APD) and disodium dichloromethylene bisphosphonate (Cl2MDP) on rat macrophage mediated bone resorption in-vitro. J Clin Invest 1982; 70: 927-933.

33. Bijvoet OLM, Frijlink WB, Jie K, van der Linden H, Meyer CJLN, Mulder H, van Paassen HC, Reitsma PH, te Velde J, de Vries E, van der Wey JP. APD in Paget's disease of bone. Role of the mononuclear phagocyte system? Arthr Rheum 1980; 23: 1193-1204.
34. Cecchini M, FelixR, Fleisch H, Cooper PH. Effects of bisphophonates on proliferation and viability of mouse bone-marrow derived macrophages. J Bone Miner Res 1987; 2: 135-142
35. Lerner UH, Larsson Å. Effects of four bisphosphonates on bone resorption, lysosmal enzyme release, protein synthesis and mitotic activities in mouse calvarial bones in vitro. Bone 1987; 8: 179-189
36. Boonekamp PM, Löwik CWGM, van der Wee-Pals LJA, van Wijk-van Lennep M, Bijvoet OLM. Enhancement of the inhibitory action of APD on the transformation of osteoclast precursors into resorbing cells after dimethylation of the amino group. Bone Mineral 1987; 2: 29-42 .
37. Löwik CWGM, van der Pluym G, van der Wee-Pals LJA, Bloys van Treslong-de Groot H, Bijvoet OLM. Migration and phenotypic transformation of osteoclast precursors into mature osteoclasts: the effects of a bisphosphonate. J Bone Mineral Res 1988; 2: 185-192.
38. Hughes DE, MacDonald BR, Hortton MA, Russell RGG, Gowen M. Bisphosphonates inhibit the formation of osteoclast-like cells in human marrow cultures. J clkin Invest 1989; (in press)
39. Horton MA. Osteoclast specific antigens. ISI Atlas of Science: Immunology 1988; 0894-3745: 35-43
40. Raisz LG. Local and systemic factors in the pathogenesis of osteoporosis. New Engl J Med 1988; 318: 818 - 828.
41. Jaworski ZGF, Duck B, Sekaly G. Kinetics of osteoclasts and their nuclei in evolving secondary Haversian systems. J Anat 1981; 133: 397-405
42. Reitsma PH, Bijvoet OLM, Potokar M, van der Wee-Pals LJA, van Wijk-van Lennep M. Apposition and resorption of bone during oral treatment with (3-amino-1-hydroxypropylidene)-1,1-bisphosphonate (APD). Calcif Tissue Int 1983; 35: 357-361.
43. Reitsma PH, Bijvoet OLM, Verlinden-Ooms H, van der Wee-Pals L. Kinetic studies of bone and mineral metabolism during treatment with (3-amino-1-hydroxypropylidene)-1,1-bisphosphonate (APD) in rats. Calcif Tissue Int 1980; 32: 145-157.

Do Dermal Losses Explain The Difference between Absorbed and Excreted Calcium in Normal Subjects on High Calcium Intakes?

B.E.C. Nordin

Division of Clinical Chemistry, Institute of Medical and Veterinary Science; Department of Pathology, University of Adelaide, South Australia

In previous publications [1,2] we have calculated the mean calcium requirement of young normal adults at about 550 mg/day based on 212 balances on 85 subjects collected from the literature [3]. The calcium requirement was shown to be determined by two independent relationships - that between calcium intake and net calcium absorption on the one hand, and that between net calcium absorption and urinary calcium excretion on the other. From the slope of urinary calcium on absorbed calcium, we were able to show that these two variables reached equality at a mean value of about 150 mg/day; below that value, urinary calcium exceeded absorbed calcium, and above that value absorbed calcium exceeded urinary calcium. From the relationship between absorbed calcium and calcium intake, we were able to show that an intake of about 550 mg daily would be required to provide the absorbed calcium of 150 mg required to meet the urinary losses. One of the unanswered questions arising from this analysis was why calcium balance should become positive in normal subjects at calcium intakes over 550 mg; one would rather expect a calcium balance of zero when calcium intake was adequate and expect additional calcium simply to be lost in the faeces and urine.

We have now found it possible to present the calcium intake, absorption and excretion in a single figure (see below) which may serve to answer this question.

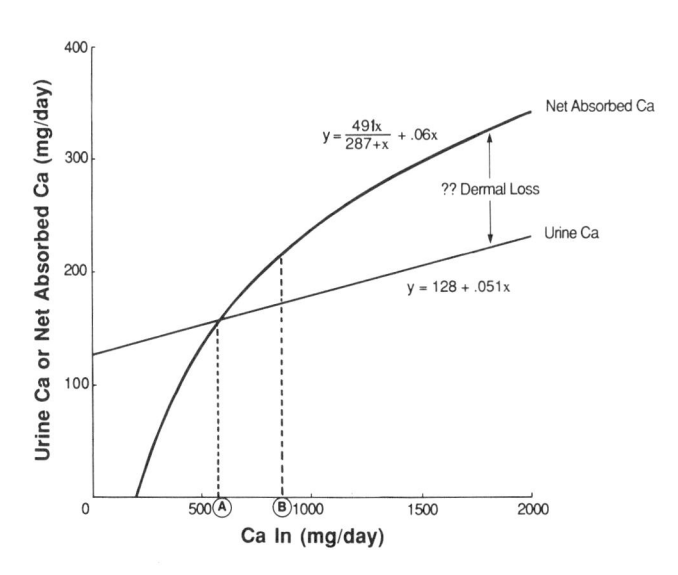

$$y = \frac{491x}{287+x} + .06x$$

?? Dermal Loss

$$y = 128 + .051x$$

As the figure shows, the slope of urinary calcium on dietary calcium has a coefficient of 0.05, i.e. urinary calcium rises at the rate of 5% of dietary intake. Absorbed calcium is a more complexed function of dietary calcium because of its two components - active transport and diffusion. However, the equation shown on the figure contains a final term of 0.06 which represents a diffusion slope of about 6%, i.e. after active transport is saturated, calcium absorption rises as 6% of dietary intake. The point at which the urinary slope intercepts the absorption slope represents the dietary calcium at which absorbed and excreted calcium are equal and calcium balance is therefore zero. As indicated above, the dietary calcium at this point is about 550 mg/day and is signified by the letter A on the abscissa of the figure. Above this intake, there is a gap between the absorbed calcium and urinary calcium of about 60 mg. The diffusion line and urinary calcium line are not quite parallel (6% compared with 5%) but this difference is not significant. Does this mean that young normal adults given adequate calcium will go into positive calcium balance of 60 mg/day? This seems very unlikely.

The solution to the paradox lies in dermal losses of calcium which have been estimated laboriously but precisely by Charles et al. at about 60 mg daily [4].

We suggest that the slope of urinary on dietary calcium of about 5% represents, and is identical with the diffusion slope of absorbed on dietary calcium of about 6%, and that the difference between the net calcium absorbed and the urinary calcium represents dermal losses. If this is correct, about 60 mg must be added to the absorbed calcium required to achieve equilibrium in young normal adults which - because of the nature of the absorption curve - adds some 300 mg to the true calcium requirement (see point B on the abscissa of the figure). Far from calcium requirement being overestimated by calcium balances, as has recently been claimed [5], it seems likely that the true calcium requirement is higher than balance techniques suggest in which case the recommended allowance should be correspondingly higher as well.

REFERENCES

1. Marshall DH, Nordin BEC, Speed R. Proc Nutr Soc 35, 163-173 (1976)
2. Nordin BEC, ed. (Churchill Livingstone, Edinburgh 1976) pp 1-35
3. Nordin BEC. J Food Nutrition 42, 67-82 (1986)
4. Charles P, Taagehoj F, Jenson L, Mosekilde L, Hansen HH. Clin Sci 65, 415-422 (1983)
5. Kanis JA, Passmore R. Br Med J 298, 137-140, 205-208 (1989)

Author Index

Agnusdei, D., 269
Aloia, J. F., 213
Avioli, L. V., 17

Barenholdt, O., 147
Baylink, D. J., 187
Bijvoet, O. L. M., 331
Birchall, M. N., 45
Block, J. E., 87

Caniggia, A., 201
Chesnut, C. H., III, 122
Christiansen, C., 259

Dallal, G. E., 295
Dawson-Hughes, B., 295
Delmas, P. D., 109, 181
Dupuis, J., 181
Dusan, R., 181

Eberl, S., 277
Eisman, J. A., 277
Eriksen, E. F., 99

Farley, S. M. G., 187
Fleisch, H., 323

Gallagher, J. C., 195
Genant, H. K., 87
Gennari, C., 269
Gilligan, C., 285
Glueer, C. C., 87
Gonnelli, S., 269

Heaney, R. P., 303
Heath, H., III, 241
Horowitz, M., 23
Horsman, A., 45

Johnston, C. C., Jr., 55

Kelly, P. J., 277
Krall, E. A., 295

Libanati, C. R., 187
Lindsay, R., 127
Lore, F., 201
Lowik, C. W. G. M., 331

Mack, T. M., 161
MacIntyre, I., 233
Mamelle, N., 181
Mariano-Menez, M. R., 187
Martini, G., 201
Mazess, R. B., 63
Melsen, F., 99

Melton, L. J., III, 39
Meunier, P. J., 181
Mosekilde, Le, 99
Mosekilde, Li, 99
Morris, H. A., 23
Munk-Jensen, N., 147

Nagant de Deuxchaisnes, C., 247
Need, A. G., 23
Nordin, B. E. C., 23
Nuti, R., 201

Obel, E. B., 147
Orimo, H., 223
Overgaard, K., 259

Papapoulos, S. E., 331
Parfitt, A. M., 315
Peck, W. A., 3
Perkel, V., 187
Pocock, N. A., 277
Pors Nielsen, S., 147
Pouillers, J. M., 137

Raisz, L. G., 120
Ribot, C., 137
Riggs, B. L., 7
Righi, G., 201
Riis, B. J., 259
Ross, R. K., 161

Sambrook, P. N., 277
Schulz, E. E., 187
Shiraki, M., 223
Slemenda, C. W., 55
Smith, E. L., 285
Steiger, P., 87
Steiniche, T., 99

Tiegs, R. D., 241
Tohme, J., 127
Tremollieres, F., 137
Tudtud-Hans, L. A., 187
Turchetti, V., 201

Valkema, R., 331
Vaswani, A., 213
Vesterby, A., 99

Ward, J. J., 277

Yeates, M. G., 277
Yeh, J. K., 213

Zaidi, M., 233

Subject Index

ADFR treatment, 331
1 alpha(OH)D$_3$, 196, 223
    adverse effects, 225
    bone mass, 223, 225
    vertebral fractures, 225
Acid phosphatase, 109
Age-related fractures, 39
Albumin, 34
    serum, 23
Alkaline phosphatase, 11, 24, 110, 225
Amenorrhea, 127
Anorexia Nervosa, 129
Anticoagulants, 19
Anticonvulsant, 19

Basic multicellular units, 11, 99
Bicarbonate, 25
Biomechanical competence of bone, 99
Bisphosphonates, 323
    alkaline phosphatase, 334
    bone dissolution, 324
    bone mass, 325, 331
    bone resorption, 324, 333
    calcification, 324
    calcium absorption, 326
    mode of action, 332
    osteoblasts, 331
    osteoclasts, 325
    Paget's disease, 331
Bone biopsy, 101
Bone densitometry, 63
Bone histomorphometry, 99
Bone hypertrophy, 285
Bone loss, 295
    age-related, 7, 10, 93, 278
    body weight, 301
    involutional, 308
    spine, 298
Bone mass, 40, 147, 323
    cancellous, 316
    fluoride treatment, 181
Bone mass-risk prediction, 56
Bone mineral content, 64
Bone mineral density, 7, 67, 277
    age, 48
    athletes, 282
    femoral neck, 277
    fluoride treatment, 184
    fracture incidence prediction, 53, 55
    fracture risk, 45
    mechanical load, 282
Bone remodeling, 11, 100, 317

Bone strength, 64
Bone tissue density (BTD), 288
Breast cancer, 159, 162
BUN, 225

Cl$_2$MBP, 327
CT receptors, 247
cAMP/creatine, 205, 209
Calcitonin, 3, 13, 24, 247, 261, 269
    ACTH, 269
    ACTH-immunoreactivity, 271
    administration, 239
    analgestic effect, 270
    beta-endorfin, 269, 271
    bone mass, 264
    bone pain, 269
    bone resorption, 261
    calcium, 261
    calcium balance, 263
    calcium carbonate, 252
    cAMP production, 248
    cell motility, 235
    cortical bone, 266
    enzyme secretion, 236
    gene-related peptide, 241
    gene structure, 238
    growth hormone, 254
    human growth hormone, 265
    immunoreactive, 236
    lumbar bone, 249
    metabolic clearance rate, 243
    monoclonal antibody, 235
    oestrogen, 262
    osteoclast, 261
    Paget's disease, 269
    phosphate supplements, 265
    physical properties, 241
    prostaglandins, 269
    receptors, 255
    resistance, 264
    1,25(OH)$_2$D$_3$, 252, 261
    salmon calcitonin nasal spray, 271
    secretion, 241
        radiometric assay, 236
    side effects, 264
    sodium, 261
    total body calcium, 251
    trabecular bone, 249, 263
    vertebral fracture rate, 263
    vitamin D, 252
Calcitonine, 113

Calcium, 24, 70, 181, 264
  age-related requirement, 306
  absorption, 7, 12, 196, 201
  balance, 196
  carbonate, 295
  citrate malate, 295
  intake, 295
  loss, 306
  serum, 225
  urinary, 24, 201
Calcium-intervention trial, 300
Calorie intake, 302, 303
Chemotherapy, 19
Clodronate, 332
Coherence therapy, 315, 335
Collagen, 4
Collagen I, 113
Colles' fracture, 9, 41, 69, 261, 285
Combined replacement therapy, 172
Corticosteroid treatment, 113
Courvoisier's equation, 149, 150
Creatinine, 225
Cytokines, 333

1,25 dihydroxyvitamin D_3, 3, 12, 25, 35, 201
  alkaline phosphatase, 217
  bone mineral density, 213 216
  calcium absorption, 202
  creatine, 213, 218
  estrogen, 202
  fracture incidence, 201, 218
  hydroxyproline, 205, 217
  hypercalcemia, 204, 213
  hypercalciuria, 212
  kidney, 220
  phosphate, 205
  serum, 195
  toxicity, 219
Densitometric methods, 71
Dentinal hypoplasia, 19
Deflazacort, 18
Diuretics, 19
Diphosphonate, 11
Dorsal kyphosis
  "dowager's hump", 10
Drug administration methods, 316
  intermittent, 316
  sequential, 316
Dual-energy x-ray
  absorptiometry (DEXA), 73
Dual-photon absorptiometry
  (DPA), 72

Endometrial cancer, 159, 171
Estrogen, 3, 9, 13, 112, 127, 161, 201, 253
  bone loss, 130, 137
  bone mineral density, 141
  breast cancer, 166
  cholesterol, 144
  endometrial cancer, 166
  gallbladder disease, 165
  ischemic heart disease, 164
  osteoporotic fractures, 164
  parenteral administration, 138
  progestrogen, 130, 133
  receptors, 4
  rheumatoid arthritis, 165
  stroke, 165
Estrogen/progestin, 147
Estrogen treatment
  hospitalizations, 168
  mortality rates, 163
Etidronate, 332, 334

Falls, 8, 40, 48
Femoral neck, 45
Femoral neck density, 93
Femur fracture, 67
Fluoride, 113, 181
Fluoride-calcium therapy, 181
  bone mass, 184
  non-vertebral fractures, 183
  vetrebral bone density, 187
  vertebral fracture rate, 181, 185
Fluoride therapy
  digestive disorders, 183
  monofluorophosphate, 182
  osteoarticular pain, 181 183, 184
  sodium fluoride, 181
Fractional calcium absorption, 204
Fractures, 7
  exercise effects, 285
Fracture incidence, 55
Fracture risk, 63

Gamma-carboxyglutamic acid, 115
Genetic determinants, 278
Glucocorticoids, 18
Gompertzian diseases, 42, 43

25 hydroxyvitamin D_3, 13, 18
Hip fracture risk, 45
Hip fractures, 55, 65, 70, 285
Hormone replacement therapy, 26, 161
Hydroxylysine, 114

Hydroxylysylpyridinoline (HP), 115
Hydroxyproline, 24, 29, 114, 201, 202, 334
Hypercalcemia, 195, 201, 225
Hypercalcuria, 195, 209
Hyperparathyroidism, 263
　　primary, 106
　　secondary, 14
Hyperthyroidism, 104

Indomethacin, 292
Insulin-like growth factor-I, 13
Insulin-like growth factors, 4
Interleukin-1, 4, 9
Ionized calcium, 25

Katacalcin, 241
Klinefelter's syndrome, 129

Lithium, 19
Lysylpyridinoline, 115

Markers of bone turnover, 110
Mechanical force, 278, 285
Medroxyprogesterone, 171
Myxedema, 106

Non-Gompertzian diseases, 43

Oophorectomy, 127
Os calcis, 282
Oral contraceptives, 172
Osteoblast, 7, 292
Osteocalcin, 11, 19, 109, 110, 112, 203, 205, 209
Osteoclast, 233
Osteoclasts and calcitonin, 248
Osteonectin, 113
Osteopenia, 63, 69
Osteoporosis
　　accelerated, 24
　　epidemiology, 259
　　simple, 24
　　type I, 9, 43, 70
　　type II, 10, 43, 70
　　type III, 18

PTH, 25, 318
Parathyroid hormone, 12, 195, 202
Perimenopausal, 296

Phosphate, 318
Physical activity
　　lumbar spine bone mass, 277
Prednisolone, 18
Prednisone, 113
Premenopausal, 23
Progesterone receptors, 4
Progestin, 161
Prostaglandins, 4
Pyridinoline crosslinks, 109

Quantitative computed
　　tomography (QCT), 64, 75, 87

Recommended dietary allowances (RDAs), 304
Renal function and calcitriol, 201, 207
Rocaltrol, 196

Sequential therapy, 247
Sialoprotein I and II, 114
Single-photon absorptiometry (SPA), 71
Skinfold thickness, 34
Spine fracture, 65, 70, 93
Stress microfractures (SMF), 185

Tartrate-resistant acid
　　phosphatase (TRAP), 114
Thiazide diuretics, 30
Thyroid hormones, 18
Thyrotoxicosis, 106
Tetracycline, 99
Testosterone, 18
Trabecular bone, 9, 218
　　density (TMB), 207
　　density and fluoride, 189
　　mass, 89
　　bone remodeling, 101
Transforming growth factor beta, 4
Turner's Syndrome, 127

Ultrasound measurements, 71

Vertebral
　　ash determination, 88
　　body load, 104
　　fracture risk index (FRI), 147
Vitamin D, 71, 264

Vitamin D analogues, 196
Vitamin D_2, 181

Weightlessness, 278